CHRONIC LEUKEMIAS AND LYMPHOMAS

CURRENT CLINICAL ONCOLOGY

Maurie Markman, MD, SERIES EDITOR

CHRONIC LEUKEMIAS AND LYMPHOMAS

Biology, Pathophysiology,
and Clinical Management

Edited by

GARY J. SCHILLER, MD

UCLA School of Medicine, Los Angeles, CA

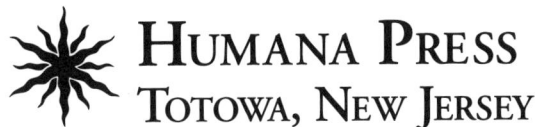

HUMANA PRESS
TOTOWA, NEW JERSEY

Library of Congress Cataloging-in-Publication Data

Chronic leukemias and lymphomas: biology, pathophysiology, and clinical management/edited by Gary J. Schiller.
        p.;cm.-- (Current clinical oncology)
    Includes bibliographical references and index.
    ISBN 0-89603-907-2 (alk. paper)
    1. Leukemia. 2. Lymphomas. I. Schiller, Gary J. II. Current clinical oncology (Totowa, N.J.)
    [DNLM: 1. Leukemia--therapy. 2. Lymphomas--therapy. 3. Lymphoproliferative Disorders--therapy. WH 250 C5555 2003]
    RC643 .C4825 2003
    616.99'419--dc21
                                                                          2002024350

PREFACE

The chronic leukemias and lymphomas represent a biologically diverse group of neoplasms characterized by relatively indolent natural history and distinct clinical features. Clinically identified by inexorable tumor progression with a propensity for an accelerated phenotype, these chronic hematologic disorders are also often associated with immune-related complications such as autoimmune thrombocytopenia, hemolytic anemia, pure erythrocyte aplasia, and dermatologic manifestations. These distinct clinical manifestations not only shed light on the immune response to these diverse neoplasms, but may also provide insight into disease biology. The purpose of *Chronic Leukemias and Lymphomas: Biology, Pathophysiology, and Clinical Management* is to describe the unique features of these chronic hematologic neoplasms—with a special emphasis on their biologic features—and to provide insights into clinical manifestations and potential targets for treatment in this new period of antineoplastic pharmacology.

Chronic lymphoproliferative neoplasms are often characterized by clonal expansion of cells demonstrating defects in apoptosis. Distinct cytogenetic and molecular abnormalities provide sensitive markers of disease, allowing for assessment of mechanisms of proliferation and cell death for a given cell population. Although the biology of malignant neoplasia is typically portrayed as a result of impairment in cellular differentiation coupled with a defect in cellular proliferation, the chronic lymphoproliferative disorders are considered models for defects in the phenotype of programmed cell death. In chronic lymphocytic leukemia, failed programmed cell death appears to be the principal disorder immortalizing the malignant precursor cell and its progeny. Presumably, molecular alterations that inhibit cell death promote the slow clonal expansion characteristic of the disease. Similar impairments of apoptosis have been described in follicular lymphomas suggesting unique targets for such therapies as the purine nucleoside analogs and monoclonal antibodies. These chronic lymphoproliferative diseases are to be contrasted with Hodgkin's disease and large cell lymphomas, disorders whose biology more closely reflects the biology of aggressive malignant neoplasias, and are also well described in this text.

In the new era of targeted therapy, another susceptible molecular feature of clonal neoplasia has been identified in chronic myelogenous leukemia. Long considered the paradigmatic myeloproliferative disease, chronic myelogenous leukemia is characterized by a distinct molecular lesion, the *bcr-abl* gene whose product confers a proliferative phenotype to the clone. Now a licensed drug, STI-571 (Gleevec) takes advantage of this unique molecular lesion, leading to a high rate of cytogenetic remission.

The other myeloproliferative disorders presumably have similar defects in cell replication. Like the chronic lymphoproliferative neoplasms, myeloproliferative diseases have a variable tendency to evolve to an accelerated phase characterized by impaired cell maturation and rapid clinical deterioration. This molecular and clinical evolution may not be inevitable, assuming that effective therapy can be initiated in the early, relatively benign clinical phase of the disease.

In the last decade, a confluence of basic and clinical research results has led to a more complex view of these so-called "indolent neoplasms." These results have also led to remarkable developments in therapy. Studies in the last ten years have led to completely different, and unanticipated, forms of therapy including unique small molecules targeted at specific genetic lesions, pro-apoptotic drugs, monoclonal antibodies, and adoptive immunotherapy. The new forms of treatment are designed to address these chronic diseases according to their unique susceptibilities, and in the process will lead to an improved understanding of the evolution of malignant neoplasia.

Gary J. Schiller, MD

CONTENTS

CONTRIBUTORS

JAMES O. ARMITAGE, MD • *Section of Hematology-Oncology, University of Nebraska Medical Center, Omaha, NE*

MARIA R. BAER, MD • *Leukemia Section, Department of Medicine, Roswell Park Cancer Institute, Buffalo, NY*

MUSTAFA BENEKLI, MD • *Leukemia Section, Department of Medicine, Roswell Park Cancer Institute, Buffalo, NY*

JAMES R. BERENSON, MD • *Division of Hematology-Oncology, Cedars-Sinai Medical Center and the University of California, Los Angeles School of Medicine, Los Angeles, CA*

R. GREGORY BOCIEK, MD • *Section of Hematology-Oncology, University of Nebraska Medical Center, Omaha, NE*

JAMIE D. CAVENAGH, MD • *Department of Hematology, St. Bartholomew's Hospital, London, UK*

CHRISTOS EMMANOUILIDES, MD • *Division of Hematology-Oncology, UCLA School of Medicine, Los Angeles, CA*

NIRAJ GUPTA, MD • *Division of Hematology-Oncology, Long Island Jewish Medical Center, New Hyde Park, NY*

SANDRA J. HORNING, MD • *Division of Oncology, Stanford University Medical Center, Palo Alto, CA*

STEVEN M. HORWITZ, MD • *Division of Hematology-Oncology, Memorial Sloan Kettering Cancer Center, New York, NY*

T. ANDREW LISTER, MD • *Cancer Research UK Department of Medical Oncology, St. Bartholomew's Hospital, London, UK*

LAUREN C. PINTER-BROWN, MD • *Department of Internal Medicine, Olive View-UCLA Medical Center, Sulmar, CA*

KANTI R. RAI, MD • *Division of Hematology-Oncology, Long Island Jewish Medical Center, New Hyde Park, NY; and Albert Einstein College of Medicine, Bronx, NY*

PETER J. ROSEN, MD • *Division of Hematology-Oncology, UCLA School of Medicine, Los Angeles, CA*

JONATHAN SAID, MD • *Department of Pathology, UCLA School of Medicine, Los Angeles, CA*

ALAN SAVEN, MD • *Division of Hematology-Oncology, Scripps Clinic and Scripps Cancer Center, La Jolla, CA*

CHARLES L. SAWYERS, MD • *Division of Hematology-Oncology, UCLA School of Medicine, Los Angeles, CA*

GARY J. SCHILLER, MD • *Division of Hematology-Oncology, UCLA School of Medicine, Los Angeles, CA*

NEIL P. SHAH, MD, PhD • *Division of Hematology-Oncology, Department of Medicine, and Molecular Biology Institute, UCLA School of Medicine, Los Angeles, CA*

NELIDA N. SJAK-SHIE, MD, PhD • *Division of Hematology-Oncology, UCLA School of Medicine, Los Angeles, CA*

ROBERT A. VESCIO, MD • *Division of Hematology and Oncology, Cedars-Sinai Medical Center and the University of California, Los Angeles School of Medicine, Los Angeles, CA*

NICOLE WENTWORTH, MD • *Division of Hematology-Oncology, Scripps Clinic, La Jolla, CA*

1 Chronic Leukemias
History, Epidemiology, and Risk Factors

Kanti R. Rai, MD and Niraj Gupta, MD

CONTENTS

HISTORY OF CHRONIC LEUKEMIAS
CHRONIC LYMPHOCYTIC LEUKEMIA (CLL)
CHRONIC MYELOGENOUS LEUKEMIA
EPIDEMIOLOGY
RISK FACTORS
REFERENCES

HISTORY OF CHRONIC LEUKEMIAS

Recognition of Leukemia as a Distinct Entity

Chronic lymphocytic leukemia (CLL) and chronic myeloid leukemia (CML) share a common history. Leukemia as a distinct entity was first described about 150 years ago. In the following years, physicians have recognized the heterogeneous spectrum of leukemia. They also developed a fuller understanding of the clinical features, natural history, and morphology of leukemia. The classification of leukemia into its various subtypes became possible in the mid-twentieth century.

The first cases of leukemia were described in 1845 by John Hughes Bennett in Scotland and Rudolph Virchow in Germany *(1,2)*. Soon after, a bitter rivalry began as each sought to take credit as the first to report this newly discovered disease. Virchow, upon microscopic examination of his patient's blood, noticed the presence of "colorless or white bodies" and coined the term "weisses blut" (white blood) to describe this disease. In 1846, after reviewing the papers by Bennett *(1)*, Craige *(3)*, and Fuller *(4)*, Virchow suggested that the increase in the colorless corpuscles in leukemia was not related to infection and that leukemia was characterized by an increase in the number of naturally occurring colorless corpuscles *(5)*. In 1847, Virchow coined the term "leukamiae" *(6)*.

From: *Current Clinical Oncology: Chronic Leukemias and Lymphomas:*
Biology, Pathophysiology, and Clinical Management
Edited by: G. J. Schiller © Humana Press Inc., Totowa, NJ

1

In 1852, Bennett published a paper on "leucocythemia," in which he described the 37 cases of leukemia reported by that time *(7)*. In 1856, Virchow suggested that the leukemias could be divided into two distinct forms: "lineal" (splenic), associated with enlargement of the spleen, and "lymphatic," associated with the enlargement of lymph nodes, with the presence of colorless corpuscles in the blood in both *(8)*. In 1857, Friedrich classified leukemias into acute and chronic forms, and tabulated their clinical and pathological features *(9)*.

Interestingly, at the same time, some physicians were unwilling to accept leukemia as a distinct entity. At a discussion in Paris, one physician said that "leukemia has no special causes, special symptoms, particular anatomic lesions or specific treatment, and I conclude that it does not exist as a distinct malady." Another remarked: "there are enough diseases without inventing new ones" *(10,11)*.

The origin of the "red" and the "colorless" corpuscles was not established until the mid-nineteenth century. In 1870, Ernest Neumann examined the bone marrow of a patient who had died of leukemia *(12)*. He described it as "dirty yellow...greenish, like pus"—unlike the normal red marrow. Neumann postulated that the bone marrow was the site of production of colorless corpuscles. In 1879, Gowers pointed out that in patients with leukemia, anemia may be caused either by decreased production or increased destruction of the red cells *(13)*. In 1891, Paul Ehrlich reported his remarkable work of developing the tri-acid staining method to study the dried blood smears, making it possible to establish a clear distinction between the lymphoid and the myeloid cells *(14)*. Newly developed staining techniques helped to correlate the microscopic findings with the clinical features of the disease, which led to the classification of the lymphoid and myeloid leukemias. In 1898, Hirschfeld identified the non-granular cells in the bone marrow and described the process of their development into granulocytes *(15)*. Two years later, Naegeli coined the term "myeloblast" to describe these non-granular cells *(16)*.

CHRONIC LYMPHOCYTIC LEUKEMIA (CLL)

Natural Course

Toward the end of the nineteenth century and the beginning of the twentieth, various terms were coined to describe the lymphoproliferative disorders, and there was confusion about the relationship between lymphoid leukemias and lymphoma. In 1893, Kundrat used the term "lymphosarcoma" to describe a condition that usually affected the lymph nodes or mucous membrane *(17)*. In 1903, Turk grouped the lymphatic leukemias and the lymphosarcomas under the term "lymphomatosis" and suggested that lymphosarcomas can be differentiated from leukemia by the local invasiveness and the absence of a leukemic blood picture in the former *(18)*.

In 1909, Sir William Osler reported his experience with leukemia patients at the Johns Hopkins University and referred to two types of leukemias: "splenomedullary" and "lymphatic" *(19)*. Chronic lymphatic leukemia in his series constituted about 22% of all leukemias with survival periods ranging from 3 to 11 yr. In 1924, Minot and Issacs published the first detailed clinical report on patients with CLL, who had a median survival of about 40 mo *(20)*. This may have been the first detailed description of the natural history of CLL. In 1938, Leavell reviewed the incidence of CLL and the various factors that influence the duration of survival with this disease *(21)*. In 1939, Wintrobe and Hasenbush published detailed clinical data on 86 patients with CLL, emphasizing the early phase of the disease *(22)*. In 1960, Hayhoe published a meticulous update on the clinical aspects of CLL in his book entitled "Leukemia" *(23)*. In 1966, Boggs et al. published a comprehensive review of diagnostic criteria, clinical features, and response to therapy and survival data of about 140 patients seen in Wintrobe's department in Salt Lake City, Utah *(24)*. Also in 1966, Galton reported his observation that the rate of increase in the lymphocyte count in blood correlated with the natural course of CLL: over a period of time, patients with a rapid increase of lymphocyte count had a poorer prognosis compared to patients with a stable count *(25)*. In 1967, Dameshek proposed a method to stratify CLL patients depending upon the extent of abnormality in the blood counts, disease-related symptoms, and enlargement of the lymph nodes, spleen, and liver *(26)*. Dameshek also reported that CLL was characterized by an accumulation of functionally incompetent lymphocytes rather than abnormal proliferation of these cells. In 1973, Hansen presented the details of clinical features of a large series of patients with CLL treated in a single institution in Denmark *(27)*.

Pathophysiology

In 1972, Aisenberg et al. and Preud'homme et al. almost simultaneously, but independently of each other, demonstrated the presence of immunoglobulins on the surface of CLL cells, indicating that CLL was a disorder of the B-lympho-cytes *(28,29)*. Further developments in this field led to the understanding of the phenotype of CLL lymphocytes and recognition of CLL as a monoclonal disorder, in which the leukemic cells are arrested at the intermediate stage of differentiation, and thus explain the accumulation of naïve B-lymphocytes *(30,31)*. Subsequent advances in immunological techniques and flow cytometry have helped to establish the characteristic phenotypic profile of the malignant B-lymphocyte, which is considered diagnostic of CLL *(32)*. These advances include recognition of co-expression of CD5 and CD23 on leukemic B-cells expressing CD20 and CD19.

In 1999, Damle et al. and Hamblin et al. made an important advance in our understanding of the immunopathology of CLL *(33,34)*. CLL lymphocytes in all patients with this disease were previously considered to originate from the "vir-gin"/pre-germinal-center B-lymphocytes, but these observations proved that there may be two types of CLL: one, without somatic mutation of IgV genes on the surface of the leukemic cells, indicating that the leukemic cells in those patients originated from the pre-germinal center stage, and the second, with somatic mutations of IgV genes, suggesting a post-germinal-center transformation of the leukemic lymphocytes. The mutational status of the IgV genes appears to correlate with the prognosis: patients with IgV gene somatic mutations have a favorable outcome compared to the patients without IgV mutations (33,34).

Unlike CML, there is no pathognomonic chromosomal abnormality in CLL. The chromosomal studies in CLL became feasible about two decades ago (approx 1980) with the discovery of polyclonal B-cell activators, which are also mitogenic for leukemic B-lymphocytes (35). Conventional giemsa-banding techniques failed to provide a consistent and reproducible data on cytogenetic abnormalities in CLL because of difficulties in determining whether a cell with a normal karyotype represented a normal or leukemic lymphocyte. However, with the application of fluorescent in situ hybridization (FISH) technique, it is now possible to analyze chromosomal abnormalities in CLL. A report from Dohner et al. reveals that about 80% of the CLL patients have a chromosomal abnormality (36).

Staging Systems and Prognostic Factors

A wide range of survival times seen in CLL in the earlier reports and a heterogeneous clinical course of patients with CLL highlight the need to have a uniform staging system with reliable prognostic factors. In 1975, Rai et al. presented a staging system based on readily measurable clinical and laboratory features (37). Binet et al. described another staging system in 1981 (38). Several other staging systems have also been described (39–42); however, the Rai and the Binet systems are most widely used in clinical practice.

Treatment

Chlorambucil has been the cornerstone of treatment of CLL, since the first report of its effectiveness by Galton et al. in 1961 (43). In 1961, Osgood had suggested that a combination of whole-body radiation and regularly spaced radioactive phosphorous could result in long-term control of chronic leukemias (44). The development of newer purine analogs such as fludarabine (45–47) and monoclonal antibodies (Mabs) against lymphocyte markers, especially CD-20 (rituximab) and CD-52 (alemtuzumab), has opened the newest chapter in the treatment of CLL (48,49).

CHRONIC MYELOGENOUS LEUKEMIA
Natural Course

In 1924, Minot and Issacs presented a review of 166 patients with CML (50). They reported that the majority of the patients were diagnosed between the third and the fifth decade, with a slight male predominance. Minot and Issacs also studied the therapeutic effects of radiation therapy in CML, and observed that the median survival for patients treated with radiation was 3.5 yr compared to 3.05 yr for untreated patients. In 1953, Tivey reported on the prognostic factors and survival affecting CML and CLL *(51)*. In 1976, Kardinal et al. from the Western Cancer Study Group reviewed the data on CML patients diagnosed between 1960 and 1974 from 22 participating institutions *(52)*. They published an extensive review of clinical features and response to treatment in 536 patients with this disease. Kardinel et al. noted that the younger patients and females had a better prognosis. Philadelphia chromosome was detected in 100 of the 110 patients tested.

Pathophysiology

The clinical and morphological features of CML were well-known by the middle of the twentieth century, but little was known about its pathogenesis. The discovery of Philadelphia chromosome (Ph[1]) by Nowell and Hungerford in 1960 heralded a new era in the field of hematology *(53)*. Fialkow et al. suggested that CML is a clonal disorder and that the defect lies with the pluripotent stem cell, early in the process of differentiation *(54)*. In 1973, Rowley *(55)* observed that the Philadelphia chromosome was formed by a reciprocal translocation between the long arms of chromosomes 9 and 22 t (9;22). In the early 1980s, Heisterkamp et al. showed that the abelson (abl) proto-oncogene located on the long arm of chromosome 9 was involved in the Ph[1] translocation, and that the breakpoints on chromosome 22 were clustered in a small DNA sequence, which was later named breakpoint cluster region (bcr) *(56,57)*. Further studies revealed that the reciprocal translocation between the chromosomes 9 and 22 resulted in a chimeric bcr-abl gene that encodes for an abnormal protein with a molecular weight of 210Kd, and had increased tyrosine kinase activity *(58,59)*. In 1990, the development of a disease resembling human CML in mice, after transfecting the murine hematopoietic cells with a retroviral construct containing bcr/abl sequences, established the leukemogenic potential of this fusion protein *(60)*. The discovery of Philadelphia chromosome also paved the way for developing new therapeutic agents and the detection of residual disease in assessing the efficacy of various therapies. Chronic myelogenous leukemia thus became a model in modern medicine, with a single chromosomal aberration resulting in the development of a disease.

Staging Systems and Prognostic Factors

In contrast to CLL, there is no single widely used staging system in clinical practice for CML. Several models have been proposed to stratify CML patients into high, medium, and low-risk categories *(61–64)*. The Sokal score proposed in 1984 is based on age, spleen size, platelet count, percentage of blasts, and basophils.

Treatment

In 1865, Lissauer administered Fowler's solution (1% arsenous oxide) to a patient with possible CML, and apparently had an appreciable response *(65)*. In

1902, Pusey used radiation for the treatment of leukemia *(66)*, and radiation therapy became the treatment of choice for treating leukemias for the next few decades. However, it was soon realized that radiation therapy was unable to deliver long-term remissions *(50)*. In 1946, Goodman et al. used derivatives of nitrogen mustard to treat patients with chronic leukemias and lymphoid disorders, and they noticed a reduction in the white-blood-cell (WBC) count and regression of lymphadenopathy *(67)*. However, these responses were short-lived. The results of these trials provided the impetus for the development of other alkylating agents.

The efficacy of busulfan, a sulfonic acid alkylating agent in CML, was first reported by Galton in 1952 *(68)*. It remained the mainstay of treatment of CML until the introduction of hydroxyurea in the late 1960s. Hydroxyurea, a cell-cycle-specific agent and ribonucleotidase inhibitor, was found to achieve a rapid but short-term disease control in CML *(69)*. In 1983, Talpaz et al. reported on the efficacy of interferon (IFN) in CML, and observed hematologic as well as cytogenetic remission in some cases *(70)*. Subsequently, low-dose cytarabine (Ara-C) was added to interferon, resulting in higher remission rates *(71)*.

Inability to achieve a cure or long-term remissions in CML led to exploration of bone-marrow transplant (BMT) as a therapeutic modality for CML. In 1983, Fefer et al. *(72)* were the first to report the successful results of syngeneic BMT in CML patients, and thus, allogeneic BMT (Allo-BMT) became the curative option for the CML patients who had an HLA-matched sibling donor *(73,74)*. The discovery of signal-transduction inhibitors led to the development of orally administered STI-571 (Gleevec), which has been shown to induce hematologic and cytogenetic responses *(75)*.

EPIDEMIOLOGY

Incidence Patterns

CLL

CLL is the most common leukemia in the adult population of Western countries. It accounts for about 30% of all leukemias in the United States. It is estimated that approx 8100 new cases of CLL will be diagnosed in the United States in 2001, and about 4600 patients will succumb to their disease during the same year *(76)*. The incidence of CLL in males is higher than females in the United States, regardless of race. The male-to-female ratio of CLL in the United States is approx 2:1. B-cell CLL constitutes about 95% of all CLL cases. There is a variation in the age-adjusted incidence among different racial groups in the United States. The SEER data from 1973 to 1997 shown in Fig. 1 indicate an overall decline in the incidence of CLL in whites as well as blacks. The incidence is lower in Hispanics and Asians. CLL is rarely seen before the age of 30, and there is a steady rise in the incidence of CLL after that age. Age-specific SEER program

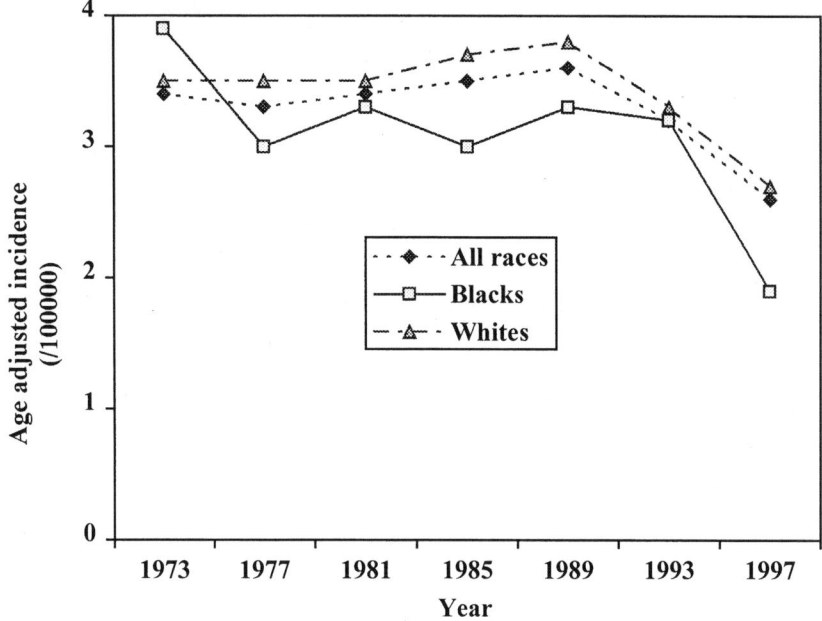

Fig. 1. Change in the age-adjusted incidence rate of CLL from the SEER data 1973–1997 in the United States.

data from 1993 to 1997 shows an incidence of 9.4 and 41.9 per yr per 100,000 population in the age group of 50–59 and 70–79 yr, respectively (Fig. 2).

CML

Chronic myelogenous leukemia accounts for about 18% of all leukemias in the United States. It is estimated that about 4700 cases of CML will be diagnosed in 2001 in the United States, and about 2300 CML patients will die of their disease. The age-specific incidence of CML is between 1.2 and 6.6 per yr per 100,000 population between the age group of 10–29 and 40–59 yr, respectively (Fig. 3). The incidence of CML is higher in males than females (1.8;1) in all age groups. Unlike CLL, the incidence of CML for both sexes combined has been consistently higher among blacks compared to whites in the United States. However, the recent SEER data indicate that this gap is shrinking (Fig. 4).

Global Variation

CLL

The prevalence of CLL differs by more than 30-fold among various populations all over the world, the greatest among all the leukemias. The incidence of CLL is higher in Canada, the United States, Europe, and Australia as compared to South American and Asian and African countries (Table 1). The incidence of

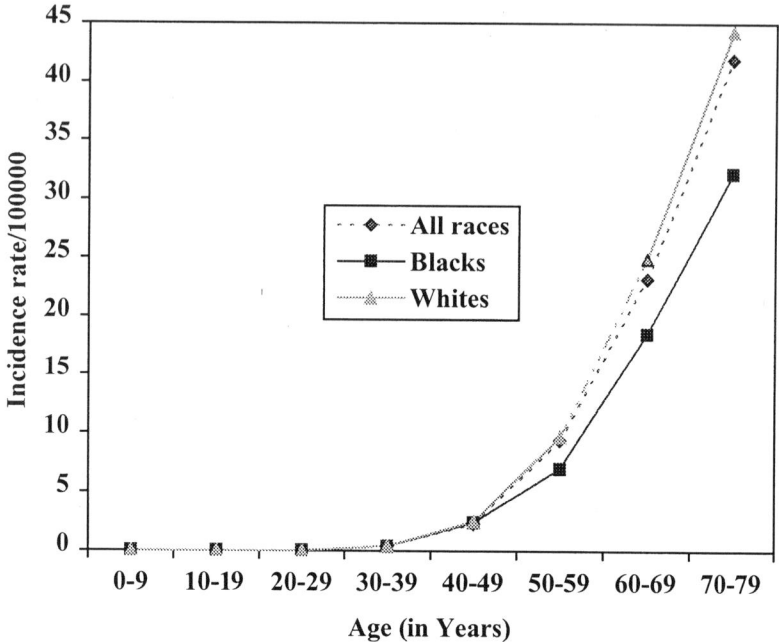

Fig. 2. Change in age-specific incidence rates by race of CLL in theUnited States. Based on the SEER data 1973–1997.

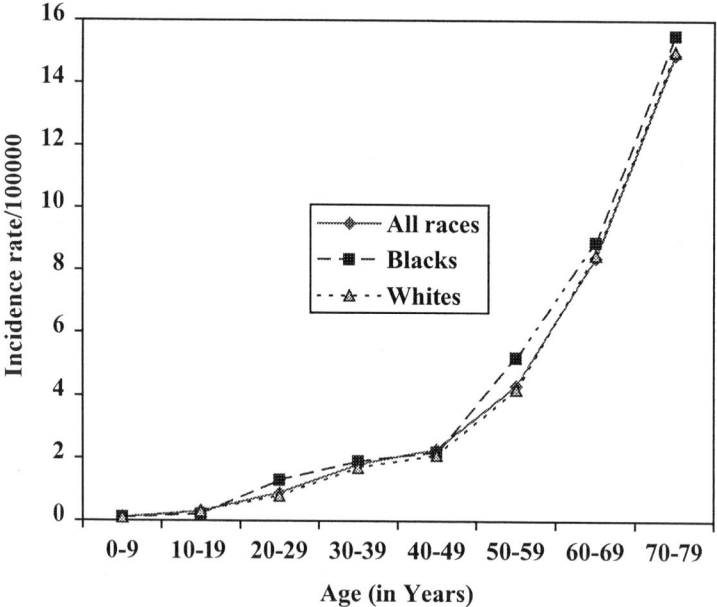

Fig. 3. Change in the age specific incidence rate of CML by race in the United States. Based on SEER data from 1973–1997.

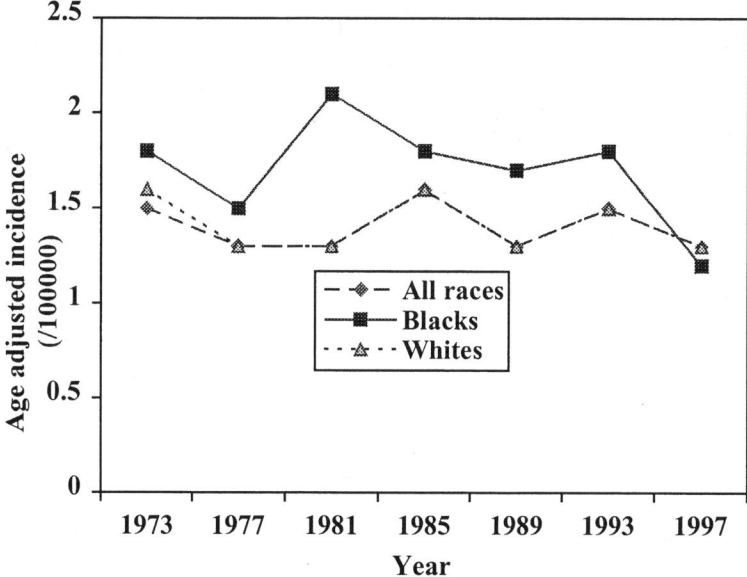

Fig. 4. Change in the age-adjusted incidence rate of CML in the United States. Based on the SEER data from 1973–1997.

CLL is consistently higher among males than females in most of the countries worldwide.

CML

In comparison to CLL, the CML shows lesser international variation (Table 2). The age-adjusted rates differ by fivefold or less among different populations, and have the least variation in the worldwide incidence among all the leukemias. The incidence of CML is high in Canada, the United States, Denmark, and Germany, and is relatively low in Spain, Poland, China, and India. Although there appears to be a male predominance, the gender difference is relatively smaller than CLL.

Secular Trends

CLL

A population-based study examining the epidemiological aspects of leuke-mias in a relatively stable population group was conducted among the residents of Olmsted County, Minnesota *(77)*. The annual incidence of CLL per 100,000 population almost doubled from 2.6 in the 1935–1944 period to 5.4 in the 1975–1984 period. The major increase was seen in people older than 50 yr of age. The recent SEER data shows that the incidence of CLL dropped by 19.4% among whites and blacks over the last 25 yr, between 1973 and 1997.

Table 1
Worldwide Incidence Rate of CLL per/100,000 in 45–85-yr Age-Group*

	Male	Female
North America		
Canada (Ontario)	17.97	10.93
USA—Los Angeles (black)	12.9	5.3
Los Angeles (whites)	15.3	11.1
Europe		
Germany (Saarland)	10.45	6.18
Spain (Zaragoza)	5.8	4.3
Denmark	15.4	9.0
UK (England and Wales)	11.1	6.7
Poland (Warsaw)	4.8	2.5
Oceana		
Australia (New South Wales)	11.6	7.0
New Zealand (Non-Maori)	13.8	8.8
Asia		
India (Bombay)	1.4	0.88
China (Shanghai)	0.71	0.26
Japan (Miyagi)	0.43	0.23
South/Central America		
Colombia (Cali)	2.0	0.71
Brazil (Goiana)	2.9	0.97
Peru (Lima)	1.0	0.46
Africa		
Uganda (Kyadondo)	0	0
Zimbabwe (Harrare)	3	4.2

*Based on *Cancer Incidence in Five Continents* (CI5VII). Ferlay et al., IARC, 1997.

The 5-yr relative survival rate for CLL in the United States between 1974 and 1976 was 68.5%, which improved to 71.4% between 1989 and 1996. The mortality in CLL patients increased by 11.3% during the same time period. The apparent increase in mortality resulting from CLL may be explained by the fact that CLL is being increasingly diagnosed in the rapidly growing elderly population, and there is an increase in mortality in this population because of other comorbid conditions.

Table 2
Worldwide Incidence Rate of CML per/100,000 in 45–85-yr Age-Group*

	Male	Female
North America		
Canada (Ontario)	5.0	3.4
USA—Los Angeles (black)	5.8	3.4
Los Angeles (whites)	6.0	3.6
Europe		
Germany (Saarland)	5.1	3.5
Spain (Zaragoza)	2.7	2.1
Denmark	4.1	2.5
UK (England and Wales)	4.2	3.0
Poland (Warsaw)	1.7	1.9
Oceana		
Australia (New South Wales)	5.7	3.3
New Zealand (Non-Maori)	5.3	3.7
Asia		
India (Bombay)	1.9	1.4
China (Shanghai)	1.5	1.0
Japan (Miyagi)	2.0	1.1
South/Central America		
Colombia (Cali)	2.3	2.1
Brazil (Goiana)	1.4	0.81
Peru (Lima)	1.5	1.3
Africa		
Uganda (Kyadondo)	0.94	0.97
Zimbabwe (Harrare)	1.8	0.68

*Based on *Cancer Incidence in Five Continents* (CI5VII). Ferlay et al., IARC, 1997.

CML

The SEER data shows that the incidence rate of CML declined by 11.4% between 1973 and 1997. This drop in the incidence of CML may be partly explained by the reclassification of chronic myelomonocytic leukemias with myelodysplastic syndromes. The 5-yr relative survival rate for CML in the United States between 1974 and 1976 was 22.4% and it improved to 32.7% between 1989 and 1996. The survival rate in CML was found to be slightly higher in Caucasian females than males, whereas the gender difference was smaller among the African-American patients. There was an overall drop in the CML mortality between 1973 and 1997 by 10.4%, with a 9.4% and 12.5% decline in males and females, respectively.

RISK FACTORS

The etiology and definitive risk factors for leukemia remain elusive. Large, systematically conducted epidemiological studies all over the world, coupled with advanced laboratory methods, have provided some clues to the possible risk factors associated with the development of leukemia.

Occupational Factors

Several studies have hinted about the leukemogenic potential of benzene and related compounds in occupationally exposed workers *(78–81)*. The relative risk for developing leukemia after benzene exposure ranges from 1.9 to 10. Although AML was the most common leukemia observed with exposure to benzene, reports of the development of CML—and rarely, CLL—have also been cited. However, most of the studies had a very small number of CLL cases, with inadequate evaluation of exposure levels.

A higher incidence of CLL is seen in some groups of workers in the rubber industry *(82)*. The chemicals used in this industry that are linked to the development of CLL include carbon tetra-chloride, carbon disulfide, acetone, and ethylacetate, although this subgroup of workers are chronically exposed to multiple chemicals *(83)*. The duration and level of exposure to these chemicals appear to correlate with the risk of developing leukemia *(84)*.

An increased incidence of CML has been reported among welders. Priston-Martin and Peters reviewed the occupational history of 130 patients with CML and 130 controls, and observed that 22 patients with CML had worked as welders in the past *(85)*. The welders who developed CML were exposed to welding fumes, smoke, gases, solvents, paints, and asbestos, and thus no specific agent could be identified as having a definite leukemogenic role.

A small increase in CLL and CML has also been seen in workers in plants that produce and process styrene monomers and butadiene *(86,87)*. The results of various studies evaluating the risk of developing chronic leukemia in petroleum workers have been contradictory *(88,89)*. A slight excess of CLL is reported in underground workers, tailors, and printers, and CML is slightly more prevalent in automobile mechanics and brewery workers *(90,91)*.

The association between farming and the development of chronic leukemias remains unclear. Several epidemiological studies conducted in the United States and abroad to evaluate the incidence of chronic leukemia among the farmers have provided conflicting results *(92–98)*. Agricultural workers are commonly exposed to pesticides, herbicides, fertilizers, diesel fuel and exhaust, and infectious agents associated with livestock, and thus it is difficult to implicate exposure to any specific chemical as the causative agent. It has been suggested that the misclassification of leukemias coupled with recall bias may partly explain the inconsistent results *(99)*. The National Academy of Sciences thoroughly evaluated the health effects of herbicides, and concluded that there was insufficient evidence to suggest a causal relationship between exposure to herbicides (2,4-D; 2,4,5-T and its contaminant) and leukemia *(100)*.

Radiation

IONIZING RADIATION

Ionizing radiation is a well-recognized and extensively studied risk factor for the development of leukemias. The leukemogenic effects of the ionizing radiation have been studied in atomic bomb survivors and those who have been exposed to radiation for diagnostic, therapeutic, and occupational reasons.

The study of atomic bomb survivors in Japan over the last 50 yr has provided invaluable information regarding radiation-induced leukemogenesis. The information is based on the incidence and mortality studies of a cohort of approx 100,000 atomic bomb survivors and their controls since the 1950s *(101–104)*. An increased incidence of acute leukemias and CML was observed in atomic bomb survivors, but there was no increase in the incidence of CLL. The leukemias developed within 3 yr of the bombing, and reached a peak 5–10 yr after exposure. The incidence of leukemia was directly related to the exposure dose of radiation in all age groups, and the highest incidence was seen among the people who lived close to the hypocenter, thus receiving the highest dose. The annual incidence rate of CML in people younger than 15 yr of age for the period 1950–1955 was 66.3 per 100,000, compared to the annual incidence rate for that time period for all types of leukemia of about 3 per 100,000 in the controls. Although the incidence of CML plateaued over the first decade of follow-up, the incidence of solid tumors and acute leukemias continued to rise.

An increased incidence of leukemia among the patients who received therapeutic radiation for malignant and non-malignant disorders has also been observed. In a landmark study by Court-Brown and Doll, about 15,000 patients with ankylosing spondylitis who were treated with radiation between 1935 and 1954 were followed for almost 50 yr and the updated results were published in 1994 *(105,106)*. Seven patients were diagnosed with CML, and seven had CLL. The increased incidence of leukemia persisted for about 25 yr after the treatment and thereafter. There was no evidence of an increased risk of developing leukemia, similar to what was seen in the atomic bomb survivors. Similarly, no leukemia deaths were observed in a Swedish study *(107)* of 836 patients with ankylosing spondylitis who were not treated with radiation therapy, thus indirectly confirming the conclusions of the prior studies.

An international case-controlled study of approx 30,000 women treated with radiation therapy for carcinoma of the cervix reported that the relative risk for all leukemias rose twofold, and the relative risk for CML was 4.2 *(108)*. A twofold risk of developing leukemia was also noted in a study of 100,000 patients with invasive uterine cancer treated with radiation therapy from 1935 to 1985, with a 1.4–3.7-fold increased risk of CML *(109)*.

Studies in the beginning of the twentieth century reported a higher mortality resulting from leukemia among the radiologists *(110,111)*. Although acute myeloid leukemia was often seen, the risk for CML was also slightly increased in this population group. A higher incidence of all leukemias (except CLL) was also seen in a cohort of about 27,000 Chinese medical X-ray workers followed between 1950 and 1980 *(112)*. A relative risk of 2.3 for the development of CML was noted. On the other hand, a 29-yr follow-up of US army radiology technicians from 1946 to 1974 failed to show any increase in leukemia deaths *(113)*. Newer and sophisticated shielding devices for radiology personnel may have contributed to the decreased incidence of leukemia in this group.

A higher incidence of leukemia was observed during the 22-yr follow-up study of about 3000 US military soldiers exposed to an above-ground nuclear detonation in 1957, code named "Smoky." Ten soldiers were diagnosed with leukemia, and four had CML *(114)*. However, another study of 46,000 soldiers involved in one or more atmospheric nuclear tests between 1951 and 1958 showed no significant increase in the risk of leukemia, suggesting that other factors may have contributed to the results obtained in the previous study *(115)*.

NON-IONIZING RADIATION

Exposure to non-ionizing radiation in the form of low-frequency electromagnetic field (EMF) induced by the generation and transmission of electricity has caused a considerable public concern, and has been linked to the development of various malignancies *(116–118)*. Studies from Sweden and New Zealand have indicated an increased incidence of CML or CLL among radio and television repairmen, electricians, linemen, and power station workers. However, a large study of workers employed at major electric power companies in the United States did not show a significant increase in leukemia mortality or in the incidence of specific leukemia cell types *(119)*. Lack of data on exposure to magnetic fields in most studies and the possibility of concurrent exposure to other chemicals makes it difficult to establish a causal relationship between non-ionizing radiation and the development of leukemia.

HEREDITARY/HOST FACTORS

CLL has the highest familial incidence compared to all other types of leukemia, suggesting a genetic component to the etiology. In 1937, Ardashnikov studied 33 pedigrees with familial leukemia, and noticed an increased incidence of lymphatic leukemia *(120)*. In his remarkable work, Gunz conducted a detailed analysis of the family histories of 909 patients with leukemia to evaluate the role of familial influence on the development of leukemia *(121)*. A history of leukemia in one or more relatives was seen in about 8% of the patients. Fifty-nine cases of leukemia were diagnosed in about 42,000 relatives. This represented a four-fold increase in the risk of leukemia among the first-degree relatives, and a 2.3-fold risk in the distant relatives. There was a markedly increased incidence of familial cases of CLL compared to CML. The concordance for subtype of leukemia between the proband and family members suggested a hereditary role in the development of leukemia.

The incidence of CLL is lower in the Asian countries such as China and Japan compared to Western countries. The lower incidence of CLL seen in the Japanese settled in Hawaii similar to the native Japanese, as compared to the American population, hints at a genetic component in the development of CLL *(122)*.

Pedigree analysis of CLL families usually reveals no definite pattern of inheritance. There is also no known well-defined single-gene disorder that predisposes to the development of CLL. However, it is possible that the conventional pedigree analysis may not reveal the role of heredity in complex disorders such as leukemia.

CML has been rarely reported in multiple members of the same families. In a Swedish study of 942 patients with hematopoietic disorders, 36 families with multiple cases of leukemia were identified *(123)*. The incidence of familial CML was lower compared to CLL, similar to that reported in other studies. In a patient with CML who had an identical twin, no evidence of CML was found in the unaffected twin, suggesting that the Ph chromosome is acquired rather than inherited *(124)*.

An association between the HLA antigens and CLL has been suggested by some investigators. However, others observed different results *(125–127)*. Recently, Posthuma et al. from the European Blood and Marrow Transplant Registry have suggested that the expression of HLA-B8 and HLA-D4 was associated with a lower risk of developing CML *(128,129)*. Technical difficulties in defining HLA subtypes and a heterogeneity of various subtypes of leukemia may be responsible for the inconsistencies of HLA association with leukemia.

Chronic myelogenous leukemia has been reported in association with certain chromosomal disorders, including, Turner's syndrome, Klinefelter's syndrome, and XYY syndrome *(130–133)*. Patients with Von Recklinghausen's (Type-1) neurofibromatosis have also been noted to have a higher incidence of juvenile CML *(134)*.

Viruses

Unlike the association of human T-cell leukemia virus (HTLV-1) with the development of acute T-cell leukemia *(135)*, there is no conclusive evidence of an association between chronic leukemia and viruses such as HTLV-II, feline leukemia virus, bovine leukemia virus, human herpes virus 6 (HHV-6), Epstein-Barr virus (EBV), and cytomegalovirus (CMV) *(136–138).*

REFERENCES

1. Bennett JH. Case of hypertrophy of the spleen and liver in which death took place from suppuration of the blood. *Edinburgh M & SJ* 1845;64:413.
2. Virchow R. *Weisses Blut. Froriep's Notizen* 1845;36:151.
3. Craigie J. Case of the disease of the spleen, in which death took place as a consequence of the presence of purulent matter in the blood. *Edinburgh M & SJ* 1845;64:400.
4. Fuller HW. Particulars of a case in which enormous enlargement of the spleen and liver, together with dilatation of all the blood vessels of the body were found coincident with a peculiarly altered condition of the blood. *Lancet* 1846;2:43.
5. Virchow R. weisses Blut und Milztumoren. I. *Med Ztg* 1846;157–163.
6. Virchow R. weisses Blut und Milztumoren II. *Med Ztg* 1847;16: 9–15.
7. Bennett JH. Leucocythaemia, or *White Cell Blood, in Relation to the Physiology and Pathology of the Lymphatic Glandular System.* Sutherland and Knox, Edinburgh, 1852.
8. Virchow R. Die leukamie. In: *Gesammelte Abhandlungen zur wiessenschaftlichen Medizin.* Meidinger Sohn Comp, Frankfurt, 1856;190.
9. Friedreich N. Ein neuer Fall von Leukamie. *Arch Path Anat* 1857;12:37.
10. Cahen. Discussion. *Bull Soc Méd Hop Paris* 1856;3:55.
11. Barthez F. Procés—Verbal de la Seance du 9 Janvier (Discussion on Leukocythemia). *Bull et mém Soc Méd Hop Paris* 1856;3:55.
12. Neumann E. Ein Fall von Leukamie mit Erkrankung des Knochenmarks. *Arch d Heilk* 1870;11:1.
13. Gowers WR. Splenic leucocythaemia. In: Reynolds JR, ed. *System of Medicine*, Lippincott, London, 1879;5:216.
14. Ehrlich P. *Farbenanalytische Untersuchungen zur Histologie und Klinik des Blutes.* A. Hirschwald, Berlin, 1891.
15. Hirschfeld H. Die generalisiertealeukamische Myelose und ihre Stellung im System der leukamischen Erkrankungen. *Zentralbl Klin Med* 1898;80:126.
16. Naegeli O. Ueber rothes knochenmark und myeloblasten. *Dtsch Med Wochenschr* 1900;26:287.
17. Kundrat H. Ueber Lympho-Sarkomatosis. *Wien Klin Wochenschr* 1893;211:234.
18. Turk W. Ein System der Lymphomatosen. *Wien Klin Wochenschr* 1903;16:1073.
19. Osler W. Leukaemia. The Principles and Practice of Medicine. D. Appleton, New York, 7th ed., 1909:pp. 731–738.
20. Minot BG, Issacs R. Lymphatic Leukemia: age, incidence, duration and benefit derived from irradiation. *Boston Med and Surgical J* 1924;191:1–9.
21. Leavell BS. Chronic Leukemia: a study of incidence and factors influencing the duration of life. *Am J Med Sci* 1938;196:329–340.
22. Wintrobe MM, Hasenbush LL. Chronic Leukemia: the early phase of chronic leukemia, the results of treatment and the effects of complicating infections; a study of eighty six adults. *Arch Int Med* 1939;64:701–718.
23. Hayhoe FGJ. Chronic lymphocytic leukemia: clinical aspects. In: *Leukemia: Research and Clinical Practice.* Little Borwn, Boston, 1960,:pp. 262–287.
24. Boggs DR, Sofferman SA, Wintrobe MM, Cartwright GE. Factors influencing the duration of survival of patients with chronic lymphocytic leukemia *Am J Med* 1966;40:243–254.
25. Galton DAG. The pathogenesis of chronic lymphocytic leukemia. *Can Med Assoc J* 1966;94:1005–1010.

26. Dameshek W. Chronic Lymphocytic Leukemia—An accumulative disease of immunological incompetent lymphocytes *Blood* 1967;29:566–584.
27. Hansen MM. Chronic Lymphocytic Leukemia: clinical studies based on 189 cases followed for a long time. *Scand J Haematol* 1973;(Suppl 18):1–286.
28. Aisenberg AC, Bloch KJ. Immunoglobulins on the surface of neoplastic lymphocytes. *N Engl J Med* 1972;287:272–276.
29. Preud'homme JL, Seligmann M. Surface bound immunoglobulins as a cell marker in human lymphoproliferative disease. *Blood* 1972;40:777–794.
30. Geisler CH Larsen JK, Hansen NE, Christensen BE, Lund B, Nielson H, et al. Prognostic importance of flow cytometric immunophenotyping of 540 consecutive patients with B-cell chronic lymphocytic leukemia. *Blood* 1991;78:1795–1802.
31. Freeman AJ, Nadler NM. Immunologic markers in B-cellchronic lymphocytic leukemia. In: Cheson BD, ed. Chronic Lymphocytic Leukemia: Scientific Advances and Clinical Developments. Marcel Dekker, New York, pp. 1–32.
32. Cheson BD, Bennette JM, Grever M, Kay N, Keating MJ, O'Brien S, et al. National Cancer Institute-sponsored working group guidelines for chronic lymphocytic leukemia: revised guidelines for diagnosis and treatment. *Blood* 1996;87:4990–4997.
33. Damle RN, Wasil T, Fais F, Ghiotto F, Valetto A, Allen SL, et al. Ig V gene mutation status and CD38 expression as novel prognostic indicators in CLL. *Blood* 1999;94:1840–1847.
34. Hamblin T, Davis Z, Gardiner A, Oscier DG, Stevenson FK. Unmutated Ig VH genes are associated with a more aggressive form of CLL. *Blood* 1999;94:1848–1854.
35. Gahrton G, Robert KH, Friberg K, Zech L, Bird AG. Nonrandom chromosomal aberrations in CLL revealed by polyclonal B cell stimulation. *Blood 1*980;56:640–647.
36. Dohner H, Stilgenbauer S, Benner A, Leupolt E, Krober A, Bullinger L, et al. Genomic aberrations and survival in chronic lymphocytic leukemia. *N Engl J Med* 2000;343:1901–1906.
37. Rai KR, Sawitsky A, Cronkite EP, Chanana AD, Levy RN, Pastermack S. Clinical staging of chronic lymphocyticleukemia. *Blood* 1975;46:219–234.
38. Binet JL, Auquier A, Dighiero G , Chastang C, Piguet H, Goasguen J, et al. A new prognostic classification of chronic lymphocytic leukemia derived from a multivariate survival analysis. *Cancer* 1981;48:198–206.
39. Jaksic B, Vitale B. A new parameter in chronic lymphocytic leukemia. Br J Haematol 1981;49:405–413.
40. Baccarani M, Cavo M, Gobbi M, Lauria F, Tura S et al. Staging of chronic lymphocytic leukemia. *Blood* 1982;59:1191–1196.
41. Rozman C, Montserrat E, Feliu E, Granena A, Marin P, Nomdedeu B, et al. Prognosis of chronic lymphocytic leukemia: a multivariate survival analysis of 150 cases. *Blood* 1982; 59:1001–1007.
42. Mandelli F, De Rossi G, Mancini P, Alberti A, Cajazzo A, Grignani F, et al. Prognosis in chronic lymphocytic leukemia: a retrospective multicenter study from the GIMEMA Group. *J Clin Oncol* 1987;5:398–406.
43. Galton DAG, Wiltshaw E, Szur I, et al. The use of chlorambucil and steroids in the treatment of chronic lymphocytic leukaemia. Br J Haematol 1961;7:73–81.
44. Osgood EE. Treatment of Chronic Leukemia. *J Nucl Med* 1964; 5:139.
45. Grever MR, Kopecky KJ, Coltman CA, Files JC, Greenberg BR, Hutton JJ, et al. Fludarabine monophosphate: a potentially useful agent in chronic lymphocytic leukemia. *Nouv Rev Fr Hematol* 1988;30:457–459.
46. Keating MJ. Fludarabine Phosphate in the treatment of chronic lymphocytic leukemia. *Semin Oncol* 1990;17:49–62.
47. Keating MJ, Kantarjian H, O'Brien S, Koller C, Talpaz M, Schachner J, et al. Fludarabine: a new agent with marked cytoreductive activity in untreated chronic lymphocytic leukemia. *J Clin Oncol* 1991;9:44–49.

48. Keating MJ, Byrd J, Rai KR, Flinn I, Jain V, Binet JL, et al. Multicenter study of Campath-1H in patients with CLL refractory to fludarabine. *Blood* 1999;94 (Suppl 1):705a.
49. Emmerich B, Huhn D, Peschal C, Wilhelm M, Schilling C, Bentz M, et al. Treatment of CLL with the anti-CD 20 antibody rituximab. *Blood* 1999;94 (Suppl 1):309b.
50. Minot BG, Buckman TE, Issac R. Chronic myelogenous leukemia. *J Am Med Assoc* 1924;82:1489–1494.
51. Tivey H. The prognosis factors for survival in chronic granulocytic and lymphocytic leukemia. *Ann Intern Med* 1953;72:68–93.
52. Kardinal CG, Bateman JR, Weiner J. Chronic granulocytic leukemia. Review of 536 cases. *Arch Intern Med* 1976;136(3):305–313.
53. Nowell PC, Hungerford DA. A minute chromosome in human chronic granulocytic leukemia. *J Natl Cancer Inst* 1960;25:85–109.
54. Fialkow PJ, Gartler SM, Yoshida A. Clonal origin of Chronic myelocytic leukemia in man. *Proc Natl Acad Sci USA* 1967;58:1468–1471.
55. Rowley JD. A new consistent chromosome abnormality in CML identified by quinacrine fluorescence and giemsa staining. *Nature* 1973; 243:290–293.
56. Heisterkamp N, Stephenson JR, Groffen J, et al. Localization of the C-abl oncogene adjacent to a translocation breakpoint in chronic myelocytic leukemia *Nature* 1983;306: 239–242.
57. Groffen J, Stephenson JR, Heisterkamp N, de Klein A, Bartram CR, Grosveld G. Philadelphia chromosome breakpoints are clustered within a limited region, bcr, on chromosome 22. *Cell* 1984;36:93–97.
58. Konopka JB, Watanabe SM, Witte O. An alteration of the human C-abl protein in K562 leukemia cells unmasks associated tyrosinase activity. *Cell* 1984; 37:1025–1042.
59. Heisterkamp N, Stam K, Groffen J, de Klein A, Grosveld G, et al. Structural organization of the bcr gene and its role in the Ph. translocation. *Nature* 1985;315:758–761.
60. Daley GQ, Van Etten RA, Baltimore D. Induction of CML leukemia in mice by the P210 bcr/abl gene of the Philadelphia chromosome. *Science* 1990; 247:824–830.
61. Tura S, Baccarani M, Corbelli G. Staging of chronic myeloid leukaemia. *Br J Haematol* 1981;47:105–119.
62. Cervantes F, Rozman C. A multivariate analysis of prognostic factors in CML. *Blood* 1982;60:1298–1304.
63. Sokal JE, Cox EB, Baccarani M, Tura S, Gomez GA, Robertson JE. Prognostic discrimination in "Good Risk" chronic granulocytic leukemia. *Blood* 1984; 63:789–799.
64. Kantarjian HM, Smith TL, McCredie KB, Keating MJ, Walters RS, Talpaz M, et al. Chronic myelogenous leukemia. A multivariate analysis of the association of patient characteristics and therapy with survival. *Blood* 1985;66:1326–1335.
65. Lissauer H. Zwei Falle Von Leukamie. *Berl Clin Wochenschr* 1865;2:403.
66. Pusey WA. Report of cases treated with roentgen rays. *J Am Med Assoc* 1962; 8:911–919.
67. Goodman LS, Wintrobe MW, Dameshek W, et al. Nitrogen mustard therapy. Use of methyl-bis (beta-chloroethyl) amine hydrochloride and pris (beta-chloroethyl) amine hydrochloride and tris (beta-chloroethyl amine hydrochloride) for Hodgkin's disease, lymphosarcoma, leukemia and certain allied and miscellaneous disorders. *J Am Med Assoc* 1946;105:475–476.
68. Galton DAG. Myleran in chronic myeloid leukaemia. *Lancet* 1953;1:208.
69. Fishbein WN, Carbone P, Freireich EJ. Clinical trials of hydroxyurea in patients with cancer and leukemia. *Clin Pharmacol Ther* 1964;5:574.
70. Talpaz M, McCredie KB, Mavligit GJ, Gutterman JU. Leukocyte-Interferon-induced myeloid cytoreduction in chronic myeloid leukemia. *Blood* 1983;62:689–692.
71. Guilhot F, Chastang C, Michallet M, Guerci A, Haroussean JL, Maloisel F, et al. Interferon 2b combined with cytarabine vs interferon alone in chronic myelogenous leukemia. *N Engl J Med* 1997;337:223–228.
72. Fefer A, Cheever MA, Greenberg PD, Appelbaum FR, Boyd LN, Bucker LD, et al. Treatment of chronic granulocytic leukemia with chemoradiotherapy and transplantation of marrow from identical twins. *N Engl J Med* 1982;306:63–68.

73. Clift RA, Thomas ED, Buckner CD, Doney K, Fefer A, Neiman PE, et al. Treatment of chronic myelogenous leukemia in chronic phase by bone marrow transplant. *Lancet* 1982;2:623–625.
74. Goldman JM, Apperley JF, Jones L, Marcus R, Goolden AW, Batchelor R, et al. Bone marrow transplantation for patients with chronic myeloid leukemia. *N Engl J Med* 1986;314:202–207.
75. Druker BJ, Kantarjian H, Sawyers CL, Resta D, Reese S, Ford J, et al. Activity of an ABL specific tyrosine kinase inhibitor in patients with BCR-ABL positive acute leukemias, including chronic myelogenous leukemia in blast crisis. *Blood* 1999;94:697a.
76. Greenlee RT, Hill-Harmon MB, Murray T, Thun M. Cancer statistics, 2001. *CA Cancer J Clin* 2001;51:15–36.
77. Call TG, Phyliky RL, Noel P, Habberman TM, Beard CM, O'Fallon WM, et al. Incidence of CLL in Olmsted county, Minnesota, 1935 through 1989, with emphasis on changes in initial stage at diagnosis. *Mayo Clin Proc* 1994;69:323–328.
78. Vigliani EC, Forni A. Benzene and leukemia. *Environ Res* 1976;11:122–127.
79. Rinsky RA, Smith AB, Horning R, Filloon TG, Young RJ, Okun AH, et al. Benzene and leukemia: an epidemiologic risk assessment. *N Engl J Med* 1987; 316:1044–1050.
80. Bond GG, Mclaren EA, Baldwin CL, Cook RR. An update of mortality among chemical workers exposed to benzene. *Br J Ind Med* 1986;43:685–691.
81. Infante PF, Rinsky RA ,Wagoner JK, Young RJ. Leukemia in benzene workers. *Lancet* 1977;2:76–78.
82. Delzell E, Monson RR. Mortality among rubber workers VII. Aerospace workers. *Am J Ind Med* 1984;6:265–271.
83. Checkoway H, Mathew RM, Shy CM, Watson JE, Tankersley WG, Wolf SH, et al. Radiation, work experience and cause specific mortality among workers at an energy research laboratory. *Br J Ind Med* 1985;42:525–533.
84. McMichael AJ, Spirtas R, Gamble JF, Tousey PM. Mortality among rubber workers. Relationship to specific jobs. *J Occup Med* 1976;18:178–185.
85. Priston-Martin S, Peters JM. Prior employment as a welder is associated with the development of chronic myeloid leukemia. *Br J Cancer* 1988;58:105–108.
86. Ott MG, Kolesar RC, Scharnweber HC, Schneider EJ, Venable JR. A mortality survey of employees engaged in the development or manufacture of styrene-based products. *J Occup Med* 1980;22: 445–460.
87. Wong O. A. Mortality Study and a case control study of workers potentially exposed with styrene in reinforced plastics and composites industry. *Br J Ind Med* 1990;47:753–762.
88. Wongsrichanalai C, Delzell E, and Cole P. Mortality from leukaemia and other diseases among workers at a petroleum refinery. *J Occup Med* 1989;31:106–111.
89. Wong O, Raabe GK. Critical review of cancer epidemiology—petroleum industry employees, with a quantitative meta-analysis by cancer site. *Am J Ind Med* 1987;15:283–310.
90. Gilman PA, Ames RG, Mc Cawley MA. Leukemia risk among US white male coal miners. *J Occup Med* 1985;27:669–671.
91. Linet MS, Malker HS, McLaughlin JK, Weiner JA, Stone BS, Blot WJ, et al. Leukemias and occupation in Sweden a registry based analysis. *Am J Ind Med* 1988;14:319–330.
92. Blair A, Zahm SH. Cancer among farmers. *Occup Med* 1991;6:335–354.
93. Blair A, White D. Leukemia cell types and agricultural plateaus in Nebraska. *Arch Environ Health* 1985;40:211–214.
94. Pearce NE, Sheppard RA, Howard JK, et al: Leukemia among New Zealand agricultural workers: a cancer registry-based study. *Am J Epidemiol* 1980;126,402–409.
95. Blair A, White DW. Death certificate study of leukemia among farmers from Wisconsin. *J Natl Cancer Inst* 1981;66:1027–1030.
96. Linos A, Kyle RA, O'Fallon WM, Kurland LT, et al: a case control study of occupational exposures and leukemias. *Int J Epidemiol* 1980;9:131–135.

97. Donham KJ, Berg JW, Savin RS. Epidemiologic relations of the bovine population and human leukemias in Iowa. *Am J Epidemiol* 1980;112:80–91.
98. Brown LM, Blair A, Gibson R, Everett GD, Cantor KP, Schuman LM, et al. Pesticide exposure and other agricultural risk factors for leukemias among men in Iowa and Minnesota. *Cancer Res* 1990;50;6585–6591.
99. Blair A, Zahm SH. Methodological issues in exposure assessment for case-control studies of cancer and herbicides. *Am J Ind Med* 1990;18:285–293.
100. Veterans and Agent Orange: Health effects of herbicides used in Vietnam. National Academy of Sciences, Washington, DC, 1994.
101. Ichimaru M, Ichimaru T, Mikami M, Yamoda Y, Ohkita T. Incidence of leukemia in a fixed cohort of A-bomb survivors and controls. Hiroshima and Nagasaki. Oct 1950-Dec 1978 RERF, technical report 1981;pp. 13–81.
102. Preston D, Kusumi S, Tomonaga M, et al. Cancer incidence in A-bomb survivors III. Leukemia, lymphoma and myeloma, 1950-1982. *Radiat Res* 1994;137 (Suppl) S68–S97.
103. Shimizu Y, Kato H, Schull W, et al. Studies of the mortality of A-bomb survivors mortality, 1950-1985, Part 2. Cancer mortality based on recently revised doses (DS86). *Radiat Res* 1990;122:120–141.
104. National Research Council Committee on Biological effects of Ionizing Radiation. The effects on population exposure to low levels of ionizing radiation. (BEIR IV). Washington, DC, Nat Acad Press, 1990.
105. Smith PG, Doll R. Mortality among patients with ankylosing spondylitis after a single treatment course with X-ray. *Br Med J* 1982;284:449–460.
106. Weiss HA, Darby SC, Doll R. Cancer mortality following x-ray treatment for ankylosing spondylitis. *Int J Cancer* 1994;59:327.
107. Weiss HA, Darby SC, Fearn T, Doll R. Leukemia mortality after X-ray treatment for ankloysing spondylitis. *Radiat Res* 1995;142:1–11.
108. Boice JD Jr, Blettner M, Kleinerman RA, Stovall M, Moloney WL, Engholm G, et al. Radiation dose and leukemia risk in patients treated for Cancer of the cervix. *J Natl Cancer Inst* 1987;79:1295–1311.
109. Curtis RE, Boice JD, Stovall M, Bernstein L, Holowaty E, Karjalainens S, et al. Relationship of leukemia risk to radiation dose following cancer of the uterine corpus. *J Natl Cancer Inst* 1994;86:1315–1324.
110. Seltser R, Sartwell PE. The influence of occupational exposure on the mortality of American radiologist and other medical specialists. *Am J Epidemiol* 1965; 101:188–198.
111. Smith PG, Doll R. Mortality from cancer and all causes among British radiologists. *Br J Radiol* 1981;54:187–194.
112. Wang JX, Inskip PD, Boice JD, Li BX, Zhang JV, Fraumeni JF. Cancer evidence among medical diagnostic x-ray workers in China 1950-85. *Int J Cancer* 1990; 45:889–895.
113. Jablon S, Miller RW. Army technologist: 29 year follow up for cause of death. *Radiology* 1978;126:677–679.
114. Caldwell GG, Kelley D, Zack M, Falk H, Heath CW. Mortality and Cancer frequency among military nuclear test (Smoky) participants 1957 through 1979. *J Am Med* Assoc 1983;250: 620–624.
115. Robinette CD, Jablon S, Preston TL. Mortality of nuclear weapons test participants medical follow up Agency. National Research Council Washington DC, National Academy Press, 1985.
116. Milham S. Mortality from leukemias in workers exposed to electrical and magnetic fields. *N Engl J Med* 1982;307:249.
117. Pearce N, Reif J, Fraser J. Case-control studies of cancer in New Zealand electrical workers. *Int J Epidemiol* 1989;18:55–59.
118. Tynes T, Andresen A, Landmark F. Incidence of Cancer in Norwegian workers potentially exposed to electromagnetic fields. *Am J Epidemiol* 1995;141:123–134.

119. Savitz DA, Loomis DP. Magnetic field exposure in relation to leukemia and brain cancer mortality. *Am J Epidemiol* 1995;41:123–134.
120. Ardashnikov SN. The genetics of leukemia in man. *J Hyg* 1937; 37:286–302.
121. Gunz FW, Gunz JP, Veale AM, Chapman CJ, Houston IB. Familial leukemia: a Study of 909 families. *Scand J Haematol* 1975;15:117–131.
122. Nishiyama H, Mokuno J, Inoue T. Relative frequency and mortality rate of various type of leukemia in Japan. *Gann* 1969;60:71–81.
123. Eriksson M, Bergstrom I. Familial malignant blood disease in the country of Jamtland, Sweden. *Eur J Haematol* 1987; 38:241–245.
124. Goh KO, Swisher SW, Herman EC. Chronic myelocytic leukemia and identical twins: additional evidence of the Philadelphia chromosome. *Arch Intern Med* 1967;120:214–219.
125. Jeannet M, Magnion C. HLA antigens in malignant diseases. *Transplant Proc* 3 1971;1301.
126. Linet MS, Bias WB, Dorgan J, McCaffrey LD, Humphrey RL. HLA antigens in chronic lymphocytic leukemias. *Tissue Antigens* 1988;31:71–78.
127. Dyer PA, Ridway JD, Flanagan NG. HLA-A, B and DR antigens in chronic lymphocytic leukemias. *Dis Mark* 1986;4:231–237.
128. Posthuma EF, Falkensburg JH, Apperley JF, Gratwohl A, Roosnek E, Hertenstein B, et al. HLA-B8 and HLA-A3 coexpressed with HLA-B8 are associated with a reduced risk of the development of chronic myeloid leukemia. The chronic leukemia working party of the EBMT. *Blood* 1999;93:3863–3865.
129. Posthuma EF, Falkensburg JH, Apperley JF, Gratwohl A, Hertenstein B, Schipper RF, et al. HLA-D4 is associated with a diminished risk of the development of chronic myeloid leukemia. Chronic Leukemia Working Party of the EBMT. *Leukemia* 2000;14:859–862.
130. Hageneijer A. Clinical abnormalities in CML. *Bailliere's Clinical Hematology* 1987;1: 963–981.
131. Chaganti R, Bailey RB, Jhanwar SC, et al. Chronic myelogenous leukemia in the monosomic cell line of a fertile tumor syndrome mosaic (45X/46,XX). *Cancer Genet Cytogenet* 1982;5:215–221.
132. Chaganti R, Jhanwar SC, Arlin ZA, et al. Chronic myelogenous leukemia in an XYY male. *Cancer Genet Cytogenet* 1982;5:223–226.
133. Oguma N, Takemoto M, Oda K, Tanaka K, Shigeta C, Sakatani K, et al. Chronic myelogenous leukemia and Klinefelters syndrome. *Eur J Haematol* 1989;42:207–208.
134. Clark RD, Hutter JJ. Familial neurofibromatosis and juvenile chronic myelogenous leukemia. *Hum Genet* 1982;60:230–232.
135. Blattner WA. Human Retrovirology: HTLV. Raven Press, New York, 1990, pp. 1–484.
136. Linet MS. The Leukemias: Epidemiologic Aspects. Oxford University Press, New York, 1985, pp. 14–27.
137. Foon KA, Rai KR, Gale RP. Chronic lymphocytic leukemia: new insights into biology and therapy. *Ann Intern Med* 1990;113:525–539.
138. Clark DA, Alexander FE, McKinney PA, Roberts BE, O'Brien C, Jarrett RF, et al. The sero-epidemiology of human herpes viruses- from a case-control study of leukemia and lymphoma. *Int J Cancer* 1990;45:829–833.

2 Chronic Lymphocytic Leukemia
Diagnosis and Management

Jamie D. Cavenagh, MD and T. Andrew Lister, MD

INTRODUCTION

CLL is characterized by the gradual accumulation of malignant lymphocytes in the bone marrow, blood, lymph nodes, liver, and spleen. Thus, the major clinical features are the sequelae of bone marrow failure and the compressive syndromes that result from gross enlargement of lymphoid organs. In addition, CLL is associated with humoral and cell-mediated immunodeficiencies as well

From: *Current Clinical Oncology: Chronic Leukemias and Lymphomas:
Biology, Pathophysiology, and Clinical Management*
Edited by: G. J. Schiller © Humana Press Inc., Totowa, NJ

as a greatly enhanced risk of autoimmune cytopenias—particularly autoimmune hemolytic anemia (AIHA).

The pathogenesis of CLL is dominated by the gradual, yet seemingly inexorable, accumulation of leukemic cells in the bone marrow and lymph nodes. This process results largely from an intrinsic failure of physiological programmed cell death or apoptosis rather than from an increased proliferative rate (1,2). The fact that CLL cells cannot die also explains their inherent resistance to conventional chemotherapy. Indeed, at the present time, CLL is best considered an incurable disease, and therapeutic interventions are largely aimed at improving bone-marrow function and resolving those complications resulting from enlargement of lymphoid organs rather than eradicating or curing the disease.

The course of CLL exhibits a striking degree of clinical heterogeneity. Unfortunately, for many patients, CLL is a clinically progressive disease that results in death within 1–2 yr from initial diagnosis. For others, in contrast, the disease is extraordinarily indolent and results in no reduction in life expectancy. Since contemporary management options range from simple observation to high-dose therapy with allogeneic bone-marrow transplantation (Allo BMT), a major challenge in the care of patients with CLL is to select appropriate interventions for each affected individual.

EPIDEMIOLOGY

CLL is the most common type of leukemia in adults, comprising 25% of all cases diagnosed in North America and Europe. Its incidence increases with age with a median age of 55 yr at diagnosis, and is more common in males (male:female ratio 2:1). The incidence of CLL varies geographically, and is much less common in the Far East (3).

ETIOLOGY

The etiology of CLL is uncertain. Interestingly—unlike virtually all other hemopoietic malignancies—exposure to ionizing radiation does not appear to be causative (4). There is an increased risk of CLL in first-degree relatives of patients with CLL and other B-cell malignancies, and the phenomenon of anticipation is observed within affected kindreds (5,6).

CLINICAL AND LABORATORY FEATURES

The cardinal clinical and laboratory features of CLL are summarized in Table 1.

Anemia can be multifactorial in CLL, and potential mechanisms include bone-marrow failure caused by leukemic infiltration, AIHA, hypersplenism, pure red-cell aplasia (PRCA), the effects of chemotherapy, and coincident hematinic deficiency. All of these possibilities should be considered when assessing the CLL patient with anemia, since important alternative causes of anemia caused by

Table 1
The Clinical and Laboratory Features of CLL

Bone-marrow failure (anemia, thrombocytopenia, and neutropenia)
Lymphadenopathy
Hepatosplenomegaly
Hypersplenism
Autoimmune disorders (AIHA, ITP, PRCA)
Positive Direct Antiglobulin Test (15–35% of cases)
Systemic symptoms (sweats, weight loss)
Hypogammaglobulinemia (recurrent bacterial infections)
T-cell immunodeficiency (shingles, Pneumocystis carinii)
Transformation to an aggressive lymphoma (Richter's Transformation)
Paraprotein (rare)

iron deficiency, such as colon cancer, occur in a similar age group. Autoimmune cytopenias, most commonly AIHA, are particularly common in CLL. Only a minority of patients with a positive direct antiglobulin test (DAGT) will develop hemolysis, although approximately 4–5% of CLL patients will develop clinically significant AIHA at some stage of their disease (7,8). The pathogenic high-affinity IgG autoantibodies responsible for AIHA are polyclonal, and therefore are not the product of the CLL clone itself (9). Rather, the autoimmune disorders associated with CLL result from a dysregulated immune system, which is itself a fundamental feature of CLL.

In approx 3% of patients with CLL, an aggressive diffuse large-cell lymphoma develops (Richter's syndrome) (10). Usually, this presents with asymmetric or discordant lymph-node enlargement, often with progressive systemic symptoms. The prognosis for this group of patients is poor, with a median survival of less than 6 mo. The clonal relationship of such lymphomas to the underlying CLL has been investigated by analyzing the sequence of the rearranged immunoglobulin genes in both lymphoma and CLL. The majority of cases of Richter's syndrome appear to result from clonal evolution of the CLL clone itself (11). Presumably, the accumulation of further genetic abnormalities results in a dramatic alteration in the biological and clinical phenotype of the disease. Similar events are well-documented in CML during the transition to blast crisis. However, 30–40% of cases of Richter's syndrome are clonally distinct from the preceding CLL (11). It is possible that these cases are analogous to the lymphomas that arise in other states of immunodeficiency, such as the post-transplant lymphoproliferative disorders (10). Certainly, in the rarer Hodgkin's disease variant of Richter's syndrome, the malignant Reed-Sternberg cells contain EBV, which is known to be central to the development of many lymphomas that arise in the setting of chronic immunosuppression (12).

THE NORMAL CELLULAR COUNTERPART OF B-CLL

Although CD5+ B-cells are relatively rare in the adult, they are found in high numbers in fetal and neonatal blood. Essentially, the antibodies produced by these naïve cells are the expression of the germline immunoglobulin repertoire, since no antigen exposure with consequent somatic hypermutation has occurred before birth. These naturally occurring antibodies are polyspecific, bind with low affinity, and generally react with autoantigens (e.g., IgG) as well as with microbial epitopes *(13,14)*. The autoreactive germline repertoire is highly conserved phylogenetically, and persists into adult life so that all normal individuals possess low levels of auto-antibodies. It is probable that in early life, these act as a first line of defense against invading microbes and function as templates upon which the antigen-driven somatic hypermutation machinery can operate in order to produce high-affinity antibodies characteristic of secondary immune responses *(15)*.

In adults, CD5+ B-cells with many of these features are found, in low numbers, in blood, primary follicles, and the mantle zone surrounding secondary follicles. CD5+ mantle-zone B-cells share many features with B-CLL cells such as the absence of extensive somatic hypermutation and the production of polyreactive autoantibodies. However, unlike mantle-zone B-cells, CLL cells express very low-level SmIg and high levels of bcl-2. Therefore, the precise normal counterpart of the CLL cell remains uncertain *(13)*.

Very weak expression of surface-membrane immunoglobulin, as well of other important signaling molecules such as CD22, are characteristic features of CLL that are shared by anergic B-cells. It has been hypothesized that in CLL, the malignant cell can be operationally defined as an anergic self-reactive CD5+ B-cell committed to the production of autoantibodies *(1,13)*.

The most important information about the cellular derivation of CLL derives from the analysis of the Ig V_H gene mutation status. Hamblin et al. found that approx 50% of CLL cases had unmutated V_H genes indicative of a naïve B-cell of origin *(16)*. The remainder had somatically mutated V_H genes characteristic of B-cells that had been exposed to the follicular microenvironment. Importantly, Ig gene mutation status correlated with certain clinical features. Unmutated cases tended to have atypical cytology, advanced stage with progressive disease, and inferior survival. Indeed, patients with stage A disease had very different median survivals in the two groups: unmutated 95 mo, mutated 293 mo. There have also been reports that trisomy 12 is associated with unmutated, and 13q⁻ with mutated status. Very similar findings have been reported by Damle et al., who also correlated unmutated V_H gene status with CD38 positivity *(17)*.

It is now clear that there are two subsets of B-CLL. The first is a malignancy derived from naïve B-cells, although the precise normal counterpart is still uncertain. The second is a malignancy of somatically mutated memory B-cells, and is associated with a significantly more favorable outcome. It seems highly

Table 2
Chromosomal Abnormalities in CLL as Detected
by Conventional Metaphase Cytogenetics

Abnormality	Frequency	Comments
Trisomy 12	33%	Atypical cytology
		Poor outcome
Del 13q	15%	Similar prognosis to cases with
		normal karyotype
Del 11q23	11%	Extensive lymphadenopathy
		Poor prognosis
		Deletions may occur at sites of
		CCG trinucleotide repeats
Del 6q	5%	
t(11;14)	2%	Probably cases of MCL

likely that these striking differences in prognosis will in turn relate to the presence of other established genetic abnormalities such as *p53* or ataxia telangiectasia mutated gene (ATM) inactivation. Current research is directed at determining whether particular cytogenetic abnormalities are correlated with unmutated or mutated phenotypes.

CYTOGENETIC ABNORMALITIES IN CLL

Early cytogenetic analyses in CLL were restricted by the fact that the malignant cells intrinsically have a low proliferative rate. Even with the use of potent B-cell mitogens, chromosomal abnormalities were only found in approx 50% of cases with admixed normal T-cells accounting for most normal metaphases *(18,19)* (Table 2). It was found that the presence of a cytogenetic abnormality by itself, as well as the percentage of abnormal metaphases in a particular case, correlated with poor survival. In addition, complex clonal abnormalities were associated with particularly poor outcomes. Interestingly, unlike the situation in CML or follicular lymphoma (FL), clonal cytogenetic evolution was not a feature of disease progression, although *p53* inactivation may well prove to be associated with transformation.

Importantly, the presence of clonal abnormalities was strongly associated with advanced disease and with cases with a higher percentage of prolymphocytes *(20,21)*. Therefore, it can be argued that the association of abnormal metaphase cytogenetics with poor prognosis results simply from an increased likelihood of detecting any clonal abnormality in those cases which are more clinically advanced, with a higher proliferative rate. Whatever the case, the abnormalities detected by conventional cytogenetics successfully identified regions of interest

Table 3
Chromosomal Abnormalities in CLL Detected by Interphase FISH

Abnormality	Frequency	Implicated Gene
Del 13q	55%	?
Del 11q	18%	ATM
Trisomy 12	16%	?
Del 17p	7%	p53
Del 6q	6%	?
14q32 rearrangements	4%	IgH translocations with multiple potential oncogenes
t(11;14)	0%	bcl-1

that could be analyzed in more detail using more sensitive tests such as interphase FISH. This technique does not rely on the presence of metaphases, and is thus independent of proliferative rate.

Using interphase cytogenetics, Dohner et al. analyzed 325 patients with CLL *(22)*. In all, 82% of the cases were abnormal. Of these, approx 65% had one, 25% had two, and 10% had more than two abnormalities (Table 3). Several striking observations are made in this study. First, cytogenetic abnormalities occur in the vast majority of cases of CLL. Second, 13q− is by far the most common abnormality in CLL. Third, the proportion of cases with trisomy 12 is significantly lower than would be expected by extrapolation of data derived from conventional cytogenetics. Also, trisomy 12 was not associated with a poor prognosis in the analysis, although this remains a contentious issue. Fourth, 14q32 translocations appear to be rather unusual events in CLL in contradistinction to myeloma—for example, in which such IgH rearrangements are nearly universal. Fifth, no cases with a t(11;14) were found. Earlier series often reported a 2–5% incidence of t(11;14), and the most likely explanation for this discrepancy is that these were misdiagnosed cases of mantle-cell lymphoma (MCL).

The correlation with clinical data showed that 17p− and 11q− were both associated with more advanced and 13q− with less advanced disease. The data was analyzed in such a way as to generate a hierarchical model of genetic subgroups: 17p−, 11q− but not 17p−, trisomy 12 but not 17p− or 11q−, normal karyotype and 13q− alone). These are associated with different clinical outcomes (Table 4). However, using multivariate analysis, only 17p− and 11q− retained prognostic importance along with age, Binet stage, LDH, and white-blood-cell count (WBC).

MOLECULAR ABNORMALITIES IN CLL

Although there is increasing knowledge about the cytogenetic abnormalities that occur in CLL, their precise pathogenetic molecular consequences are largely

Table 4
Cytogenetic Abnormalities and Prognosis

Karyotype	Median survival (mo)	
17p−	32	mo
11q−	79	mo
Trisomy 12	114	mo
Normal	111	mo
13q−	133	mo

unknown. Indeed, *bcl-2* overexpression, which occurs in 85% of cases, is not a consequence of any known chromosomal translocations, as is the case with the t(14;18) characteristic of FL *(2)*. In CLL, possible mechanisms include hypomethylation of the bcl-2-promoter region *(23)* or production of basic fibroblast growth factor (bFGF) by the CLL cells themselves *(24)*, which in turn induces *bcl-2* expression. Whatever the case, bcl-2 is a negative regulator of apoptosis although it is likely that the *bcl-2:bax* ratio is more critical in setting the precise threshold for programmed cell death. Indeed, in CLL, a high bcl-2:bax ratio correlates with progressive disease and resistance to treatment *(25,26)*.

Usually *p53* mutations accompany 17p deletions, are found in 12–25% of cases of CLL, and are strongly associated with advanced disease and Richter's transformation *(27)*. *ATM* is another gene that may function as a classical tumor-suppressor gene in CLL. *ATM* is located at 11q22-11q23, which is the region deleted in CLL. Inherited homozygous *ATM* mutations result in ataxia telangiectasia, which is itself associated with a greatly increased risk of lymphoid neoplasia and acquired homozygous *ATM* mutations are also known to occur in T-PLL. Schaffner et al. analyzed 22 cases of B-CLL with monoallelic deletions of 11q22–23, and found that 5 of 22 also possessed point mutations in the remaining allele *(28)*. Furthermore, germline mutations in *ATM* have been found at a much higher frequency in patients with CLL than in the general population *(29)*. Taken together, these observations suggest that *ATM* may function as a classical tumor-suppressor gene in a subset of patients with CLL, although it is possible that another tumor-suppressor gene at 11q23 is operative in CLL.

Since 13q− is a frequent abnormality in CLL, it is another likely site for a tumor-suppressor gene. The entire minimal region of deletion (MDR) has now been sequenced and analyzed. The MDR contains two pseudogenes and three transcribed genes (*CAR*, *Leu1*, and *Leu2*). However, no mutations have been found in these genes in 20 cases of CLL with 13q− *(30)*. These findings suggest that the 13q- MDR does not actually harbor a classical tumor-suppressor gene, although it is possible that haploinsufficiency of one of these genes may be involved in the pathogenesis of CLL.

Table 5
Minimal Criteria for a Diagnosis of CLL (NCI Working Group)

1. Peripheral-blood lymphocytosis $>5 \times 10^9/L$
2. Lymphocytes must be morphologically mature-appearing with less than 55% atypical cells (prolymphocytes or lymphoplasmacytoid cells)
3. Greater than 30% lymphocytes in a normocellular or hypercellular bone-marrow aspirate (bone-marrow not absolutely required for diagnosis)
4. Monoclonal light-chain expression
5. Expression of B-lineage markers (at least one of CD19, CD20, and CD23)
6. CD5 expression

The advent of gene-expression profiling will undoubtedly have a major impact on efforts to unravel the molecular phenotypes of CLL. Currently available data demonstrate that the expression profile of CLL is analogous to that of resting B-cells, although there are additional genes expressed by CLL, the so-called CLL signature. Notably, there is a complete lack of gene expression typical of germinal center B-cells *(31)*. A more detailed analysis of gene expression is currently underway, and will undoubtedly further highlight differences between mutated and unmutated cases, and also shed light on the molecular basis of drug resistance.

THE DIAGNOSIS OF CLL

CLL can be defined as a neoplasm of small, round B-lymphocytes found in the peripheral blood, bone marrow, and lymph nodes. Guidelines for diagnosis and treatment of CLL have been published and subsequently revised by an NCI-sponsored Working Group *(32,33)*. The major purpose of these guidelines was to facilitate comparisons between clinical trials. The minimal criteria for a diagnosis of CLL are listed in Table 5. The International Working Group on CLL and The French-American-British Cooperative Group have published very similar diagnostic criteria *(34,35)*.

In the great majority of cases, a diagnosis of CLL can easily be made after examination of a peripheral blood smear and cell-marker analysis. Occasionally, bone-marrow biopsy, lymph-node histology, cytogenetics, or molecular studies are required in order to distinguish CLL from rarer lymphoproliferative disorders. On a peripheral-blood smear, CLL cells appear small and uniform with scanty cytoplasm and clumped nuclear chromatin, giving rise to a mosaic or 'cracked mud' appearance. Characteristically, numerous smear cells are also present. The bone marrow is infiltrated in an interstitial, nodular, or diffuse pattern, and lymph nodes are effaced by monomorphic small lymphocytes with scattered, paler-appearing proliferation centers containing larger nucleolated

Table 6
The Characteristic Immunophenotype of CLL

κ or λ light-chain restriction
Weak SmIg
IgM or IgM/IgD SmIg
CD5
CD23
Pan-B markers (with normal levels of intensity): CD19, CD24, CD79a
Pan-B markers (with reduced levels of intensity): CD20, CD22, CD79b
Lack of expression: FMC7, CD11c, CD25

cells known as prolymphocytes or paraimmunoblasts. Occasionally, patients will present with lymph-node involvement without significant blood or marrow involvement. Nevertheless, CLL and small-cell lymphocytic lymphoma (SLL) are biologically the same entity, and the WHO classification highlights the fact that CLL and SLL are one disease at different stages *(36)*.

The immunophenotype of CLL is highly characteristic. Surface-membrane immunoglobulin (SmIg) is usually of IgM or IgM/IgD isotype, is very weakly expressed, and can sometimes be undetectable. By definition, there is κ or λ light-chain restriction. Almost universally, there is co-expression of CD5 and CD23. CD5 is conventionally considered as a T-lineage antigen, but is also expressed by approx 10–15% of normal blood B-cells, which may be the normal cellular counterpart of CLL. CD23 is the low-affinity FcR that is expressed by activated B-cells and eosinophils, by cases of CLL but rarely by other B-cell malignancies. Pan B-lineage markers such as CD19, CD24, and CD79a are expressed at normal levels, whereas others such as CD20, CD22, and CD79b are characteristically expressed at very low levels. Antigens that are expressed by other B-cell lymphoproliferative disorders such as FMC7 (most B-cell malignancies) or CD11c and CD25 (hairy cell leukemia) (HCL) are typically absent in CLL (Table 6). The characteristic spectrum of antigen expression in CLL has encouraged the development of a highly predictive scoring system for its positive identification and discrimination from other leukemias *(37,38)* (Table 7).

The FAB group recognized two types of atypical CLL, which together are termed CLL of mixed cell type *(35)*. In CLL/PL, prolymphocytes account for 10–55% of circulating cells, whereas if there are more than 55% prolymphocytes, a diagnosis of B-PLL is made. The other variety of atypical CLL is characterized by a spectrum of small to large lymphocytes, but with less than 10% prolympho-cytes. Two groups have reported that atypical CLL tends to be a more aggressive disease with an earlier requirement for therapy and a shorter survival *(39,40)*. In addition, trisomy 12 and abnormalities of *p53* may be more common in atypical CLL *(39,41)*. These findings must be reanalyzed along with immunoglobulin gene

Table 7
A Scoring System for the
Immunophenotypic Diagnosis of CLL

Marker	Score
Weak SmIg	+1
CD5+	+1
CD23+	+1
FMC7−	+1
CD22 weak or −*	+1

A score of 4/5 or 5/5 confirms CLL.
*As an alternative to CD22, negativity for CD79b can score +1. This refinement results in greater discrimination between CLL and other B-cell malignancies.

mutation status, since it seems probable that atypical cytology, the presence of trisomy 12 by conventional metaphase cytogenetics, and *p53* abnormalities may be surrogate markers for an unmutated genotype or an increased proliferative rate.

THE DIFFERENTIAL DIAGNOSIS OF CLL

In the great majority of cases, the characteristic cytology and immunophenotype of CLL result in the rapid and unequivocal recognition of this entity. In addition, in those cases with atypical morphology, the immunophenotype usually makes a diagnosis of CLL relatively straightforward (Table 7). A variety of reactive conditions can produce a peripheral-blood lymphocytosis but the clinical scenario is usually suggestive (e.g., infectious mononucleosis). Yet if any doubt remains after appropriate investigations (such as testing for the presence of heterophile or EBV-specific antibodies), immunophenotyping will rapidly exclude a clonal B-cell disorder.

A relatively large number of B- and T-cell neoplasms can result in peripheral-blood lymphocytosis. The acute lymphoblastic leukemias (ALLs) are readily distinguished by their blastic morphology, but if any doubt persists, immunophenotyping will readily distinguish these disorders from mature, post-thymic B-cell malignancies. Similarly, Burkitt's lymphoma in the leukemic phase has a characteristic morphology, phenotype, and cytogenetics.

Although collectively rare, the most frequently encountered mature T-cell leukemias are T-prolymphocytic leukemia, Sézary syndrome, adult T-cell leukemia-lymphoma, and T-cell large granular lymphocyte (T-LGL) leukemia. These leukemias have characteristic morphologies and display a mature T-cell phenotype (CD3+, CD4/8+), and are thus readily distinguishable from B-cell neoplasms.

Table 8
Chronic B-Cell Leukemias in the Differential Diagnosis of CLL

B-CLL/SLL
B-cell prolymphocytic leukemia
Lymphoplasmacytic lymphoma
Splenic marginal zone B-cell lymphoma with circulating villous lymphocytes
Hairy cell leukemia
Follicular lymphoma
Mantle cell lymphoma

Therefore, in routine clinical practice, the major entities that can be confused with CLL include other types of peripheral B-cell lymphoid malignancies with a propensity to involve the blood (Table 8). A unifying feature that helps to distinguish B-CLL from other entities is the highly characteristic immunophenotype of CLL. The bulk of the other peripheral B-cell neoplasms express a "consensus" phenotype with typically strong expression of the pan-B antigens CD19, CD20, CD22, CD24, and CD79a/b, as well as strong FMC7 and SmIg. Weak expression of CD20, CD22 and CD79b is highly characteristic of B-CLL, as is the co-expression of CD23 and CD5.

B-PLL typically presents in elderly men with a high WBC and splenomegaly. The leukemic cells have a characteristic cytological appearance with a prominent, central nucleolus and express the consensus B-cell leukemia immunophenotype with negativity for CD23 and CD5. Lymphoplasmacytic lymphoma occasionally presents in leukemic phase. The diagnosis is suggested by typical lymphoplasmacytic cytology, and the consensus immunophenotype, and often by the presence of a serum paraprotein.

HCL seldom presents diagnostic difficulties in view of its characteristic clinical and laboratory features. Typical HCL presents with pancytopenia and massive splenomegaly along with typical hairy cells in the blood and monocytopenia. A highly predictive HCL scoring system has been developed in which a score of one is given for positivity with CD25, CD11c, HC2, and CD103 *(42)*. Virtually all cases of HCL will have a score of 3–4/5. Two other disorders are associated with the presence of 'hairy cells' in the blood, namely variant hairy cell leukemia (HCL-V) and splenic marginal B-cell lymphoma with circulating villous lymphocytes (SLVL). HCL-V typically presents with a higher count than HCL and has typical cytology with a hairy cytoplasm, but a prominently nucleolated nucleus and preserved monocyte numbers. The HCL score is typically 0–2/4, with CD11c most often expressed. SLVL presents with splenomegaly and lymphocytosis, with the malignant cells demonstrating 'polar' villi rather than the circumferential 'hairs' of HCL and HCL-V.

The two entities that most often must be differentiated from CLL are FL in leukemic phase and mantle cell lymphoma (MCL). FL typically presents with prominent lymphadenopathy and bone-marrow infiltration, but can occasionally be leukemic. The circulating cells have typical centrocytic cytology and are small—often the size of normal red cells—with inconspicuous but deep nuclear clefting and minimal amounts of cytoplasm. They possess the consensus phenotype, and the majority are also CD10+. The bone marrow is infiltrated in a characteristic paratrabecular pattern, but if any doubt remains, the lymph-node histology will distinguish FL, as will the presence of a t(14;18). MCL usually presents with lymphadenopathy, but frequently involves the gastrointestinal tract and bone marrow, with circulating malignant cells. The leukemic cells are often heterogeneous in appearance, and, this lack of homogeneity is often the first clue to a diagnosis of MCL. The immunophenotype of MCL conforms largely to the consensus phenotype, with the important exception of CD5 positivity. This feature accounts for the occasional difficulty in distinguishing MCL from CLL, and in the past, cases of MCL were probably misdiagnosed as CLL. Again, if doubt persists, lymph-node histology and detection of the characteristic t(11;14) with resulting cyclin D1 expression can confirm a diagnosis of MCL. Cyclin D1 expression can be identified by flow cytometry or immunocytochemistry. It is of significant clinical importance to distinguish MCL from CLL, because the former has a particularly poor clinical outcome, for which intensive and experimental therapies are appropriate.

In summary, CLL can usually be easily distinguished from other leukemic B-cell malignancies. In those rare cases in which the clinical features, cytology, pattern of bone-marrow infiltration, and immunophenotype cannot provide a definitive diagnosis, then lymph-node biopsy and cytogenetic analysis are likely to increase diagnostic certainty.

STAGING OF CLL

The major staging systems for CLL (Rai and Binet) were originally devised 20–25 years ago, and the fact that these systems are still widely used is an indication of their overall clinical utility and robust nature. The Rai clinical staging system was first published in 1975, with formal modifications made in 1987 *(43,44)* (Table 9). The modified system was introduced to assist in the design of prospective trials, and its use is recommended by the NCI Guidelines for the diagnosis and treatment of CLL. It is important to remember that when anemia or thrombocytopenia is immune in etiology, the patient should not be assigned to stage III/IV, because these stages refer to cytopenias that result from bone-marrow failure rather than autoimmune destruction. The Binet staging system consists of three stages *(45)*. Stage C disease is defined by anemia or thrombocytopenia resulting from bone-marrow failure, whereas stages A and B are defined according to the

Table 9
Rai Clinical Staging Systems

Risk Group[b]	Stage[a]	Description
Low	0	Lymphocytosis only
Intermediate	I	Lymphocytosis plus enlarged nodes
	II	Lymphocytosis plus enlarged liver or spleen with or without enlarged nodes
High	III	Lymphocytosis plus anemia (Hb <11 g/dL) with or without enlarged nodes, liver, or spleen
	IV	Lymphocytosis plus thrombocytopenia (Plats <100 × 10^9/L) with or without anemia, enlarged nodes, liver, or spleen

[a]Original Rai system (1975).
[b]Modified Rai system (1987).

Table 10
Binet Clinical Staging System

Stage	Clinical features
A	<3 palpable lymphoid areas
B	3 or more palpable lymphoid areas
C	Anemia (<10 g/dL) or thrombocytopenia (<100 × 10^9/L)

number of palpably enlarged lymphoid areas. For these purposes, five lymphoid areas are described: cervical, axillary, and inguinal nodes, and spleen and liver (Table 10). There have been various attempts to devise new staging systems, including the IWCLL's proposal to integrate the Rai and Binet systems *(46)*, but none of these have achieved widespread acceptance.

PROGNOSTIC FACTORS IN CLL

By far the most important prognostic factor in CLL is clinical stage, whether defined by the Rai or Binet systems *(43–45)* (Table 11). The prognostic significance of clinical stage is of major importance, and many putative prognostic factors have failed to maintain statistical significance after multivariate analysis. Nevertheless, it remains impossible to predict outcomes for individual patients regardless of their clinical stage, because the natural history of CLL is so highly variable.

After multivariate analysis, only a few variables retain prognostic power above that provided by clinical stage, and these include age, sex, and lymphocyte doubling time (LDT). A number of studies have identified increasing age as indica-

Table 11
Survival in CLL According to Clinical Stage

Rai Clinical Staging System

Stage	Median survival (yr)
0	>12
I	8.5
II	6
III	1.5
IV	1.5

Modified Rai Clinical Staging System

Risk Group (Rai stage)	Median survival (yr)
Low (0)	>10
Intermediate (I/II)	7
High (III/IV)	1.5

Binet Clinical Staging System

Stage	Median survival (yr)
A	>10
B	5
C	2

tive of inferior outcome, although it is difficult to allow for the influence of co-existing morbidities. For instance, one study demonstrated a clear survival disadvantage associated with advancing age (age <50 yr, median survival 7.1 yr; age >50 yr, median survival 4.1 yr) *(47)*. However, there was no difference in survival after adjustment for non-CLL mortality. Intriguingly, female patients survive longer than male patients of equivalent stage, for unknown reasons. Galton was the first to suggest that LDT was a poor prognostic indicator *(48)*, and Montserrat subsequently reported that patients with a LDT of less than 12 mo had an overall survival of less than 5 yr whereas at the time of publication, the survival of those with a LDT of over 12 mo had not yet been reached *(49)*. Importantly, although there was a weak correlation of LDT with stage, the prognostic power of LDT was independent of stage. Utilizing the prognostic importance of the LDT, Montserrat was able to identify a subgroup of patients with stage A disease who had a particularly favorable outcome. Such patients with smoldering CLL must fulfill the following criteria: stage A disease, non-diffuse bone-marrow infiltration, hemoglobin >13 g/dL, lymphocytes <30 × 10^9/L, and LDT >12 mo *(50)*. These patients are most unlikely to progress (approx 15% risk at 5 yr) and have life expectancies equivalent to age-matched controls without CLL.

Various groups have suggested that the pattern of bone-marrow infiltration in CLL has prognostic importance. In a retrospective analysis, Rozman et al. found that patients with a non-diffuse pattern of infiltration had a better survival rate than patients with a diffuse pattern *(51)*. However, the difference was only significant in those patients with stage B disease. Similarly, in a prospective analysis of untreated patients, Desablens et al. found no difference in survival in patients with stage A or B disease with diffuse and non-diffuse infiltration *(52)*. Therefore, although there are somewhat contradictory findings, it would appear that the prognostic significance of the pattern of bone-marrow infiltration adds little to that supplied by clinical stage alone. Indeed, it seems probable that diffuse marrow infiltration is strongly associated with advanced stage itself, and this in turn defines prognosis. Other variables, such as the levels of soluble intercellular adhesion molecule-1 (ICAM-1) or soluble CD23, have been reported to have prognostic importance, but their contribution, beyond that supplied by clinical stage, remains uncertain *(53,54)*. Of these biological variables, serum $\beta2$-microglobulin ($\beta2M$) may well be the most important, since high levels have been associated with shortened survival within each of the three modified Rai clinical stages *(55)*. Further large prospective studies are required to formally assess the significance of these biological variables, and are not presently used to routinely guide therapeutic strategies.

The importance of cytogenetic abnormalities is addressed in the preceding section 'Cytogenic Abnormalities in CLL.' Perhaps the most significant development in our current understanding of the biology of CLL is that there appear to be two distinct types of CLL, one with unmutated and the other with mutated Ig VH genes *(16,17)*. These findings have been discussed previously, but are likely to have major importance in defining prognosis for individual patients. Among patients with stage A disease, those with unmutated, pre-germinal-center CLL have a survival of 95 mo whereas those with mutated, post-germinal-center have a survival of 293 mo *(16)*. The finding that there are two variants of CLL, as defined by Ig V_H gene mutation status, has potentially major implications. It is imperative to determine the importance of mutation status for prognosis within each clinical stage and to dissect out its relationship with other cytogenetic and molecular abnormalities as well as with response to therapy. Mutation status is likely to become increasingly important as a prognostic indicator and to direct new therapeutic strategies—particularly for younger patients with early-stage disease.

In summary, at the present time it is fair to say that clinical stage is overwhelmingly the most important prognostic indicator in CLL. No other disease-related variables have found a universally applicable role in predicting outcome. However, the fundamental observation that Ig V_H gene-mutation status divides CLL into two distinct disease groups is likely to have far-reaching implications for the understanding and management of CLL.

THE TREATMENT OF CLL

In the 1950's, chlorambucil was first shown to have activity in CLL by reducing the lymphocyte count, improving bone-marrow function, and reducing the size of the lymph nodes, liver, and spleen *(56)*. This drug, with or without prednisolone, remains the most commonly used agent in CLL, despite a large number of trials of alternative and combination regimes. Response rates, which have been variably defined, range from 38–75% *(57)* and although small studies have suggested a higher response rate with the combination of chlorambucil and prednisolone *(58)*, there is no clear evidence to suggest that the addition of a steroid is beneficial. Indeed, although chlorambucil can relieve symptoms related to progressive CLL, there is no definitive proof that it actually prolongs survival. Chlorambucil has been used in a variety of ways, including continuous daily therapy, and as pulsed or intermittent high-dose schedules. Again, no advantage to any particular regime is evident *(57)*.

Treatment of Early CLL

One important question is whether therapy should be instituted in the early stages of the disease, before clear symptomatic indications for treatment have appeared. Although initial randomized studies had already demonstrated no benefit from early treatment *(59)*, the definitive trials investigating the utility of early treatment were performed by the French Cooperative Group on CLL *(60,61)*. Two consecutive trials investigated daily chlorambucil and pulsed chlorambucil with prednisolone vs no treatment. In all, 1535 patients were treated, with follow-up periods of 11 and 6 yr, respectively. Although treatment with chlorambucil delayed the time to disease progression, there was no difference in overall survival between the treated and untreated groups. Importantly, 49% of the untreated group did not progress or require therapy on prolonged follow-up of up to 11 yr or more.

These results clearly demonstrate that early treatment does not prolong survival of stage A patients. Furthermore, exposure to alkylating agents may result in unwanted complications, such as myelodysplasia or acute myelogenous leukemia (AML). In the first French trial, an increased rate of secondary epithelial cancers was noted, although the second and successive studies have not confirmed this finding. It is also possible that early exposure to chlorambucil may result in acquired drug resistance, which would result in reduced efficacy of therapy at a future date when it is required for symptomatic reasons.

Recommendations for the Initiation of Therapy in CLL

It is generally accepted that patients with stage A disease should be monitored without intervention until there is evidence of disease progression. Most patients with stage C disease will benefit from therapy at diagnosis, although a minor-

Table 12
NCIWG Criteria for Initiating Treatment on a Protocol

1. A minimum of any one of the following disease-related symptoms must be present:
    a. Weight loss >10% within the previous 6 mo
    b. Extreme fatigue (cannot work or unable to perform usual activities)
    c. Fevers >100.5° F for > 2 wk without evidence of infection
    d. Night sweats without evidence of infection
2. Progressive marrow failure: developing or worsening anemia or thrombocytopenia that is not autoimmune in nature
3. Autoimmune anemia or thrombocytopenia that is poorly responsive to steroid therapy
4. Progressive splenomegaly (>6 cm below the costal margin)
5. Massive nodes or clusters (>10 cm in longest diameter) or progressive lymphadenopathy
6. Progressive lymphocytosis with an increase of >50% over a 2 mo period or an anticipated LDT of less than 6 mo

ity—as with many patients with stage B disease—can simply be monitored without treatment until progressive or symptomatic disease develops. If there is doubt about the need for intervention, it is advisable to delay therapy and to review the situation after 1–2 mo of observation.

The NCI-sponsored Working Group has published clear guidelines for the definition of progressive or active disease, and these should be followed in clinical trials so that comparative analyses between studies are possible (32,33) (Table 12). They can also be applied to general clinical practice, although each case must be considered based on its own merits.

Treatment of CLL with Alkylator-Based Multi-Agent Therapies

A number of clinical trials have attempted to determine whether combination regimes are more effective than single-agent chlorambucil in the treatment of advanced-stage or progressive CLL. In 1985, Montserrat et al. published the results of a randomized study comparing chlorambucil and prednisolone with cyclophosphamide, vincristine, and prednisone (COP) (62). Although the response rate was higher for the chlorambucil arm in this study (59% vs 31%, $p < 0.01$), there was no difference in overall survival. Similar results were observed by the French Cooperative Group, in which patients with stage B disease were randomized to treatment with chlorambucil or COP (63). In this study, there was no difference in the overall median survival of approx 5 yr. Again, an ECOG randomized trial of chlorambucil and prednisolone vs (COP) showed equivalent response rates (72% vs 82%) and survival (64).

The addition of an anthracyclene has also been investigated. An early report suggested that mini-CHOP was superior to COP in stage C patients (65). Overall 3-yr survival was significantly higher in the CHOP arm (71% vs 28%), which resulted in early closure of the trial. However, this was a small study, and the outcome of patients in the COP arm was unusually poor. Subsequently, two further studies comparing CHOP with chlorambucil and prednisolone failed to show any advantage with CHOP, although in both the response rate was higher in the anthracyclene-containing arm (66,67).

Thus, a recurring theme is that although these more intensive, multi-agent regimes result in higher response rates, they fail to improve survival. This conclusion is confirmed by a meta-analysis of 10 randomized trials comparing chlorambucil with a variety of combination chemotherapies (68). Indeed, there is no compelling evidence to suggest that any particular combination of chlorambucil and prednisolone, COP, or CHOP, offers any major advantage as the initial treatment for CLL.

Treatment with Purine Analogs

Of the three purine analogs currently available, fludarabine has been used most extensively in the treatment of CLL. The pivotal phase II studies were performed at the MDACC, and reported response rates of 38–57% in previously treated patients and 78% in treatment naïve patients (69–71). These single-center results suggest that fludarabine is the most active single agent currently available for the treatment of CLL. Many of the practical difficulties associated with the conventional intravenous (iv) administration of fludarabine can be overcome with the recently developed oral form of the drug (72). However, it remains to be seen whether it is equally effective when administered in this way. There is less clinical experience with 2-CDA and deoxycoformycin in CLL, and no comparative trials with fludarabine have been performed.

Fludarabine is metabolized to fluoro-ara-A that is resistant to the enzyme adenine deaminase, which is found at high levels within T- and B-cells. The phosphorylated metabolite accumulates within cells, inhibits DNA and RNA synthesis, inhibits ribonucleotide reductase, and results in apoptosis (73). The drug causes significant T-cell depletion, with the greatest effect on CD4+ T-cells. Thus, the drug leads to significant immunosuppression, and indeed, this effect has been successfully used in non-myeloablative conditioning regimes for allogeneic stem-cell transplantation (74). This effect has led to concerns about the potential for a high incidence of infective complications following fludarabine treatment, particularly with pathogens associated with cellular immunodeficiency, such as Pneumocystis carinii and varicella zoster. However, it is likely that only the combination of fludarabine with steroids has a significant effect in this regard (69).

Table 13
Results of the European Trial of Fludarabine vs CAP Chemotherapy

	Fludarabine	CAP	
Previously untreated patients			
CR	23%	17%	NS
Overall RR	71%	60%	NS
Median response duration	NYR	6.9 mo	$p < 0.0001$
Median OS	NYR	52.5 mo	$p = 0.087$
	Fludarabine	*CAP*	
Previously treated patients			
CR	13%	6%	NS
Overall RR	48%	27%	$p = 0.036$
Median response duration	10.8 mo	6 mo	NS
Median OS	24.3 mo	24.4 mo	NS

Three major randomized, prospective phase III trials have compared fludarabine with conventional treatments. The European Trial randomized a total of 196 patients with either untreated stage B or C disease or relapsed disease to treatment with 6–10 cycles of fludarabine or CAP chemotherapy *(75)*. Fludarabine was better tolerated, with significantly less nausea, vomiting, and alopecia than in the CAP arm. Furthermore, there was no difference in the infection rate between the two arms, although fludarabine had to be stopped in 5% of patients because of the development of autoimmune cytopenias. Overall, the response rate was higher for fludarabine-treated patients (60% vs 44%, $p = 0.023$). Results for the two groups of patients are shown in Table 13. Fludarabine resulted in a higher response rate in previously treated patients and prolonged remission duration in previously untreated patients, with a trend toward prolonged overall survival in this group.

The second 'French' study compared six cycles of treatment with fludarabine vs ChOP (mini-CHOP) or CAP in 938 previously untreated patients with stage B or C disease *(76)*. The CAP arm was closed early because of a significantly reduced response rate, and the interim results as published in abstract form are summarized in Table 14. Treatment with fludarabine resulted in higher initial response rates, but this was not translated into longer progression-free or overall survival. Notably, there was no increase in the rate of autoimmune cytopenia in the fludarabine arm.

The third study of this type, conducted by the US Intergroup, compared fludarabine with chlorambucil in previously untreated patients *(77)*. A third arm with combined fludarabine and chlorambucil was stopped early because of

Table 14
Preliminary Results of the French Trial of Fludarabine vs CHOP vs CAP

Fludarabine	CHOP	CAP		
RR	41%	30%	15%	$p = 0.006/0.0001$
PFS	30 mo	28 mo	27 mo	NS
Median OS	74 mo	68 mo	70 mo	NS

Table 15
Results of the US Intergroup Study of Fludarabine vs Chlorambucil

	Fludarabine	Chlorambucil	
CR	20%	4%	$p < 0.001$
RR	63%	37%	$p < 0.001$
PFS	20 mo	14 mo	$p < 0.001$
Median OS	66 mo	56 mo	NS

excess toxicity. A total of 509 patients with Rai stage III/IV or I/II with active disease were treated for up to 12 monthly cycles of therapy. The chlorambucil was given monthly at a dose of 40 mg/m^2. The results of this study are summarized in Table 15. Patients with primary treatment failure were allowed to cross over to the other arm. For chlorambucil treatment failures, there was a subsequent 46% response rate to fludarabine, whereas for patients who failed fludarabine, only 7% responded to chlorambucil. The authors conclude that fludarabine resulted in higher complete and overall response rates and in prolonged response duration. However, this did not result in a prolongation of overall survival, perhaps because of the relative success of fludarabine as salvage therapy in patients who failed chlorambucil.

What are the general conclusions that can be drawn from these three studies? First, fludarabine results in a higher response rate and longer response duration than alkylator-based regimes in previously untreated patients with CLL. However, this superiority has not resulted in prolonged survival, and this is a result—at least in part—to the clear efficacy of fludarabine as a salvage therapy. Yet, the achievement of higher response rates with fludaribine is highly encouraging, and is stimulating further clinical investigation designed to improve on this success. Such strategies include the use of fludarabine in combination with other agents, and the use of high-dose therapy with stem-cell support to consolidate remission.

Combination Therapy with Fludarabine and Cyclophosphamide

In vitro studies have indicated that the combination of cyclophosphamide and fludarabine is likely to be synergistic. Normally, the DNA interstrand crosslinks induced by alkylating agents are rapidly repaired. However, the addition of

Table 16
New Therapeutic Targets in CLL

Target	Example of drug
Histone deacetylase inhibition	Depsipeptide
Protein kinase C inhibition	Staurosporine derivatives
Protein kinase C activation	Bryostatin
Cyclin-dependent kinase inhibition	Flavopiridol
Phosphodiesterase inhibition	Theophylline
Anti-angiogenesis	Thalidomide
Proteosome inhibition	PS-341

fludarabine results in significant inhibition of crosslink repair, presumably because of its ability to directly inhibit DNA repair enzymes (78,79). Two single-center studies have investigated the clinical efficacy of this combination in vivo.

Flinn et al. studied the combination of cyclophosphamide (600 mg/m^2 on d 1) with fludarabine (20 mg/m^2 on d 1–5) supported by granulocyte-colony-stimulation factor (G-CSF) in a variety of previously untreated indolent lymphoid malignancies. For the 17 patients with CLL, 51% and 41% achieved a complete remission (CR) and partial remission (PR) respectively (80). A larger number of patients with CLL at various stages have been treated at the MDACC with a slightly different regime comprised of cyclophosphamide at doses ranging from 300–500 mg/m^2 for 3 d and fludarabine at 20 mg/m^2 for 3 d (81). Excess toxicity was observed at the higher cyclophosphamide doses, and the majority of patients were therefore treated at the lowest dose level. For the previously untreated patients, the total response rate (RR) was 88%, with 35% achieving CR. Although the CR rate was not significantly higher than the 27% rate observed with fludarabine as a single agent in the Intergroup Study (77), a potentially important observation was that only 8% of the patients with CR had detectable CD5+ B-cells in the marrow by flow cytometry. The suggestion is that the combination regime results in a better quality of remission in responding patients.

The potential value of these findings has not yet been established in prospective randomized studies. Certainly, the ability to induce remissions associated with the elimination of disease by the most sensitive techniques is encouraging. Indeed, such responses are likely to be the most favorable platforms from which to launch high-dose therapies with the intent of cure, since such approaches are known to be most effective in the setting of minimal disease.

Potential New Therapies for CLL

A variety of biological therapies are currently under development for the treatment of CLL. The underlying concept is that these agents will interfere with molecular or biological targets that are operative in CLL. It is beyond the scope of this chapter to review these promising agents in any detail, but further information can be found in a recent comprehensive review *(82)*. Examples of such potential targets and drugs are provided in Table 16.

Two monoclonal antibodies (MAbs) have been examined in CLL. Anti-CD20 has shown only marginal activity when administered in a conventional fashion (375 mg/m^2 weekly for 4 wk) with a response rate of only 12% *(83)*. Intuitively, this is not surprising, since CD20 is expressed only at low levels by CLL cells. Attempts to overcome this problem have included using the drug at significantly higher concentrations or with a 3x weekly dosage regime *(84,85)*. Although high response rates have been observed, the considerable cost associated with such strategies means that this approach is unlikely to be widely applicable.

Anti-CD52 (CAMPATH-1H) has shown promise in CLL, with response rates of 42% in previously treated patients *(86)*. Notably, responses were more marked in blood and bone marrow than lymph nodes. In a large pivotal study (CAM211), patients with fludarabine-refractory CLL showed a 33% response rate *(87)*. CD52 is expressed by T- and B-lymphocytes as well as by monocytes. A major concern is that its use will result in clinically significant immunosuppression. Indeed, in a series of 56 treated patients, 7% experienced CMV reactivation, and one death resulted *(88)*.

How these new treatments will impact on the treatment of CLL remains uncertain, and there is a clear need for well-planned trials investigating their use both as single agents and in combination with established therapies. Nevertheless, it is highly encouraging that these new agents under development offer distinct modes of action and considerable potential for the future.

AUTOLOGOUS STEM-CELL TRANSPLANTATION IN CLL

Autologous stem-cell transplantation can be curative in a proportion of patients with relapsed Hodgkin's disease and aggressive non-Hodgkin's lymphomas. These results have encouraged the investigation of this treatment strategy in CLL, with conflicting results. The MDACC experience was that, in a group of heavily pretreated patients, transient remissions at best were achieved following high-dose therapy with stem-cell rescue *(89)*. However, investigators at the DFCI, have reported superior results in a group of 12 patients with poor-prognosis CLL *(90)*. Ten of 12 patients achieved a CR after autografting with cyclophosphamide/total body irradiation (TBI) conditioning. These patients were generally treated earlier in the natural history of their disease, and were treated with conventional chemotherapy to a state of complete remission or minimal disease prior to high-dose therapy. The bone-marrow harvests were also purged with a cocktail of anti-B-cell MAbs. Of the first five patients who achieved a CR, all remained in CR for a median of 25 mo (range 6–31 mo). Perhaps most importantly, all three patients with prolonged follow-up showed the absence of a clonally rearranged immunoglobulin gene by Southern blot analysis.

A retrospective analysis of 321 patients with CLL who have undergone autologous transplantation has been performed by the EBMT *(91)*. Overall, there was a transplant-related mortality rate of 6%. Improved survival was correlated with a shorter interval from diagnosis to transplant, CR status at the time of transplant, and the use of TBI in the conditioning regime. No benefit was observed from in vitro purging.

In summary, there are indications that high-dose therapy with autologous stem-cell transplantation results in molecular remissions in CLL, and it is possible that these favorable responses will result in long-term survival. It is also evident that this approach is most likely to be of benefit early in the course of the disease, and in the presence of minimal residual disease at the time of transplant. Important questions remain concerning the role of purging, the most appropriate conditioning regime, patient selection, and, most significantly, the impact on overall survival. These questions can only be answered definitively in prospective randomized trials.

THE ROLE OF ALLOGENEIC STEM-CELL TRANSPLANTATION (ALLO SCT) IN CLL

In the light of the success of Allo SCT in a variety of hematological malignancies, this treatment modality has been investigated in patients with CLL. Retrospective analyses of conventional ablative transplants have been reported, the largest from the EBMT/IBMTR *(89,90,92,93)*. The majority of patients in these series had advanced, often chemorefractory, disease and transplant-related mortality ranged from 35–46%. Nevertheless, overall survival ranged from 46% to 62% at 3–5 yr. Furthermore, in those cases that were analyzed, molecular remissions were often achieved at intervals greater than 6 mo following transplantation, suggesting that a graft vs leukemia effect (GVL) may be operative in CLL *(89)*. The most convincing evidence that a GVL effect is operative in hematological malignancies derives from observing responses to the cessation of immunosuppressive therapy or the administration of donor lymphocyte infusions in the setting of persistent or relapsing disease following Allo SCT *(94)*. There are only anecdotal reports of such responses for CLL, and in all cases, GVL has been associated with GVHD *(95–97)*. Therefore, it remains to be seen whether there is a specific GVL effect in CLL that can be separated from GVHD.

In an update of the MDACC series, which included ablative and non-ablative transplants, the 3 yr overall and disease-free survivals were 47% and 34%, respectively *(98)*. The outcome was significantly better for patients with chemosensitive disease and for those who had received fewer lines of chemotherapy. Of particular interest is the observation that survival following nonablative transplants was equivalent to that following conventional SCT. In view of the reduced toxicity of such transplants, this treatment should be investigated in both younger and older patients with CLL.

At present, it can be concluded that the precise role of Allo SCT in CLL remains uncertain. There is only limited evidence to support the existence of a GVL effect in CLL, and further information is required concerning the efficacy of donor lymphocyte infusions to clarify this issue. As is the case with many hematological malignancies, it is likely that Allo SCT will be most effective in early-stage chemosensitive disease, but these issues must be formally addressed in prospective studies.

THE TREATMENT OF YOUNGER PATIENTS WITH CLL

The management of younger patients presents special difficulties, because life expectancy is likely to be reduced by up to 20 yr overall in this subgroup of patients with CLL (99). Estimates of the proportion of younger patients with CLL have varied from 6–20% with youth usually defined as less than 55 yr of age (100,101). A representative series of 204 younger patients showed that, in general, the presenting features and response to therapy were similar to those in older patients. Of this group, 34% had smoldering CLL and an identical median overall survival of 10 yr (101). However, an important point is that, for younger patients, death was much more likely to result from CLL itself rather than any other extraneous comorbidity. In this series, younger patients with CLL had a higher male-to-female ratio than older patients (2.85 vs 1.29) and a greater risk of developing Richter's syndrome (5.9% vs 1.2%), although other reports have not confirmed these differences (102). In addition, only dynamic parameters such as active disease (as defined by the NCI criteria) and a short LDT were prognostically significant. In contrast to older patients, on multivariate analysis, the stage of disease had no prognostic importance. Two subgroups were easily identifiable—60% of younger patients had progressive disease with a median survival from the time of initial therapy of only 5 yr. The remaining 40% had long-lasting stable disease, which did not require therapy and was associated with 94% survival at 12 yr from diagnosis.

This study and others clearly indicate that young patients with CLL who do not have conventional indications for treatment should be managed expectantly. However, for the group with progressive disease, innovative therapies with or without stem-cell transplantation are appropriate within the context of clinical trials.

AUTOIMMUNE DISEASE AND ITS TREATMENT IN CLL

A characteristic feature of CLL is the frequent development of both autoimmune disease and immunodeficiency. The autoimmune phenomena that occur in CLL are largely restricted to hemopoietic tissues with autoimmune hemolytic anemia (AIHA), immune thrombocytopenia (ITP) and pure red-cell aplasia (PRCA) observed with decreasing frequency *(103)*. The intriguing co-existence of immunodeficiency with autoimmunity is also observed in a number of other primary and acquired immunodefiency states, such as common variable immunodeficiency, X-linked immunodeficiency with hyper IgM, and HIV infection. The hyper IgM syndrome is caused by inherited defects of the gene for CD40-ligand (CD154) and is characterized by profound immunodeficiency and a greatly increased risk of immune hematological abnormalities *(104)*. The interaction of CD154 with CD40 present on antigen-presenting cells (APC) is required for the generation of normal secondary immune responses that are characterized by isotype-class switching and somatic hypermutation. Intriguingly, CD4+ T-cells from patients with CLL appear to have an acquired CD154 deficiency and fail to express this immunoregulatory molecule after CD3 ligation. Furthermore, the addition of CLL cells results in decreased CD154 expression in vitro by normal activated CD4+ T-cells *(105)*. These similarities between the hyper IgM syndrome and CLL suggest that the acquired CD154 deficiency characteristic of CLL is likely to be central to the immunodeficiency and autoimmunity observed in CLL. Furthermore, transduction of CLL cells with CD154 may be a novel strategy for circumventing the defective immune responses seen in CLL, and may allow for restoration of effective anti-tumor activity *(106)*.

Whatever the case, AIHA is the most common immune disorder found in CLL, and its occurrence poses particular challenges to management. Highly variable incidence rates for AIHA have been observed, ranging from 3–37% *(103)*. It has been reported that AIHA may be related to advanced-stage disease, and indeed, the NCI guidelines suggest that AIHA or ITP that is poorly responsive to steroid therapy is indicative of active disease, and is thus an indication for the initiation of chemotherapy *(32,33)*. However, it is important to emphasize that in the vast majority of cases AIHA is caused by polyclonal autoantibodies that are not the product of the CLL clone itself *(107)*. Rather, they are the result of the disturbed immunoregulatory pathways that are characteristic of CLL, particularly the imbalance and deficiency of CD4+ T-cell subsets. In this regard, it has long been noted that AIHA can be triggered by the initiation of chemotherapy, whether this is in the form of alkylating agents *(108)* or purine analogs *(109,110)*. A number of reports have suggested that fludarabine is especially likely to result in AIHA and in the European Cooperative Study autoimmune cytopenias developed in 5% of patients of patients treated with fludarabine, but none treated with CAP *(75)*.

Mauro and colleagues retrospectively analyzed their large cohort of patients with CLL for the occurrence of AIHA *(111)*. AIHA developed in 4.3% (52 of 1203) of their patients, and in 90% of cases was associated with active CLL, although 75% of instances occurred in previously untreated cases of CLL. Using multivariate analysis, AIHA was associated with increasing age, male sex, and a high lymphocyte count. By itself, AIHA had no detrimental effect on survival. It is clear from this large study that AIHA is associated with CLL itself, and most cases occur prior to therapy. Furthermore, there was no difference in frequency between patients treated with chlorambucil and fludarabine, although both groups received concurrent prednisolone in this study. Therefore, it seems likely that the triggering effect of drugs such as fludarabine, which are themselves potent immunosuppressive agents, results from a further disturbance of immuno-regulatory mechanisms in addition to those caused by the disease itself.

The relative rarity of autoimmune blood disorders associated with CLL means that most therapeutic strategies are informed by largely anecdotal reports, and there is a distinct lack of evidence-based guidelines to assist the physician. Nevertheless, the generally accepted practice is to treat coexistent AIHA, ITP, and PRCA in a similar manner to that adopted for idiopathic cases *(103)*. Thus, the mainstay of treatment remains the use of steroids in conventional doses with the use of immunosuppressive agents as second-line agents. Similarly, there is not enough evidence to provide firm guidelines about the efficacy of splenectomy in such cases. Our practice is to treat autoimmune disorders in their own right and to reserve specific CLL-directed therapies for patients who have alternative conventional indications for therapy or who fail standard immunomodulatory treatments. The increased risk of opportunistic infections is a particular concern in patients treated with steroids and other immunosuppressive agents, and careful clinical evaluation of this group of patients is warranted. The role of prophylactic antimicrobials remains unproven, and indeed, in the series reported by Mauro et al., prophylactic cotrimoxazole, did not improve survival *(111)*. In summary, despite the introduction of new therapies for CLL, the disease remains incurable. There is an urgent need to assess treatment strategies with the aim of curing patients with CLL.

REFERENCES

1. Calligaris-Cappio F, Hamblin TJ. B-cell chronic lymphocytic leukemia: a bird of a different feather. *J Clin Oncol* 1999;17:399–408.
2. Reed JC. Molecular biology of chronic lymphocytic leukemia. *Semin Oncol* 1998;25:11–18.
3. Finch SC, Linet MS. Chronic Leukemias. Balliere's *Clin Haematol* 1992;5:27.
4. Finch SC, Finch CA. Summary of the studies at ABCC-RERF concerning the late hematological effects of atomic bomb exposure in Hiroshima and Nagasaki. RERF Technical Report. 1988;23–88:5.
5. Horwitz M. The genetics of familial leukemia. *Leukemia* 1997;11:1347–1359.
6. Yuille MR, Houlston RS, Catovsky D. Anticipation in familial chronic lymphocytic leukemia. *Leukemia* 1998;12:1696–1698.
7. Hamblin TJ, Oscier DG, Young BJ. Autoimmunity in chronic lymphocytic leukemia. *J Clin Pathol* 1986;39:713–718.
8. Mauro FR, Foa R, Cerretti R, et al. Autoimmune hemolytic anemia in in chronic lymphocytic leukemia: clinical, therapeutic and prognostic factors. *Blood* 2000;95:2786–2792.

9. Kipps T, Carson DA. Autoantibodies in chronic lymphocytic leukemia and related systemic autoimmune diseases. *Blood* 1993;81:2475–2487.
10. Giles FJ, O'Brien SM, Keating MJ. Chronic lymphocytic leukemia in (Richter's) transformation. *Semin Oncol* 1998;25: 117–125.
11. Bessudo A, Kipps TJ. Origin of high-grade lymphomas in Richter syndrome. *Leuk Lymphoma* 1995;18:367–372.
12. Momose H, Jaffe ES, Shin SS, et al. Chronic lymphocytic leukemia/small lymphocytic lymphoma with Reed-Sternberg-like cells and possible transformation to Hodgkin's disease. Mediation by Epstein-Barr virus. *Am J Surg Pathol* 1992;16:859–867.
13. Caligaris-Cappio F. B-chronic lymphocytic leukemia: a malignancy of anti-self B-cells. *Blood* 1996;87:2615–2620.
14. Schroeder HW, Dighiero G. The pathogenesis of chronic lymphocytic leukemia: analysis of the antibody repertoire. *Immunol Today* 1994;15:288–294.
15. Pritsch O, Maloum K, Dighiero G. Basic biology of autoimmune phenomena in chronic lymphocytic leukemia. *Semin Oncol* 1998;25:34–41.
16. Hamblin TJ, Davis Z, Gardiner A, et al. Unmutated Ig VH genes are associated with a more aggressive form of of chronic lymphocytic leukemia. *Blood* 1999;94:1948–1854.
17. Damle RN, Wasil T, Fais F, et al. Ig V gene mutation status and CD38 expression as novel prognostic indicators in chronic lymphocytic leukemia. *Blood* 1999;94:1840–1847.
18. Juliusson G, Oscier DG, Fitchett M, et al. Prognostic subgroups in B-cell chronic lymphocytic leukemia defined by specific chromosomal abnormalities. *N Engl J Med* 1990;323:720–724.
19. Juliusson G, Oscier DG, Gahrton G for the International Working Party on Chromosomes in Chronic Lymphocytic Leukemia. Second international compilation of data on 662 patients. *Leuk Lymphoma* 1991;5 (Suppl):21–25.
20. Han T, Henderson ES, Emrich LJ, et al. Prognostic significance of karyotypic abnormalities in B-cell chronic lymphocytic leukemia: an update. *Semin Hematol* 1987;24:257–262.
21. Bird ML, Ueshima Y, Rowley JD, et al. Chromosome abnormalities in B-cell chronic lymphocytic leukemia and their clinical correlations. *Leukemia* 1989;3:182–186.
22. Dohner H, Stilenbauer S, Benner A, et al. Genomic aberrations and survival in chronic lymphocytic leukemia. *N Engl J Med* 2000;343:1910–1916.
23. Hanada M, Delia D, Aiello A, et al. Bcl-2 gene hypomethylation and high-level expression in B-cell chronic lymphocytic leukemia. *Blood* 1993;82:1820–1828.
24. Konig A, Menzel T, Lynen S, et al. Basic fibroblast growth factor (bFGF) upregulates the expression of bcl-2 in B-cell chronic lymphocytic leukemia cell lines resulting in delaying apoptosis. *Leukemia* 1997;11:258–265.
25. Aguilar-Santelises M, Rottenberg ME, Lewin N, et al. Bcl-2, bax and p53 expression in B-cell chronic lymphocytic leukemia in relation to in vitro survival and clinical progression. *Int J Cancer* 1996;69:114–119.
26. Pepper C, Bentley P, Hoy T. Regulation of clinical chemoresistance by bcl-2 and bax oncoproteins in B-cell chronic lymphocytic leukemia. *Br J Haematol* 1996;95:513–517.
27. Fenaux P, Preudhomme C, Lai JL, et al. Mutations of the p53 gene in B-cell chronic lymphocytic leukemia: a report on 39 cases with cytogenetic analysis. *Leukemia* 1992;6:246–250.
28. Schaffner C, Stilgenbauer S, Rapplod GA, et al. Somatic ATM mutations indicate a pathogenic role of ATM in in B-cell chronic lymphocytic leukemia. *Blood* 1999;94:748–753.
29. Stankovic T, Weber P, Stewart G, et al. Inactivation of ataxia telangiectasia mutated gene in B-cell chronic lymphocytic leukemia. *Lancet* 1999;353:26–29.
30. Migliazza A, Bosch F, Komatsu H, et al. Nucleotide sequence, transcription map and mutation analysis of the 13q14 chromosomal region deleted in B-cell chronic lymphocytic leukemia. *Blood* 2001;97:2098–2104.
31. Staudt LM. Gene expression physiology and pathophysiology of the immune system. *Trends in Immunology* 2001; 22:35–41.

32. Cheson BD, Bennett JM, Rai KR, et al. Guidelines for clinical protocols for chronic lymphocytic leukemia: report of the NCI-sponsored Working Group. *Am J Hematol* 1988;29:152–159.
33. Cheson BD, Bennett JM, Grever M, et al. National Cancer Institute-sponsored working group guidelines for chronic lymphocytic leukemia: revised guidelines for diagnosis and treatment. *Blood* 1996;87:4990–4997.
34. International Workshop on chronic lymphocytic leukemia: recommendations for diagnosis, staging and response criteria. *Ann Intern Med* 1989;236:1989–1995.
35. Bennett JM, Catovsky D, Daniel M-T, et al. Proposals for the classification of chronic (mature) B and T lymphoid leukaemias. *J Clin Pathol* 1989;42:567–584.
36. Harris NL, Jaffe ES, Diebold J, et al. World Health Organization classification of neoplastic diseases of the hematopoietic and lymphoid tissues: Report of the clinical advisory committee-Airlie House, Virginia, November 1997. *J Clin Oncol* 1999;17:3835–3849.
37. Matutes E, Owusu-Ankomah K, Morilla R, et al. The immunological profile of B-cell disorders and proposal of a scoring system for the diagnosis of CLL. *Leukemia* 1994;8:1640–1645.
38. Moreau EJ, Matutes E, A'Hern RP, et al. Improvement of the chronic lymphocytic leukemia scoring system with the monoclonal antibody SN8 (CD79b). *Am J Clin Path* 1997;108:278–282.
39. Criel A, Verhoef G, Vlietinck R, et al. Further characterization of morphologically defined typical and atypical CLL: a clinical, immunophentypic, cytogenetic and prognostic study on 390 cases. *Br J Haematol* 1997;97:383–391.
40. Oscier DG, Matutes E, Copplestone A, et al. Atypical lymphocyte morphology: an adverse prognostic factor for disease progression in stage A CLL independent of trisomy 12. *Br J Haematol* 1997;98:934–939.
41. Lens D, Dyer MJ, Garcia-Marco JM, et al. P53 abnormalities in CLL are associated with excess of prolymphocytes and poor prognosis. *Br J Haematol* 1997;99:848–857.
42. Matutes E, and Catovsky S. The value of scoring systems for the diagnosis of biphenotypic leukaemia and mature B-cell disorders. *Leukemia and Lymphoma* 1994;3 (Suppl. 1):11–14.
43. Rai KR, Sawitsky A, Cronkite EP, et al. Clinical staging of chronic lymphocytic leukemia. *Blood* 1975;46:219–234.
44. Rai KR. A critical analysis of staging in CLL. In: Gale RP, Rai KR, eds. Chronic lymphocytic leukemia: recent progress and future directions. UCLA Symposia on Molecular and Cellular Biology, New Series, Vol 59, Alan R. Liss, New York, 1987, p. 253.
45. Binet JL, Auquier A, Dighiero G, et al. A new prognostic classification of chronic lymphocytic leukemia derived from a multivariate survival analysis. *Cancer* 1981;48:198–206.
46. International Workshop on chronic lymphocytic leukemia: recommendations for diagnosis, staging and response criteria. *Ann Intern Med* 1989;110:236–241.
47. Molica S, Brugiatelli M, Callea V, et al. Comparison of younger versus older B-cell chronic lymphocytic leukemia patients for clinical presentation and prognosis. A retrospective study of 53 cases. *Eur J Haematol* 1994;52:216–221.
48. Galton DAG. The pathogenesis of chronic lymphocytic leukemia. *Can Med Assoc J* 1966;94:1005–1010.
49. Montserrat E, Sanchez-Bisono J, Vinolas N, et al. Lymphocyte doubling time in chronic lymphocytic leukemia: analysis of its prognostic significance. Br J Haematol 1986;62:567–575.
50. Montserrat E, Vinolas N, Rverer JC, et al. Natural history of chronic lymphocytic leukemia: on the progression and prognosis of early stages. *Nouv Rev Fr Hematol* 1988;30:359–361.
51. Rozman C, Montserrat E, Rodriguez-Fernandez JM, et al. Bone marrow histological pattern—the best single prognostic parameter in chronic lymphocytic leukemia: a multivariate survival analysis. *Blood* 1984;64:642–648.
52. Desablens B, Claisse JF, Piprot-Choffat C, et al. Prognostic value of bone marrow biopsy in chronic lymphocytic leukemia. *Nouv Rev Fr Hematol* 1989;31:179–182.

53. Molica S, Levato D, Dell'Olio M, et al. Clinico-prognostic implications of increased levels of soluble CD54 in the serum of B-cell chronic lymphocytic leukemia patients. Results of a multivariate survival analysis. *Haematologica* 1997;82:148–151.
54. Sarfati M, Chevret S, Chastang C, et al. Prognostic importance of serum soluble CD23 level in cell chronic lymphocytic leukemia, *Br J Haematol* 1996;88:4259–4264.
55. Keating M, Lerner S, Kantarjian H, et al. The serum beta2-microglobulin level is more powerful than stage in predicting response and survival in chronic lymphocytic leukemia. *Blood* 1995;86(Suppl 1):606a.
56. Galton DAG, Wiltshaw E, Szur L, et al. The use of chlorambucil and steroids in the treatment of chronic lymphocytic leukaemia. *Br J Haematol* 1961;7:73–78.
57. Keating MJ. Chronic lymphocytic leukaemia. In: Henderson ES, Lister TA, Greaves MF, eds. *Leukemia*, 6th ed. WB Saunders Company, Philadelphia, 1996.
58. Han T, Ezdinli EZ, Emrich LJ, et al. Chlorambucil vs. chlorambucil-corticosteroid therapy in chronic lymphocytic leukaemia. *Cancer* 1973;31:502–507.
59. Catovsky D, Richards S, Fooks J, et al. CLL trials in the United Kingdom: The Medical Research Council CLL trials 1, 2 and 3. *Leuk Lymphoma* 1991;5:105–112.
60. French Cooperative Group on Chronic Lymphocytic Leukaemia: effects of chlorambucil and therapeutic decision in initial forms of chronic lymphocytic leukaemia (stage A): results of a randomised clinical trial in 612 patients. *Blood* 1990;75:1414–1420.
61. French Cooperative Group on Chronic Lymphocytic Leukaemia: chlorambucil in indolent chronic lymphocytic leukaemia. *N Engl J Med* 1998;338:1506–1514.
62. Montserrat E, Alcala A, Parody R, et al. Treatment of chronic lymphocytic leukaemia in advanced stages. *Cancer* 1985;56:2369–2371.
63. French Cooperative Group on Chronic Lymphocytic Leukaemia: a randomised trial of chlorambucil versus COP in stage B chronic lymphocytic leukaemia. *Blood* 1990;75:1422–1427.
64. Raphael B, Andersen JW, Silber R, et al. Comparison of chlorambucil and prednisone versus cyclophosphamide, vincristine and prednisone as initial treatment for chronic lymphocytic leukaemia: long-term follow-up of an Eastern Cooperative Oncology Group randomised clinical trial. *J Clin Oncol* 1991;9:770–776.
65. French Cooperative Group on Chronic Lymphocytic Leukaemia: long-term results of the CHOP regimen in Stage C chronic lymphocytic leukaemia. *Br J Haematol* 1989;73:334–339.
66. Hansen MM, Anderson E, Birgens H, et al. CHOP vs chlorambucil and prednisone in chronic lymphocytic leukaemia. *Leuk Lymphoma* 1991;5:97–103.
67. Kimby E, Mellstedt H. Chlorambucil/prednisone versus CHOP in symptomatic chronic lymphocytic leukaemias of B-cell type. A randomised trial. *Leuk Lymphoma* 1991;5:93–97.
68. CLL Trialists Collaborative Group. Chemotherapeutic options in chronic lymphocytic leukaemia: a meta-analysis of the randomised trials. *J Natl Cancer Inst* 1999;91:861–868.
69. O'Brien S, Kantarjian H, Beran M, et al. Results of fludarabine and prednisone therapy in 264 patients with chronic lymphocytic leukaemia with multivariate analysis-derived prognostic model for response to treatment. *Blood* 1993;82:1695–1700.
70. Keating MJ, Kantarjian H, Talpaz M, et al. Fludarabine—a new agent with major activity against chronic lymphocytic leukaemia. *Blood* 1989;74:19–25.
71. Keating MJ, Kantarjian H, O'Brien S, et al. Fludarabine: a new agent with marked cytoreductive activity in untreated chronic lymphocytic leukaemia. *J Clin Oncol* 1991;9:44–49.
72. Foran JM, Oscier D, Orchard J, et al. Pharmacokinetic study of single doses of oral fludarabine phosphate in patients with low-grade non-Hodgkin's lymphoma and B-cell chronic lymphocytic leukaemia. *J Clin Oncol* 1999;17:1574–1579.
73. Astrow AB. Fludarabine in chronic leukaemia. *Lancet* 1996;347:1420–1421.
74. Giralt S, Thall PF, Khouri I, et al. Melphalan and purine-containing preparative regimens: reduced-intensity conditioning for patients with hematologic malignancies undergoing allogeneic progenitor cell transplantation. *Blood* 2001;97:631–637.

75. The French Cooperative Group on CLL. Multicentre prospective randomised trial of fludarabine versus cyclophosphamide, doxorubicin and prednisone (CAP) for treatment of advanced-stage chronic lymphocytic leukaemia. *Lancet* 1996;347:1432–1438.
76. Leporrier M, Chevret S, Cazin B, et al. Randomised clinical trial comparing two anthracyclene-containing regimens (CHOP and CAP) and fludarabine in advanced chronic lymphocytic leukaemia. *Blood* 1999;94(Suppl 1):603a.
77. Rai KR, Peterson BL, Appelbaum FR, et al. Fludarabine compared with chlorambucil as primary therapy for chronic lymphocytic leukaemia. *N Engl J Med* 2000;343:1750–1757.
78. Koehl U, Li L, Nowak B, et al. Fludarabine and cyclophosphamide: synergistic cytotoxicity associated with inhibition of interstrand cross-link removal. *Proc Am Assoc Cancer Res* 1997;38:2.
79. Bellosillo B, Villamor N, Colomer, et al. In vitro evaluation of fludarabine in combination with cyclophosphamide and/or mitoxantrone in B-cell chronic lymphocytic leukaemia. *Blood* 1999;94:2836–2843.
80. Flinn IW, Byrd JC, Morrison C, et al. Fludarabine and cyclophosphamide with filgrastim support in patients with previously untreated indolent lymphoid malignancies. *Blood* 2000;96:71–75.
81. O'Brien SM, Kantarjian HM, Cortes J, et al. Results of the fludarabine and cyclophosphamide combination in chronic lymphocytic leukaemia. *J Clin Oncol* 2001;19:1414–1420.
82. Byrd JC, Waselenko JK, Keating M, et al. Novel therapies for chronic lymphocytic leukaemia in the 21st century. *Semin Oncol* 2000;27:587–597.
83. Nguyen DT, Amess J, Doughty H, et al. IDEC-C2B8 anti-CD20 (Rituximab) immunotherapy in patients with low-grade non-Hodgkin's lymphoma and lymphoproliferative disorders: evaluation of response in 48 patients. *Eur J Haematol* 1999;62:76–82.
84. O'Brien S, Kantarjian H, Thomas DA, et al. Rituximab dose escalation trial in chronic lymphocytic leukemia. *J Clin Oncol* 2001;19:2165–2170.
85. Byrd JC, Murphy T, Howard RS, et al. Rituximab using a thrice weekly dosing schedule in B-cell chronic lymphocytic leukemia and small lymphocytic lymphoma demonstrates clinical activity and acceptable toxicity. *J Clin Oncol* 2001;19:2153–2164.
86. Osterborg A, Dyer M, Bunjes D, et al. Phase II multicenter study of human CD52 antibody in previously treated chronic lymphocytic leukaemia. *J Clin Oncol* 1997;15:1567–1574.
87. Keating MJ, Byrd JC, Rai KR, et al. Mulicenter study of Campath-1H in patients with chronic lymphocytic leukaemia refractory to fludarabine. *Blood* 1999;94(Suppl 1):705a.
88. Kennedy B, Rawstron A, Richards S, Hillmen P. Campath-1H in CLL: immune reconstitution and viral infections during and after therapy. *Blood* 2000;96(Suppl 1):164a.
89. Khouri IF, Keating MJ, Vriesendorp HM, et al. Autologous and allogeneic bone marrow transplantation for chronic lymphocytic leukemia: preliminary results. *J Clin Oncol* 1994;12:748–758.
90. Rabinowe SN, Soiffier RJ, Gribben JG, et al. Autologous and allogeneic bone marrow transplantation for poor prognosis patients with B-cell chronic lymphocytic leukemia. *Blood* 1993;82:1366–1376.
91. Dreger P, van Biezen A, Brand R, et al for the Chronic Leukaemia Working Party, EBMT. Prognostic factors for survival after autologous stem cell transplantation for chronic lymphocytic leukaemia (CLL): the EBMT experience. *Blood* 2000;96(Suppl 1):482a.
92. Michallet M, Archimbaud E, Bandini G, et al. HLA-identical sibling bone marrow transplantation in younger patients with chronic lymphocytic leukemia. *Ann Intern Med* 1996;124:311–315.
93. Pavletic ZS, Arrowsmith ER, Bierman PJ, et al. Outcome of allogeneic stem cell transplantation for B-cell chronic lymphocytic leukemia. *Bone Marrow Transplant* 2000;25:717–722.

94. Champlin R. Harnessing graft-versus-malignancy: non-myeloablative preparative regimens for allogeneic haematopoietic transplantation, an evolving strategy for adoptive immunotherapy. *Br J Haematol* 2000; 111:18–29.
95. Rondon G, Giralt S, Huh Y, et al. Graft-versus-leukemia after allogeneic bone marrow transplantation for chronic lymphocytic leukaemia. *Bone Marrow Transplant* 1996;18:669–672.
96. Mehta J, Powles R, Kulkarni S, et al. Induction of graft-versus-host disease as immunotherapy of leukaemia relapsing after allogeneic transplantation: a single-center experience of 32 adults. *Bone Marrow Transplant* 1997;20:129–135.
97. deMagalhaes M, Donnenberg A, Hammert L et al. Induction of graft-vs-leukemia in apatient with chronic lymphocytic leukaemia. *Bone Marrow Transplant* 1997;20:175–177.
98. Khouri IF, Munsell M, Yajzi S, et al. Comparable survival for nonablative and ablative allogeneic transplantation for chronic lymphocytic leukemia (CLL): the case for early intervention. *Blood* 2000;96(Suppl1):205a.
99. Montserrat E, Gomis F, Vallespi T, et al. Presenting features and prognosis of chronic lymphocytic leukemia in younger adults. *Blood* 1991;78:1545–1551.
100. Catovsky D, Fooks J, Richards S. Prognostic factors in chronic lymphocytic leukemia: the importance of age, sex and response to treatment in survival. *Br J Haematol* 1989;72:141–149.
101. Mauro FR, Foa R, Giannarelli D, et al. Clinical characteristics and outcome of young chronic lymphocytic leukemia patients: a single institution study of 204 cases. *Blood* 1999;94:448–454.
102. De Lima M, O'Brien S, Lerner S, Keating MJ. Chronic lymphocytic leukemia in the young patient. *Semin Oncol* 1998;25:107–116.
103. Diehl LF, Ketchum LH. Autoimmune disease and chronic lymphocytic leukemia: autoimmune hemolytic anemia, pure red cell aplasia and autoimmune thrombocytopenia. *Semin Oncol* 1998;25:80–97.
104. DiSanto JP, Bonnefoy JY, Gauchat JF, et al. CD40 ligand mutations in X-linked immunodeficiency with hyper-IgM syndrome. *Nature* 1993;361:541–543.
105. Cantwell M, Hua T, Pappas J, Kipps TJ. Acquired CD40-ligand deficiency in and chronic lymphocytic leukemia. *Nat Med* 1997;3:984–989.
106. Wierda WG, Cantwell MJ, Woods SJ, et al. CD40-ligand (CD154) gene therapy for chronic lymphocytic leukemia. *Blood* 2000;96:2917–2924.
107. Kipps TJ, Carson DA. Autoantibodies in chronic lymphocytic leukemia and related systemic autoimmune disease. *Blood* 1993;81:2475–2800.
108. Lewis FB, Schwartz RS, Damashek W. X-radiation and alkylating agents as possible 'trigger' mechanism in the autoimmune complications of malignant lymphoproliferative disease. *Clin Exp Immunol* 1966;1:3–8.
109. Byrd JC, Weiss RB, Kweeder SL, Diehl LF. Fludarabine therapy for lymphoid malignancies is associated with hemolytic anemia. *Proc Am Soc Clin Oncol.* 1994;13: 304-309.
110. Weiss BR, Freiman, Kweder SL, et al. Hemolytic anemia after fludarabine therapy for chronic lymphocytic leukemia. *J Clin Oncol* 1998;16:1885–1890.
111. Mauro FR, Foa R, Cerretti R et al. Autoimmune hemolytic anemia in chronic lymphocytic leukemia: clinical, therapeutic and prognostic features. *Blood* 2000;95:2786–2792.

3 Hairy Cell Leukemia
Biology, Diagnosis, and Treatment

Nicole Wentworth, MD and Alan Saven, MD

CONTENTS

EPIDEMIOLOGY

Approximately 600 patients are diagnosed each year in the United States, with hairy cell leukemia (HCL), accounting for 2–3% of all adult leukemias. The median age is 52 yr at presentation, with a 4:1 male predominance. The disease is rare in Asian or African Americans, and has a higher incidence in Ashkenazi Jews, and occasional familial cases have been described *(1,2)*.

DEFINITION AND HISTORY

HCL is a rare, mature B-cell, chronic lymphoproliferative disorder characterized clinically by pancytopenia, splenomegaly, and recurrent infections. Pathologically, the abnormal cells are mononuclear cells displaying irregular cytoplasmic projections that permeate the peripheral blood, bone marrow, and spleen. Originally recognized by Ewald in 1923 as *leukämische reticuloendotheliosis (3)*, in 1958 it was first referred to as a distinct clinicopathologic entity—leukemic reticuloendotheliosis—by Bouroncle *(4)*. The term "hairy cell leukemia" was first used by Scheck and Donnelly in 1966, emphasizing the

From: *Current Clinical Oncology: Chronic Leukemias and Lymphomas:*
Biology, Pathophysiology, and Clinical Management
Edited by: G. J. Schiller © Humana Press Inc., Totowa, NJ

unusual appearance of the leukemic cells *(5)*. The treatment of HCL has evolved over the past decade and a half from the transiently effective splenectomy to newer systemic therapies. Biologic and chemotherapeutic agents—interferon alpha (IFN-α), pentostatin (2´-deoxycoformycin), and cladribine (2-chlorodeoxyad-enosine)—have dramatically improved the prognosis for patients with this disease entity.

ETIOLOGY AND PATHOGENESIS

The exact etiology of HCL has not been elucidated. A history of exposure to radiation and organic solvents may be more frequent among HCL patients *(6,7)*. The Epstein-Barr virus (EBV) has also been implicated as a possible etiologic agent in the development of HCL *(8)*; however, some investigators have refuted this virus as a causative agent *(9)*. The most common karyotypic abnormalities have been found to be clonal anomalies of chromosome 5 in 40% of patients *(10)*, most commonly trisomy 5 or pericentric inversions and interstitial deletions involving band 5q13.

The precise origin of the hairy-cell clone remains unknown. Immunophenotypic surface markers suggest a mature, but not terminally differentiated, B-cell *(11)*. Early cell-surface markers such as CD10 are absent, yet CD19 and CD21, generally lost in the terminal phases of lymphocyte maturation, are present on hairy cells. The early plasma-cell marker PCA-1 is expressed on hairy cells, suggesting a late stage of B-cell ontogeny and possibly a pre-plasma cell origin *(12)*.

Hairy cells are known to secrete cytokines. The anemia associated with HCL may be partially caused by the secretion of tumor necrosis factor-α (TNF-α), which decreases the growth of erythroid colony-forming units (CFU-E) through impaired hematopoiesis *(13)*. Additionally, macrophage colony-stimulating factor (M-CSF) *(14)* and the specific integrin receptor $\alpha_v\beta_3$ are released, which promote hairy-cell motility *(15)*.

CLINICAL FEATURES

The cardinal clinical features of HCL are splenomegaly, pancytopenia, recurrent infections, and circulating hairy cells (Table 1). At initial presentation, 25% of patients complain of fatigue and weakness, a further 25% present with symptomatic thrombocytopenia and/or leukopenia, and yet another quarter have abdominal fullness and early satiety from splenomegaly. The remainder are generally diagnosed following evaluation of incidentally found cytopenias or splenomegaly *(16,17)*.

Ninety percent of patients present with splenomegaly, which may be massive *(18,19)*. Hepatomegaly or palpable peripheral adenopathy are rarely present. With the increasing use of computerized axial tomographic (CAT) scans in patients with hematologic malignancies, approximately one-third of HCL patients have significant internal adenopathy. *(20,21)*.

Table 1
Common Clinical Features of HCL

Middle-aged to elderly males
Splenomegaly
Recurrent infections
    Bacterial: gram-positive and gram-negative
    Pneumocystis carinii pneumonia
    Atypical mycobacteria
    Toxoplasmosis
    Fungal: cryptococcus, aspergillus
Pancytopenia
Inaspirable bone marrow
TRAP-stain positive
Immunophenotype
    CD11c, CD19, CD20, CD22, CD25, and CD103 positive expression

Pancytopenia is found in 50% of patients at presentation. Thirty percent of HCL patients have an absolute neutrophil count of $<0.5 \times 10^9$/L. Most also have monocytopenia *(22)*. Because of the neutropenia, patients are at risk for infections, including Gram-positive and Gram-negative bacteria, atypical myco-bacteria, and invasive fungus. Cellular immunity is, in part, impaired secondary to decreased alpha interferon (IFN) production by peripheral-blood mononuclear cells *(23)*. Common infectious organisms in HCL patients include *Mycobacterium kansasii, Pneumocystis carinii*, Aspergillus, histoplasma, Cryptococcus, and *Toxoplasma gondii (24)*. Bacterial infections occur as a result of neutropenia, and opportunistic infections occur as a result of the cellular immune defects. In a series of 137 patients with HCL, culture-proven infections were found in 47, clinically significant infectious episodes with negative cultures were found in 48, and the remaining 48 patients had no infectious complications *(25)*.

Other laboratory abnormalities include elevated liver function tests, azotemia, and hypergammaglobulinemia (which may be monoclonal) *(26)*. Hypogammaglobulinemia is rare. Unusual connective tissue manifestations of HCL, including leukocytoclastic vasculitis, erythema nodosum, and Raynaud's phenomenon, is often secondary to the paraproteinemia *(26)* Hypocholesterolemia is not rare in advanced HCL; this is because of low concentrations of low-density lipoprotein cholesterol, which tends to resolve after successful treatment of HCL *(27,28)*.

Unusual presentations have been described. A small number of patients (3% in one series) had painful bony involvement *(29)*; this tends to occur in patients with higher tumor burdens and bone marrow that is more diffusely infiltrated with HCL. Occasionally, diffuse osteoporosis and focal or diffuse osteosclerosis may be found. Skeletal lytic lesions have also been reported *(29)*.

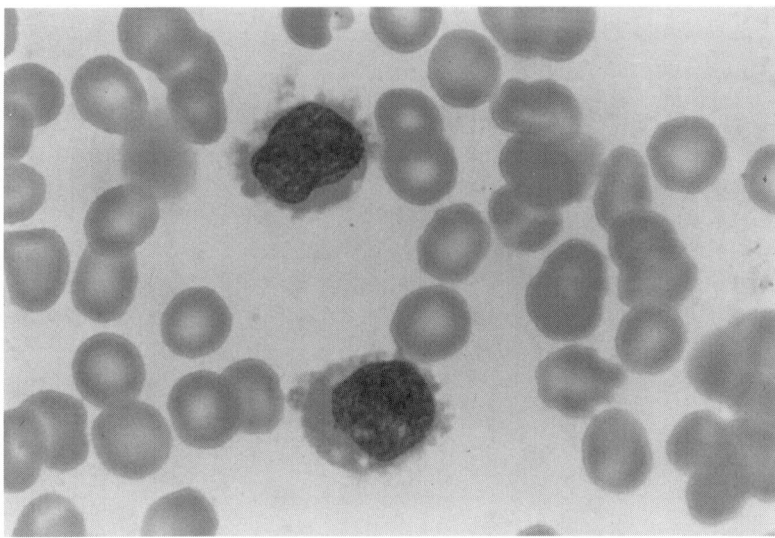

Fig. 1. Peripheral blood with circulating hairy cells. Mononuclear cells with oval to reniform nuclei; finely condensed chromatin; textured, agranular cytoplasm with delicate cytoplasmic projections (×100).

Other extremely rare complications were demonstrated in a series of 116 HCL patients followed for over two decades, including spontaneous splenic rupture, normal peripheral counts and bone-marrow examination in a patient with massive splenomegaly from hairy-cell infiltration, protein-losing enteropathy from bowel infiltration with HCL, and esophageal perforation with a fistulous tract *(30)*.

PATHOLOGIC FEATURES

Peripheral Blood

Hairy cells are mononuclear cells that have central or eccentric nuclei *(31)* (Fig. 1). The shape of the nucleus is variable: oval, round, or convoluted. Generally, the chromatin is in a generous, loose, lacy pattern, and nucleoli are usually indistinct. The hairy-cell cytoplasm is pale to blue-gray in color with fine, hair-like projections. On occasion, cytoplasmic granular rod-shaped inclusions can be seen, which correspond to the ribosomal lamellar complexes identified by electron microscopy *(32)*.

Bone Marrow

Marrow involvement with HCL may be focal or diffuse. This patchy infiltration may make it difficult to demonstrate the presence of hairy cells. Upon presentation, the marrow in HCL is generally hypercellular. Rarely, patients

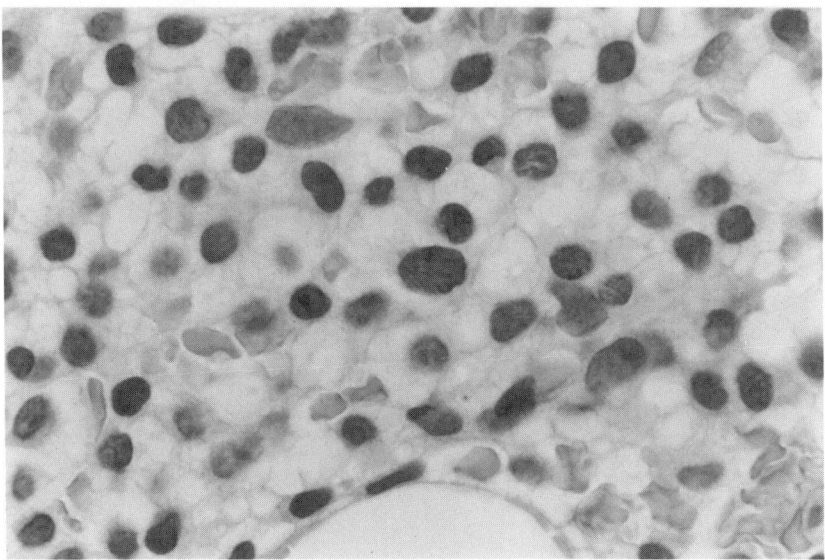

Fig. 2. Bone-marrow morphology. Lymphoid infiltrate composed of cells with copious clear cytoplasm and distinct cell borders, giving a "fried-egg" appearance (×100).

have a hypocellular marrow with scarce hairy-cell infiltration interspersed with normal areas of hematopoiesis *(31,33)*. The variable shaped hairy-cell nuclei are separated by copious amounts of cytoplasm, referred to as the "fried-egg" appearance (Fig. 2). Residual hematopoietic cells are often decreased in number.

Bone-marrow fibroblast infiltration and collagen fibrin are usually absent; however, marrow reticulin fibrosis may be marked, making the marrow characteristically inaspirable. Silver stains demonstrate increased stromal reticulin fibrils *(34)*.

Red blood cells (RBC) can extravasate into areas of hairy-cell infiltrate in the bone-marrow, appearing as red blood cell lakes, which are more characteristically found in the spleen.

Splenic, Hepatic, and Lymph-Node Infiltration

Splenomegaly is a common finding in HCL. Hairy cells infiltrate the splenic red pulp and sinuses, and the splenic white pulp often atrophies (Fig. 3). Pseudosinuses— blood-filled spaces lined by leukemic cells—may also be seen *(35)*. Hepatic infiltration also occurs; this is generally sinusoidal and portal *(35)*. Enlarged lymph nodes have both sinusoidal and interstitial patterns of involvement by HCL (Figs. 4 and 5).

Cytochemistry

The hairy-cell cytoplasm generally stains tartrate-resistant acid phosphatase (TRAP)-positive; the cytoplasm resists decolorization by tartrate because of

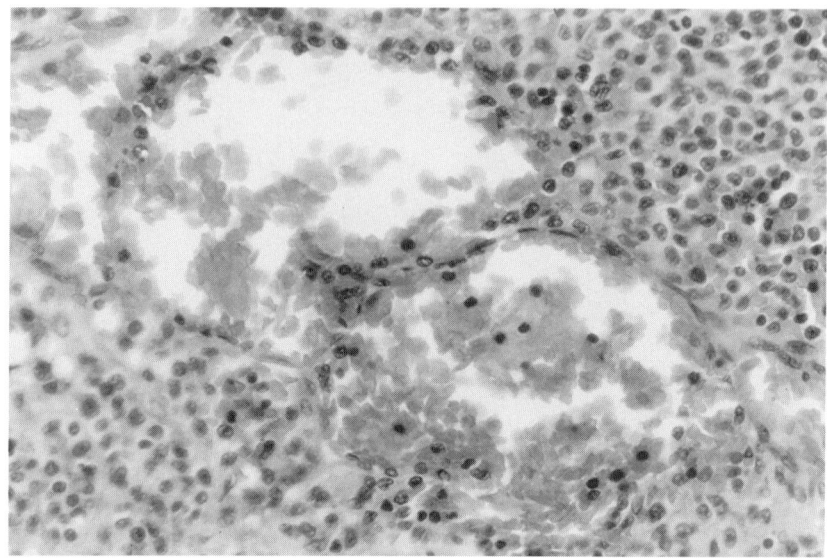

Fig. 3. Splenic pathology. HCL involving the spleen with formation of a "blood lake" (×60).

isoenzyme 5, one of seven acid phosphatase-isoenzymes found in human leuko-cytes *(36,37)*. Most hairy cells stain positively for TRAP; 90% of peripheral-blood buffy-coat smears in HCL will stain TRAP-positive *(36)*. Other diseases may display weak-to-moderate TRAP-staining, including prolymphocytic leu-kemia, non-Hodgkin's lymphoma, Sézary syndrome, and adult T-cell leukemia/lymphoma *(38)*.

Electron Microscopy

On electron microscopy, hairy cells have circumferential cytoplasmic projections with fewer and blunter microvilli than that observed in splenic marginal lymphoma with circulating villous lymphocytes (SLVL) *(39)*. Hairy cells must be contrasted from the villous lymphocytes of splenic lymphoma that also display cytoplasmic projections, but which tend to be polarized to one end of the cell *(39,40)*.

In up to one-half of HCL patients, lamella complexes may be observed by electron microscopy. These cylindrical structures are centrally hollow, with an outer sheath of multiple parallel lamellae. The intralamellar space contains ribo-somal-like granules *(41)*.

Immunophenotype

The pattern of antigen expression on HCL distinguishes it from other lymphoproliferative disorders *(42)*. The pan B-cell antigens CD19, CD20, and CD22, along with the absence of CD21, an antigen lost in B-cell maturation,

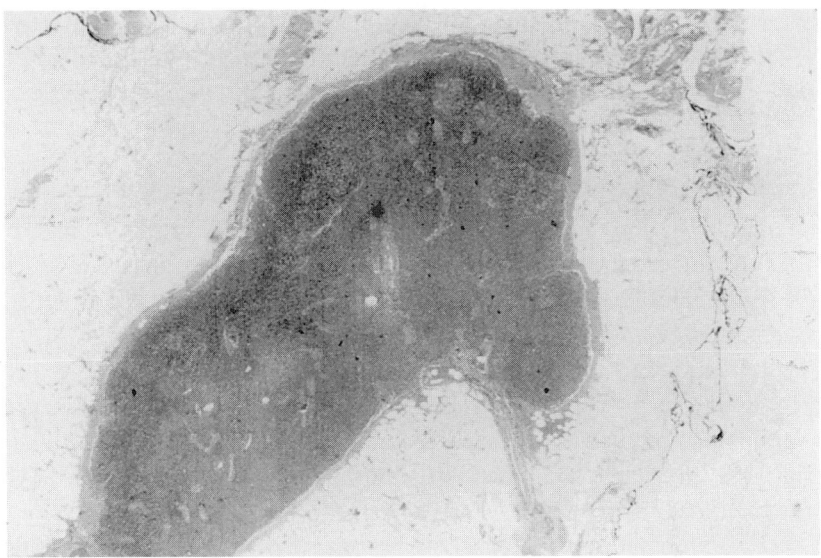

Fig. 4. Lymph-node pathology. Lymph node showing partial effacement by hairy-cell infiltration (×10).

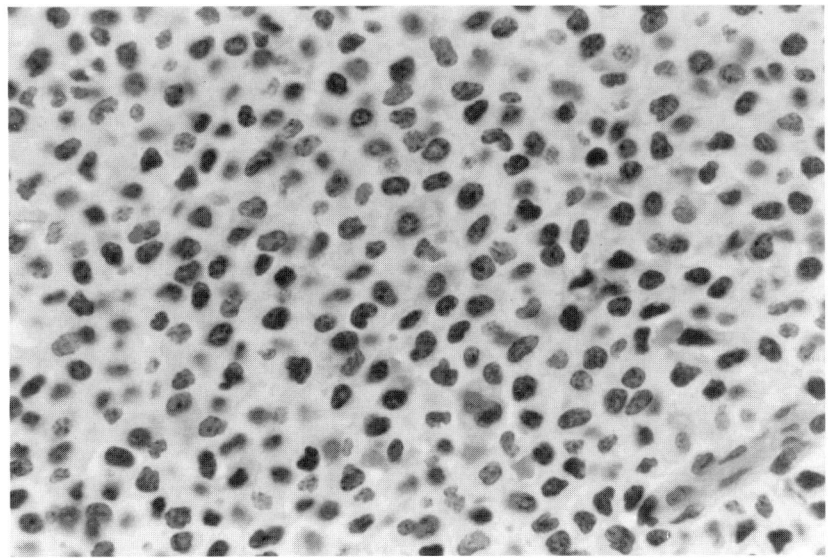

Fig. 5. Lymph-node pathology. Diffuse lymphoid infiltrate composed of cells with round to reniform nuclei and a generous cytoplasmic domain (×60).

mark the leukemic cell as a mature B-lymphocyte *(43–45)*. Distinctive to HCL is the expression of CD11c, CD22, CD25, and CD103 antigens *(46)* The CD11c antigen stains extremely bright in HCL compared to chronic lymphocytic leukemia *(CLL) (47)*; it is a 150-Kd α-chain of the 150/95 β2-integrin normally expressed on monocytes and neutrophils *(46,48)*.

HCL was the first B-cell lymphoproliferative disorder found to express the interleukin-2 (IL-2) receptor, CD25. CD25 is composed of the α-chain of the high-affinity heterodimeric IL-2 receptor. Normally, it is expressed by activated T cells *(49)* Soluble serum IL-2 receptor levels can be followed in HCL as a surrogate marker for disease activity *(50)*.

The most specific marker for HCL is CD103 (Bly-7). It is primarily expressed on intra-epithelial T-lymphocytes, and is believed to be involved in the process of lymphocyte honing and adhesion. Its molecular origin is from the αE subunit of the αEβ7-integrin, also known as the human mucosal lymphocyte-1 (HMC-1) antigen *(51–53)*.

CD22 is expressed most intensely in chronic B-cell lymphoproliferative disorders. In HCL, CD22 stains 50 times more intensely than CLL, where it only has weak expression *(42)*. In 26% of cases, the CALLA antigen, CD10, is weakly expressed. Rarely, there is weak expression of CD5, the anomalous T-cell antigen most commonly expressed in CLL *(54)*.

Peripheral-blood immunophenotypic analysis can be very useful in establishing the diagnosis of HCL. Hairy cells typically coexpress the antigens CD11c, CD25, and CD103, and the B-cell antigens CD19, CD20, and CD22 *(42)*. In one report, morphologic evaluation of the peripheral blood established the diagnosis of HCL in only 80% of patients, and flow cytometry identified circulating hairy cells in 92% of the HCL patients *(55)*.

Immunohistochemistry

Immunohistochemical staining can be helpful in both making the diagnosis of HCL as well as in the detection of minimal residual disease following successful treatment. This staining of bone-marrow samples requires processing by frozen section to detect antigens such as CD103 *(56)*. In contrast, the antigen CD20 (L26) and the monoclonal antibody DBA.44 can be evaluated on routinely processed paraffin sections *(57–59)*. DBA.44 stains positively in 30% of low-grade non-Hodgkin's lymphoma, and thus is not specific for HCL. In HCL, DBA.44 (which is yet an undefined antigen) can stain in both a cytoplasmic granular and membranous pattern. The L26 antibody, however, exhibits membranous staining only.

DIFFERENTIAL DIAGNOSIS

The differential diagnosis of HCL includes HCL-variant, splenic lymphoma with circulating villous lymphocytes, other indolent low-grade non-Hodgkin's

Table 2
Differential Diagnosis of HCL

	HCL	HCL-V	CLL	B-cell PLL	Splenic lymphoma	Low-grade non-Hodgkin's lymphoma
Splenomegaly	++	++	+/−	+++	++	+/−
Leukocyte count	low	moderate elevation	high	high	mild elevation	generally normal
Aspirable bone marrow	no	yes	yes	+/−	yes	yes
TRAP staining	yes	variable	no	no	variable	no
Immunophenotype						
CD5	+/−	−	+	+/−	+/−	+/−
CD11c	+	+	+/−	+/−	+/−	−
CD20	+	+/−	+	+	+	+
CD25	+	−	+/−	+/−	+/−	+/−
CD103	+	+/−	−	−	+/−	−

lymphomas, B-cell prolymphocytic leukemia (B-PLL), mast-cell disease, and aplastic anemia (Table 2). These diseases are differentiated by their pattern of morphology, by differences in their clinical expression, and by immunophenotypic analysis.

HCL-variant (HCL-v) is a rare disease characterized by features of both prolymphocytic leukemia and HCL (Fig. 6). The morphologic evaluation reveals a nucleus closely resembling that of a prolymphocyte, and the cytoplasm that of a hairy-cell (60). Morphologically, the hairy-cell variant cells have a higher nuclear-to-cytoplasmic ratio, more highly condensed chromatin, and larger central nucleoli than HCL cells (61). Clinically, both diseases present with massive splenomegaly. HCL-v patients frequently exhibit a profound lymphocytosis (62). TRAP staining is negative or only weakly positive in HCL-v. Unlike classic HCL, CD25 and CD10 antigens are absent in the HCL-variant, and patients have aspirable bone-marrows. Additionally, the ribosomal lamellar complexes present in HCL are absent in HCL-v (62).

The *blastic* variant of HCL, remarkable for massive splenomegaly, peripheral adenopathy, and cytopenias (63), also stains positive with TRAP. A B-cell lymphoproliferative disorder resembling HCL has been described in Japan (64). This disorder is characterized by a lymphocytosis with abnormal lymphocytes displaying long microvilli. These lymphocytes are polyclonal, CD25-negative, and only weakly TRAP-positive. Clinically, patients demonstrate splenomegaly without lymphadenopathy.

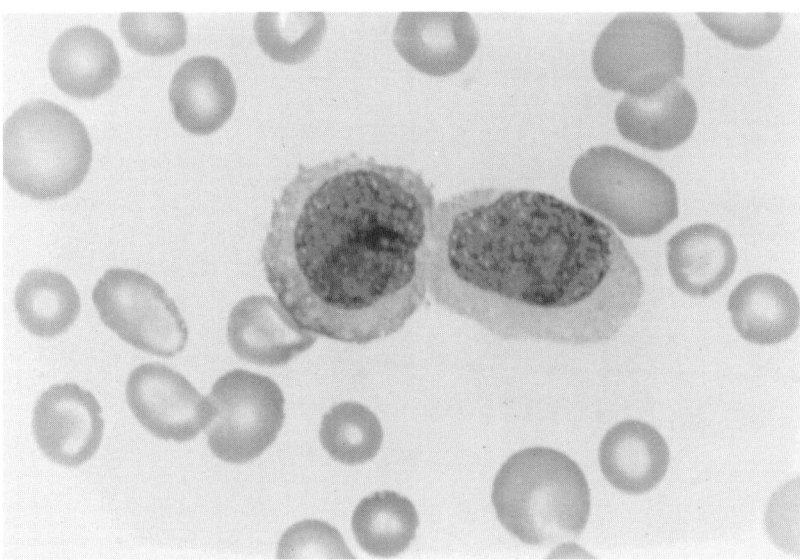

Fig. 6. Peripheral blood with HCL-variant. HCL-variant cells are larger, with a slightly greater nuclear-to-cytoplasmic ratio. HCL-variant cells have more condensed chromatin and a more prominent nucleus than typical hairy cells (×100).

Splenic lymphoma with circulating villous lymphocytes must be distinguished from HCL. Unlike cases of HCL, peripheral lymphocytosis is more common *(65)*. These lymphocytes demonstrate more subtle polar cytoplasmic projections, and the cytoplasm tends to be more basophilic and somewhat plasmacytoid *(40)*. Peripheral monocytopenia is usually absent. These abnormal lymphocytes are generally TRAP-negative, or only weakly positive *(36,66)*, CD11c-positive, and frequently CD103-negative. Splenic pathology reveals involvement of predominantly the white pulp *(65)*.

B-PLL demonstrates similarities to the prolymphocytic variant of HCL. Both present with prominent splenomegaly. TRAP staining is only focally positive, whereas in HCL TRAP-staining tends to be more diffuse. In B-PLL, the leukemic cells are generally CD11c-negative *(67)*.

Various indolent non-Hodgkin's lymphomas may also mimic HCL, including *marginal-zone lymphoma and monocytoid B-cell lymphoma (68,69)*. These lymphomas are generally TRAP-stain-negative *(70,71)*.

Systemic mastocytosis is also included in the differential diagnosis of HCL. Both disorders are characterized by bone-marrow infiltration with spindle-shaped cells. In systemic mastocytosis, immunohistochemical stains show an absence of CD20, and Giemsa stains demonstrate metachromatic granules *(72)*.

Finally, patients with *myelofibrosis* may present with cytopenias and splenomegaly, thus mimicking HCL.

TREATMENT

Indications

Because of the indolent behavior of HCL, treatment is not always mandatory at diagnosis. Generally accepted indications for initiating therapy in patients with HCL include anemia (hemoglobin <10 g/dL), neutropenia (absolute neutrophil count <1 × 10^9/L), and/or recurrent infections, thrombocytopenia (platelets <100 × 10^9/L), symptomatic splenomegaly, bulky lymphadenopathy, leukocytosis with a high proportion of leukemic cells, vasculitis, or bony involvement.

Splenectomy

With multiple effective systemic agents now available for the treatment of HCL, splenectomy is less commonly used in the primary treatment of HCL. Current indications for splenectomy include active, uncontrolled infections, thrombocytopenic bleeding, and massive and symptomatic splenomegaly, as well as failure of systemic therapies. Splenectomy rapidly reverses peripheral-blood cytopenias; 90% of patients show improvement in at least one hematologic parameter and 40–60% have normalization of blood counts *(73,74)*. Within days of splenectomy, thrombocytopenia reverses in 75% of patients *(75)*. Median length of response following splenectomy is 8.3 mo. At this time, 50% of patients require further treatment. *(76)*.

Interferon

IFN-α is an active agent against HCL, and is the disease for which it was first FDA-approved in 1986 (Table 3). Given the major activity of purine nucleoside analogs in HCL, the use of IFN is now generally reserved for HCL patients who have active infections and therefore are unable to undergo therapy with a purine nucleoside analog because of their associated severe T-cell suppression *(24,77)*. IFN is also indicated as salvage therapy in HCL patients who have failed primary treatment with a purine nucleoside analog *(78)*.

The first report of IFN activity in HCL was by Quesada and colleagues in 1984. Seven patients were treated with partially purified alpha (leukocyte) human IFN. All seven patients achieved normalization of their peripheral blood counts, and three patients had elimination of hairy cells from their bone-marrow *(79)*. In 1986, recombinant IFN-α-2b (Intron® A; Schering Corporation, Kenilworth, NY) administration was reported in 64 patients with HCL. A dose of 2 million U per square meter for 12 mo was used *(80)*. Five percent (3 of 64) of patients treated achieved complete responses, and 70% (45 of 64) achieved partial responses. Generally, 12 mo of IFN-α is utilized; longer durations of treatment do not regularly increase response rates or diminish relapse rates, but do exacerbate toxicities *(81,82)*.

A long-term study of 64 patients treated with IFN-α had a median follow-up of 92 mo *(83)*. These patients received IFN-α at 3 million U per square meter 3×

Table 3

Interferon Results in HCL

Investigators	No. of patients	Overall response rates (percentage)	Complete responses (percentage)	Partial responses (percentage)	Refs.
Quesada et al.	30	26 (87)	9 (30)	17 (57)	(131)
Foon et al.	14	13 (93)	1 (7)	12 (86)	(132)
Rai et al.	25	13 (52)	7 (28)	6 (24)	(133)
Golomb et al.	195	159 (82)	7 (4)	152 (78)	(134)
Grever et al.	159	60 (38)	17 (11)	43 (27)	(99)
Damasio et al.	64	50 (78)	8 (13)	42 (66)	(83)
Total	487	321 (66)	49 (10)	272 (56)	

weekly for 12–18 mo. Those patients who responded received maintenance therapy with 3 million U per square meter weekly until relapse. The overall response rate was 91%; 13% complete responses and 65% partial responses. The results of this study are consistent with prior reports of IFN-α use in HCL.

Recombinant IFN-α-2a (Roferon®, Hoffman-La Roche, Nutley, NJ), which has a cysteine residue at position 23, rather than arginine as in IFN-α-2b, was evaluated and demonstrated similar results in 30 HCL patients (84). Occasionally, patients may lose ongoing responsiveness to recombinant IFN-α-2a because of the development of neutralizing and binding antibodies; however, some of these patients may still respond to natural IFN-α (85).

Platelet counts begin to normalize at a median of 2 mo following IFN therapy. Anemia generally resolves at a median of 3 mo, and neutropenia at a median of 5 mo. Treatment failure occurs at a median of 18–25 mo after discontinuation of IFN (86). At relapse following IFN use, the reinstitution of IFN induced a 77% response rate (87).

The side effects most commonly associated with IFN are fever, myalgias, and fatigue. Acetaminophen generally alleviates these symptoms. An increased incidence of second malignancies in HCL patients treated with IFN-α-2b has been reported (88). Of 69 patients followed for a median of 91 mo, 13 patients (19%) developed second malignancies (6 hematologic in origin and 7 adenocarcinomas). Median survival was 8.8 mo after diagnosis of the second neoplasm.

The mechanism of action of IFN in HCL remains poorly understood. IFN stimulates natural killer (NK)-cell activity, normally suppressed in HCL (89,90). In addition, IFN-α stimulates differentiation of leukemic cell lines and has growth-inhibitory effects on lymphoma cell lines (91,92).

In summary, IFN-α is an effective agent in HCL; however, responses are generally short-lived after its discontinuation. The recommended dose of IFN-α-2b is 2 million U per square meter subcutaneously 3× weekly for 12 mo. The dose of IFN-α-2a is 3 million U per square meter subcutaneously daily for 6 mo, later adjusted to 3× a week for 6 mo.

Purine Analogs

Adenosine deaminase deficiency was first described by Giblett in 1972 *(93)*. This enzyme irreversibly catalyzes the deamination of adenosine to 2´-deoxyadenosine. The absence of adenosine deaminase results in the accumulation of the triphosphorylated derivative of deoxyadenosine, which in turn results in lymphopenia *(94)*. Thirty percent of children with severe combined immunodeficiency disease (SCID) exhibit this enzymatic deficiency. This enhanced understanding of purine biochemistry was applied as an anti-leukemic strategy through the deliberate inhibition of adenosine deaminase; 2´-deoxycoformycin (pentostatin) is a direct inhibitor of adenosine deaminase, and 2-chlorodeoxyadenosine (cladribine) is a chlorine-substituted purine deoxynucleoside *(95)*.

Pentostatin (2´-Deoxycoformycin)

Pentostatin (2´-deoxycoformycin; Nipent(r), SuperGen Inc., San Ramon, CA) was the first agent applied to the treatment of HCL that regularly induced complete responses. It is a natural product of *Streptomyces antibioticus*. The Eastern Cooperative Oncology Group (ECOG) reported on 50 HCL patients treated with pentostatin at 5 mg per square meter for 2 d every other week, which was continued until complete response *(96)* (Table 4); 32 (64%) obtained complete responses and 10 (20%) achieved partial responses *(97)*. Pentostatin was also evaluated by the European Organization for the Research and Treatment of Cancer (EORTC) in HCL patients who were resistant to or had relapsed following failed IFN-α therapy *(98)*. Pentostatin was administered at 4 mg per square meter weekly for 3 wk, then 4 mg per square meter every other week for three doses. Thirty-three percent of patients (11 of 33 patients) achieved complete responses, and 45% (15 of 33) achieved partial responses. The median response duration was 12 mo.

In the Intergroup study, untreated HCL patients were randomized to receive either IFN-α-2a at 3 million U per square meter subcutaneously 3× a week or pentostatin at 4 mg per square meter intravenously every 2 wk *(99)*. Of this group, 313 patients were randomized; 150 patients to IFN. Of the 150 IFN-treated patients, 11% (17 patients) achieved complete responses and 27% (43 patients) achieved partial responses, for an overall response rate of 38%. One hundred and fifty-four patients were randomized to pentostatin with 76% (117 of 154 patients) achieving complete responses, and 3% (4 of 154 patients) achieved partial responses. Patients randomized to pentostatin achieved higher response rates and enjoyed longer relapse-free survivals.

French investigators studied the response to and long-term follow-up of 50 HCL patients treated with pentostatin *(100)*. The majority of these patients were

Table 4
Pentostatin Results in HCL

Investigators	No. of patients	Overall response rates (precentage)	Complete responses (percentage)	Partial responses (percentage)	Refs.
Cassileth et al.	50	42 (84)	32 (64)	10 (20)	(97)
Kraut et al.	23	21 (91)	20 (87)	1 (4)	(135)
Ho et al.	33	26 (79)	11 (33)	15 (45)	(98)
Grem et al.	66	52 (79)	37 (56)	15 (23)	(136)
Grever et al.	154	121 (79)	117 (76)	4 (3)	(99)
Ribeiro et al.	50	40 (80)	22 (44)	18 (36)	(100)
Dearden et al.	165	160 (97)	135 (82)	25 (15)	(101)
Total	541	462 (85)	374 (69)	88 (16)	

pretreated; 31 with IFN, one with cladribine, and 18 with no previous therapy. The overall response rate was 96%; 44% complete responses and 36% partial responses. Overall survival was 86% at 38 mo. English investigators evaluated 165 HCL patients treated with pentostatin (101). Similar results were achieved with an overall response rate of 97%, including 82% complete responses, and 15% partial responses. Median time to relapse was 51 mo.

The long-term follow-up on 24 HCL patients who achieved complete responses following pentostatin (102) has been documented; 23 patients had a median follow-up of 82 mo and the twenty-fourth patient died from refractory disease. Of these 23 patients, 11 relapsed at a median of 30 mo. One patient developed disseminated herpes zoster at 52 mo posttreatment, but no other severe infections were recorded. Three patients developed skin cancer, and one patient developed stage 1A Hodgkin's disease.

Side effects of pentostatin include fever, nausea, vomiting, photosensitivity, keratoconjunctivitis (103,104), and severe immunosuppression (97,105,106) (CD4+ and CD8+ T-lymphocytes often decrease below 200 cells per µL). Infectious complications include disseminated zoster, E. coli, H. influenzae, S. pneumoniae, and fungal infections. These infections are generally observed soon after initiating pentostatin (104). As with other purine nucleoside analogs, the use of pentostatin should be avoided in HCL patients with active, uncontrolled infections (96).

The standard pentostatin dose for HCL patients is 4 mg per square m every other week for 3–6 mo, until maximum response is achieved.

Cladribine

Cladribine (2-chlorodeoxyadenosine [2-CdA]; Leustatin, Ortho Biotech, Raritan, NJ) treatment of HCL patients was first reported in 1990 by Scripps

Table 5
Cladribine Results in HCL

Investigators	No. of patients	Overall response rates (percentage)	Complete responses (percentage)	Partial responses (percentage)	Refs.
Saven et al.	349	341 (98)	319 (91)	22 (6)	(113)
Estey et al.	46	41 (89)	36 (78)	5 (11)	(109)
Juliusson et al.	16	12 (75)	12 (75)	0 (0)	(108)
Hoffman et al.	49	49 (100)	37 (76)	12 (24)	(111)
Tallman et al.	50	49 (98)	40 (80)	9 (18)	(110)
Dearden et al.	45	45 (100)	38 (84)	7 (16)	(101)
Blasinka-Moraniec et al.	97	93 (96)	75 (77)	18 (19)	(137)
Bastie et al.	29	28 (97)	25 (86)	3 (10)	(138)
Cheson et al.	861	541 (63)	430 (50)	111 (13)	(112)
Total	1542	1199 (78)	1012 (66)	187 (12)	

Clinic investigators (Table 5). Cladribine was administered as a single 7-d continuous intravenous infusion at 0.1 mg per kg body wt daily (107). Of 12 HCL patients, 11 achieved complete responses and one achieved a partial response.

Other investigators have documented similar results. Of 20 HCL patients treated with cladribine, 80% achieved complete responses and 20% achieved partial responses (108). Forty-six patients were treated with cladribine at the MD Anderson Cancer Center, Houston, Texas; 78% of patients achieved complete responses and 11% achieved partial responses (109). Northwestern University investigators in Chicago, Illinois treated 50 HCL patients with cladribine (110); the complete response rate was 80% and the partial response rate was 18%, for an overall response rate of 98% (110). The progression-free survival was 72% at 4 yr for all responder patients and 83% for the complete responders alone. Long Island Jewish Hospital investigators in Long Island, New York treated 49 HCL patients (111); 76% achieved complete responses and 24% achieved partial responses. Relapse-free survival was 80% at 55 mo, with an overall survival of 95% (111). Finally, the National Cancer Institute has reported the largest series of HCL patients treated with cladribine (112); 861 patients achieved an overall response rate of 87%, but the complete response rate was only 50%. The explanation for this lower complete response rate is not clear. Because the pathology was not centrally reviewed, lymphoproliferative disorders other than typical HCL may have been included (112).

The long-term follow-up of 358 cladribine-treated HCL patients at Scripps Clinic in La Jolla, California was reported (113). Of 349 HCL patients, 91% (319 patients) achieved complete responses and 7% (22 patients) achieved partial responses. The median duration of follow-up was 52 mo. Twenty-six percent (90 patients) relapsed at a median of 29 mo. For all 341 responders, the median time to treatment failure was 19% at 48 mo, 16% for complete responders, and 54% for partial responders. Fifty-three patients received a second course of cladribine; at first relapse 62% (33 patients) achieved complete responses and 26% (14 patients) achieved partial responses. Eight percent of the cladribine-treated patients developed second malignancies, with an observed to expected ratio of 1.88 (95% confidence interval, 1.24–2.74). Overall survival was 98% at 48 mo. There was no obvious plateau on the time-to-treatment-failure graph; therefore, the percentage of patients—if any—cured with cladribine could not be determined. Patients in morphologic complete response after cladribine exhibit minimal residual disease, detected by immunohistochemical staining of the bone-marrow biopsy, in 25–50% of specimens (114,115).

A report from the MD Anderson Cancer Center did not support an increased incidence of second malignancies in HCL patients (116). A Canadian study reviewed 117 HCL patients treated with systemic therapies including, but not limited to, cladribine (117). At a median follow-up time of 68 mo, 36 second malignancies were documented with a relative frequency of 2.91 for women (statistically significant) and 1.65 for men (not significant). The authors concluded that HCL patients were inherently prone to second malignancies, which were probably not treatment-related (117). Finally, 2,014 patients with HCL and CLL treated with purine nucleoside analogs were analyzed, and no increased incidence of second malignancies was recorded (118).

The most frequent acute side effect of cladribine is the onset of neutropenic fever; 42% of patients developed fever related to the disappearance of hairy cells. Fever was more common in patients with greater pretreatment HCL disease burdens. A study was performed at the Scripps Clinic in which patients undergoing cladribine treatment for HCL were first primed with filgrastim, then treated with cladribine, and thereafter received posttreatment filgrastim (119). The filgrastim-treated group had higher nadir absolute neutrophil counts and experienced a decreased number of days of severe neutropenia than the historic control group, which did not receive filgrastim. However, the percentage of febrile patients, the number of febrile days, and the frequency of admissions for antibiotics were not statistically different between the two groups. Thus, routine administration of filgrastim to HCL patients who received cladribine cannot be recommended (119).

The most common late infection following cladribine treatment in HCL was dermatomal varicella zoster (77). Cladribine, like pentostatin, depletes CD4 and CD8 T-lymphocytes, resulting in severe and protracted immunosuppression (77).

In summary, when single courses of cladribine are administered at 0.1 mg per kg body wt daily for 7 d by continuous intravenous (iv) infusion, the vast majority of patients achieve complete and long-lasting remissions with a generally favorable toxicity profile. Ongoing responsiveness to cladribine is usually demonstrated at relapse.

Fludarabine

Fludarabine (Fludara; Berlex, Wayne, NJ), a purine nucleoside analog intensively tested in CLL patients, has not achieved the same excellent response rates recorded for cladribine or pentostatin in HCL, although only evaluated in small numbers of patients. Patients with HCL-v have achieved partial responses with fludarabine *(120–122)*.

Other Systemic Agents

The chronic daily administration of chlorambucil for 6–9 mo induces partial peripheral hematologic responses. The absolute neutrophil count rarely shows substantial improvement with this therapy *(123)*. Occasionally, protracted androgen use *(124)* or lithium given to patients with HCL may be beneficial *(125)*.

Irradiation

Bony lytic lesions are generally managed with irradiation, 1500–3000 rads *(126,127)*.

Monoclonal Antibodies (MAbs)

Two different MAbs have been administered to patients with HCL. In one report, four patients with HCL received a recombinant immunotoxin composed of the variable domains of the anti-Tac (anti-CD25) MAb fused to PE38, a truncated version of the Pseudomonas exotoxin *(128)*. All four HCL patients achieved a response, one with a duration greater than 13 mo.

In a small series of patients from the MD Anderson Cancer Center, eight patients with relapsed or refractory HCL received the anti-CD20 MAb, rituximab (Rituxan; IDEC Pharmaceuticals, San Diego, CA) *(129)*. Rituximab was administered at 375 mg per square meter weekly for 8 wk. At a median follow-up of 2 mo, 80% of patients achieved a response, including two complete responses. These two studies demonstrated the feasibility and potential for the successful application of MAbs to the treatment of HCL patients.

Current and Future Perspectives

Prior to the availability of successful systemic therapies, patients with HCL had median survivals of only 53 mo *(130)*. The introduction of effective systemic treatments using IFN-α, pentostatin, and cladribine have improved long-term survival rates, and have raised the possibility of a curative strategy. Purine nucleoside analog therapy in patients with HCL has demonstrated durable, complete, and unmaintained remissions with overall survivals in excess of 95% at 4 yr *(113)*. The use of MAbs in HCL patients with only minimal residual disease following purine nucleoside analog administration may potentially improve the response rates, the response duration, and even possibly the number of patients actually being cured. The rational introduction of purine nucleoside analogs to the treatment of HCL by improved insights into adenosine deaminase deficiency, a rare pediatric disorder, serves as the paradigm for the successful application of new agents to the treatment of cancer.

REFERENCES

1. Wylis RF, Greene MH, Palretke M, Khilanani P, Tabaczka P, Swiderski G. Hairy cell leukemia in three siblings: an apparent HLA-linked disease. *Cancer* 1982; 49:538–542.
2. Egli FL, Koller B, Furrer J. Hairy cell leukemia and glucose-6-phosphatase dehydrogenase deficiency in two brothers (Letter). *N Engl J Med* 1990; 322:1159.
3. Ewald O. Die leukämische reticuloendotheliose. *Deutsches Arch Klin Med* 1923; 142:222–228.
4. Bouroncle BA, Wiseman BK, Doan CA. Leukemic reticuloendotheliosis. *Blood* 1958; 13: 609–630.
5. Schrek R, Donnelly WJ. "Hairy" cells in blood in lymphoreticular neoplastic disease and "flagellated" cells of normal lymph nodes. *Blood* 1966; 27:199–211.
6. Oleske D, Golomb HM, Farber MD, Levy PS. A case-control inquiry into the etiology of hairy cell leukemia. *Am J Epidemiol* 1985; 121:675–683.
7. Stewart DJ, Keating MJ. Radiation exposure as a possible etiologic factor in hairy cell leukemia. *Cancer* 1980; 46:1577–1580.
8. Wolf BC, Martin AW, Neiman RS, et al. The detection of Epstein-Barr virus in hairy cell leukemia cells by in situ hybridization. *Am J Clin Pathol* 1990; 136:717–723.
9. Chang KL, Chen YY, Weiss LM. Lack of evidence of Epstein-Barr virus in hairy cell leukemia and monocytoid B-cell lymphoma. *Hum Pathol* 1993; 24:58.
10. Haglund U, Juliusson G, Stellan B, Gahrton G. Hairy cell leukemia is characterized by clonal chromosome abnormalities clustered to specific regions. *Blood* 1994; 83:2637–2645.
11. Burthem J, Zuzel M, Cawley JC. What is the nature of the hairy cell and why should we be interested? [Annotation]. *Br J Haematol* 1997; 97:511–514.
12. Anderson KC, Boyd AW, Fisher DC, Leslie D, Schlossman SF, Nadler LF. Hairy cell leukemia: a tumor of pre-plasma cells. *Blood* 1985; 65:620–629.
13. Lindemann A, Ludwig WD, Oster W. High-level secretion of tumor necrosis factor-alpha contributes to hematopoietic failure in hairy cell leukemia. *Blood* 1989; 73:880.
14. Burthem J, Baker PK, Hunt JA, Cawley JC. The function of c-fms in hairy-cell leukemia: macrophage colony-stimulating factor stimulates hairy-cell movement. *Blood* 1994;83:1381–1389.
15. Burthem J, Baker PK, Cawley JC. Hairy cell interactions with extracellular matrix: expression of specific integrin receptors and their role in the cell's response to specific adhesive proteins. *Blood* 1994; 84:873–882.
16. Flandrin G, Sigaux F, Sebahoun G, Bouffette P. Hairy cell leukemia: clinical presentation and follow-up of 211 patients. *Semin Oncol* 1984; 11:458–471.
17. Catovsky D. Hairy cell leukemia and prolymphocytic leukemia. *Clin Haematol* 1977; 6:245–268.
18. Katayama I, Finkel HE. Leukemic reticuloendotheliosis. A clinicopathologic study with review of the literature. *Am J Med* 1974; 57:115.
19. Golomb HM. Hairy cell leukemia. An unusual lymphoproliferative disease: A study of 24 patients. *Cancer* 1978; 42:946.
20. Hakimian D, Tallman MS, Hogan DK, Rademaker AW, Rose E, Nemcek AA, Jr. Prospective evaluation of internal adenopathy in a cohort of 43 patients with hairy cell leukemia. *J Clin Oncol* 1994; 12:268–272.

21. Mercieca J, Matutes E, Moskovic E. Massive abdominal lymphadenopathy in hairy cell leukaemia: a report of 12 cases. *Br J Haematol* 1992; 82:547.
22. Goyette RE. Hairy cell leukemia. In: Goyette RE, ed. *Hematology: A Comprehensive Guide to the Diagnosis and Treatment of Blood Disorders.* PMIC, Los Angeles, 1997, pp. 576–582.
23. Siegal FP, Shodell M, Shah K, et al. Impaired interferon alpha response in hairy cell leukemia is corrected by therapy with 2-chloro-2'-deoxyadenosine: implications for susceptibility to opportunistic infections. *Leukemia* 1994; 8:1474–1479.
24. Kraut EH, Neff JC, Bouroncle BA, Gochnor D, Grever MR. Immunosuppressive effects of pentostatin. *J Clin Oncol* 1990; 8:848–855.
25. Golomb HM, Hadad LJ. Infectious complications in 127 patients with hairy cell leukemia. *Am J Hematol* 1984; 16:393.
26. Dorsey JK, Penick GD. The association of hairy cell leukemia with unusual immunologic disorders. *Arch Intern Med* 1982; 142:902–903.
27. Juliusson G, Vitols S, Liliemark J. Mechanisms behind hypocholesterolaemia in hairy cell leukaemia. *Br Med J* 1995; 310:27.
28. Juliusson G, Vitols S, Liliemark J. Disease-related hypocholesterolemia in patients with hairy cell leukemia. *Cancer* 1995; 76:423–428.
29. Quesada JR, Keating MJ, Libshitz HI, Llamas L. Bone involvement in hairy cell leukemia. *Am J Med* 1983; 74:228.
30. Bouroncle BA. Unusual presentations and complications of hairy cell leukemia. *Leukemia* 1987; 1:288–293.
31. Bartl R, Frisch B, Hill W. Bone marrow histology in hairy cell leukemia. *Am J Clin Pathol* 1983; 79:531–545.
32. Katayama I. Bone marrow in hairy cell leukemia. *Hematol Oncol Clin N Am* 1988; 2:585–602.
33. Burke JS. The value of the bone-marrow biopsy in the diagnosis of hairy cell leukemia. *J Clin Pathol* 1978; 70:876–884.
34. Burthem J, Cawley JC. The bone marrow fibrosis of hairy-cell leukemia is caused by the synthesis and assembly of a fibronectin matrix by the hairy cells. *Blood* 1994; 83:497–504.
35. Nanba K, Soban EJ, Bowling MC, Berard CW. Splenic pseudosinuses and hepatic angiomatous lesions: distinctive features of hairy cell leukemia. *Am J Clin Pathol* 1977; 67:415–426.
36. Yam LT, Janckila AJ, Li CY, Lam WKW. Cytochemistry of tartrate-resistant acid phosphatase: fifteen years' experience. *Leukemia* 1987; 1:285–288.
37. Li CY, Yam LT, Lam KW. Studies of acid phosphatase isoenzymes in human leukocytes: demonstration of isoenzyme specificity. *J Histochem Cytochem* 1970; 18:901–910.
38. Drexler HG, Gaedicke G, Minowade J. Isoenzyme studies in human leukemia-lymphoma cell lines. II. Acid phosphatase. *Leuk Res* 1985; 9:537.
39. Catovsky D, O'Brien M, Melo JV, Wardle J, Brozovic M. Hairy cell leukemia variant: an intermediate disease between hairy cell leukemia and B prolymphocytic leukemia. *Semin Oncol* 1984; 11:362–369.
40. Melo JV, Robinson DS, Gregory C, Catovsky D. Splenic B cell lymphoma with "villous" lymphocytes in the peripheral blood: a disorder distinct from hairy cell leukemia. *Leukemia* 1987; 1:294–299.
41. Rosner MC, Golomb HM. Ribsome-lamella complex in hairy cell leukemia. Ultrastructure and distribution. *Lab Invest* 1980; 42:236.
42. Robbins BA, Ellison DJ, Spinosa JC, et al. Diagnostic application of two-color flow cytometry in 161 cases of hairy cell leukemia. *Blood* 1993; 82:1277–1287.
43. Korsmeyer SJ, Greene WC, Cossman J, et al. Rearrangement and expression of immunoglobulin genes and expression of Tac antigen in hairy cell leukemia. *Proc Natl Acad Sci USA* 1983; 80:4522.
44. Hsu S, Yang K, Jaffe ES. Hairy cell leukemia: a B-cell neoplasm with a unique antigenic phenotype. *Am J Clin Pathol* 1983; 80:421–428.

45. Falini B, Schwarting R, Erber W, et al. The differential diagnosis of hairy cell leukemia with a panel of monoclonal antibodies. *Am J Clin Pathol* 1985; 83:289–300.

46. Visser L, Shaw A, Slupsky J, Vos H, Poppema S. Monoclonal antibodies reactive with hairy cell leukemia. *Blood* 1989; 74:320–325.

47. Hanson CA, Gribbin TE, Schnitzer B, Schlegelmilch JA, Mitchell BS, Stoolman LM. CD11c (LEU-M5) expression characterizes a B-cell chronic lymphoproliferative disorder with features of both chronic lymphocytic leukemia and hairy cell leukemia. *Blood* 1990; 76: 2360–2367.

48. Schwarting R, Stein H, Wang CY. The monoclonal antibodies alpha S-HCL-1 (alpha Leu-14) and alpha S-HCL-3 (alpha Leu-M5) allow the diagnosis of hairy cell leukemia. *Blood* 1985; 65:974.

49. de Totero D, Tazzari PL, Lauria F. Phenotypic analysis of hairy cell leukemia: "Variant" cases express the interleukin-2 receptor beta chain, but not the alpha chain (CD25). *Blood* 1993; 82:528.

50. Steis RG, Marcon L, Clark J, et al. Serum soluble IL-2 receptor as a tumor marker in patients with hairy cell leukemia. *Blood* 1988; 77:1304–1309.

51. Micklem KJ, Dong Y, Willis A, et al. HML-1 antigen on mucosa-associated T cells, activated cells, and hairy leukemic cells is a new integrin containing the β7 subunit. *Am J Clin Pathol* 1991; 139:1297–1301.

52. Flenghi L, Spinozzi F, Stein H, Krushwitz Ml, Pileri S, Falini B. A new monoclonal antibody directed against a trimeric molecule (150 kDa, 125 kDa, 105 kDa) associated with hairy cell leukemia. *Br J Haematol* 1990; 76:451–459.

53. Cepek KL, Parker CM, Madara JL, Brenner MB. Integrin alpha E beta F mediates adhesion of T lymphocytes to epithelial cell. *J Immunol* 1993; 150:3459.

54. Linde GA, Hammarstrom L, Persson MAA, Smith CI, Sundqvist VA, Wahren B. Virus-specific antibody activity of different subclasses of immunoglobulins G and A in cytomegalovirus infections. *Infect Immun* 1983; 42:237–244.

55. Oken MM, Creech RH, Tormey DC, et al. Toxicity and response criteria of the Eastern Cooperative Oncology Group. *Am J Clin Oncol* 1982; 5:649–655.

56. Perri RT, Kay NE. Large granular lymphocytes from B-chronic lymphocytic leukemia patients inhibit normal B cell proliferation. *Am J Hematol* 1989; 31:166–172.

57. Stroup R, Sheibani K. Antigenic phenotypes of hairy cell leukemia and monocytoid B-cell lymphoma. An immunohistochemical evaluation of 66 cases. *Hum Pathol* 1992; 23:172–177.

58. al Saati T, Caspar S, Brousset P, et al. Production of anti-B monoclonal antibodies (DBB.42, DBA.44, DNA.7, and DND.53) reactive on paraffin-embedded tissues with a new B-lymphoma cell line grafted into athymic nude mice. *Blood* 1989; 74:2476–2485.

59. Hounieu H, Chittal SM, al Saati T, et al. Hairy cell leukemia. Diagnosis of bone marrow involvement in paraffin-embedded sections with monoclonal antibody DBA.44. *Am J Clin Pathol* 1992; 98:26–33.

60. Sainati L, Matutes E, Mulligan S, et al. A variant form of hairy cell leukemia resistant to alpha-interferon: clinical and phenotype characteristics of 17 patients. *Blood* 1990; 76:157–162.

61. Cawley JC, Burns GF, Hayhoe RGH. A chronic lymphoproliferative disorder with distinctive features: a distinct variant of hairy cell leukemia. *Leuk Res* 1980; 4:547–559.

62. Tetreault S, Robbins BA, Saven A. Treatment of hairy cell leukemia-variant with cladribine. *Leuk Lymphoma* 1999; 35:347–354.

63. Diez-Martin JL, Li CY, Banks PM. Blastic variant of hairy cell leukemia. *Am J Clin Pathol* 1987; 87:576–583.

64. Machii T, Yamaguchi M, Inoue R, et al. Polyclonal B-cell lymphocytes with features resembling hairy cell leukemia-Japanese variant. *Blood* 1997; 89:2008–2014.

65. Sun T, Susin M, Brody J. Splenic lymphoma with circulating villous lymphocytes: report of seven cases and review of the literature. *Am J Clin Pathol* 1994; 45:39.

66. Yam LT, Li CY, Lam KW. Tartrate-resistant acid phosphatase isoenzyme in the reticulum cells of leukemic reticuloendotheliosis. *N Engl J Med* 1971; 284:357–360.
67. Slovak ML, Weiss LM, Nathwan BN. Cytogenetic studies of composite lymphomas: monocytoid B-cell lymphoma and other B-cell non-Hodgkin's lymphomas. *Hum Pathol* 1993; 24:1086.
68. Sheibani K, Burke JS, Swartz WG. Monocytoid B-cell lymphoma: clinicopathologic study of 21 cases of a unique type of low-grade lymphoma. *Cancer* 1988; 62:1531–1538.
69. Shin SS, Sahibani K. Monocytoid B-cell lymphoma. *Am J Clin Pathol* 1973; 99:421.
70. Saven A, Piro LD. Hairy cell leukemia. In: Hoffman R, ed. *Hematology: Basic Principles and Practice*. Churchill Livingstone, New York, 1995, pp. 1322–1329.
71. Traweek ST, Sheibani K. Monocytoid B-cell lymphoma. The biologic and clinical implications of peripheral blood involvement. *Am J Clin Pathol* 1992; 97:591.
72. Burke JS, Rappaport H. The differential diagnosis of hairy cell leukemia in bone marrow and spleen. *Semin Oncol* 1984; 11:334–346.
73. Mintz U, Golomb HM. Splenectomy as initial therapy in twenty-six patients with leukemic reticuloendotheliosis (hairy cell leukemia). *Cancer Res* 1979; 39:2366–2370.
74. Jansen J, Hermans J. Splenectomy in hairy cell leukemia: a retrospective multicenter analysis. *Cancer* 1981; 47:2066–2076.
75. Golomb HM, Vardiman JW. Response to splenectomy in 65 patients with hairy cell leukemia: an evaluation of spleen weight and bone-marrow involvement. *Blood* 1983; 61:349–352.
76. Golde DW. Therapy of hairy cell leukemia. *N Engl J Med* 1982; 307:495–496.
77. Juliusson G, Lenkei R, Liliemark J. Flow cytometry of blood and bone marrow cells from patients with hairy cell leukemia: phenotype of hairy cells and lymphocyte subsets after treatment with 2-chlorodeoxyadenosine. *Blood* 1994; 83:3672–3681.
78. Seymour JF, Estey EH, Keating MJ, Kurzrock R. Response to interferon-α in patients with hairy cell leukemia relapsing after treatment with 2-chlorodeoxyadenosine. *Leukemia* 1995;9:929–932.
79. Quesada JR, Reuben J, Manning JT, Hersh EM, Gutterman JU. Alpha-interferon for induction of remission in hairy cell leukemia. *N Engl J Med* 1984; 310:15–18.
80. Golomb HM, Jacobs A, Fefer A, et al. Alpha-2 interferon therapy of hairy cell leukemia: a multicenter study of 64 patients. *J Clin Oncol* 1986; 4:900–905.
81. Golomb HM, Ratain MJ, Fefer A, et al. Randomized study of the duration of treatment with interferon alfa-2b in patients with hairy cell leukemia. *J Natl Cancer Inst* 1988; 80:369–373.
82. Berman E, Heller G, Kempin S, Gee T, Tran L, Clarkson B. Incidence of response and long-term follow-up in patients with hairy cell leukemia with recombinant alpha-2a. *Blood* 1990; 75:839–845.
83. Damasio EE, Clavio M, et al. Alpha-interferon as induction and maintenance therapy in hairy cell leukemia: a long term follow-up analysis. *Eur J Haematol* 2000; 64:47–52.
84. Quesada JR, Hersh EM, Manning J, et al. Treatment of hairy cell leukemia with recombinant alpha-interferon. *Blood* 1986; 68:493–497.
85. Von Wussow P, Pralle H, Hochkeppel H, et al. Effective natural interferon-α therapy in recombinant-α-resistant patients with hairy cell leukemia. *Blood* 1991; 78:38–43.
86. Ratain MJ, Golomb HM, Vardiman JW, et al. Relapse after interferon alpha-2b therapy for hairy cell leukemia: analysis of diagnostic variables. *J Clin Oncol* 1988; 6:1714–1721.
87. Ratain MJ, Golomb HM, Vardiman JW, et al. Interferon alpha-2b therapy for hairy cell leukemia in 69 patients. A 6-year update. *Blood* 1989; 74:76:(abstract 276).
88. Kampmeier P, Spielberger R, Dickstein J, Mick R, Golomb H, Vardiman JW. Increased incidence of second neoplasms in patients treated with interferon α-2b for hairy cell leukemia: a clinicopathologic assessment. *Blood* 1994; 83:2931–2938.
89. Ruco LP, Procapio A, Maccallini V, et al. Severe deficiency of natural killer activity in the peripheral blood of patients with hairy cell leukemia. *Blood* 1983; 61:1132.
90. Lee SH, Kelley S, Chin H, Stebbing N. Stimulation of natural killer cell activity and inhibition of proliferation of various leukemic cells by purified human leukocyte interferon subtypes. *Cancer Res* 1982; 42:1312.

91. Lieberman D, Voloch Z, Aviv H, Nudel U, Revel M. Effects of interferon on hemoglobin synthesis and leukemia virus production in Friend cells. *Mol Biol Rep* 1974; 1:447–451.
92. Taylor-Papadimitriou J. Effects of interferons on cell growth and function. In: Gresser I, ed. Interferon 1980. Academic Press, New York, 1980, pp. 13–46.
93. Giblett ER, Anderson JE, Cohen F, Pollara B, Meuwissen HJ. Adenosine deaminase deficiency in two patients with severely impaired cellular immunity. *Lancet* 1972; 2: 1067–1069.
94. Cohen A, Hirshhorn R, Horowitz SD, et al. Deoxyadenosine triphosphate as a potentially toxic metabolite in adenosine deaminase deficiency. *Proc Natl Acad Sci USA* 1978; 75:472–476.
95. Carson DA, Wasson DB, Kaye J, et al. Deoxycytidine kinase-mediated toxicity of deoxyadenosine analogs toward malignant human lymphoblasts in vitro and toward murine L1210 leukemia in vivo. *Proc Natl Acad Sci USA* 1980; 77:6865–6869.
96. Spiers ASD, Moore D, Cassileth PA, et al. Remissions in hairy cell leukemia with pentostatin (2'-deoxycoformycin). *N Engl J Med* 1987; 316:825–871.
97. Cassileth PA, Cheuvant B, Spiers ASD, et al. Pentostatin induces durable remissions in hairy cell leukemia. *J Clin Oncol* 1991; 9:243–246.
98. Ho AD, Thaler J, Stryckmans P, et al. Pentostatin in resistant chronic lymphocytic leukemia. A phase II trial of the European Organization for Research and Treatment of Cancer. *Proc Am Soc Clin Oncol* 1990; 9:206.
99. Grever M, Kopecky K, Foular K. Randomization comparison of pentostatin versus inter-feron alpha-2a in previously untreated patients with hairy cell leukemia. *J Clin Oncol* 1995; 13:974.
100. Ribeiro P, Bouaffia F, et al. Long term outcome of patients with hairy cell leukemia treated with pentostatin. *Cancer* 1999; 84:65–70.
101. Dearden CE, Matutes E, Hilditch BL, Swansbury GJ, Catovsky D. Long-term follow-up of patients with hairy cell leukemia after treatment with pentostatin or cladribine. *Br J Haematol* 1999; 106:515–519.
102. Kraut EH, Grever MR, Bouroncle BA. Long-term follow-up of patients with hairy cell leukemia after treatment with 2'-deoxycoformycin. *Blood* 1994; 84:4061–4063.
103. Spiers ASD, Parekh SJ, Bishop MB. Hairy cell leukemia: Induction of complete remission with pentostatin (2'-deoxycoformycin). *J Clin Oncol* 1984; 2:1336–1342.
104. Johnston JB, Glazer RI, Pugh L, Israels LG. The treatment of hairy cell leukemia with 2'-deoxycoformycin. *Br J Haematol* 1986; 63:525–534.
105. Ho AD, Thaler J, Stryckmans P, Coiffier B, Luciani M. Pentostatin in refractory chronic lymphocytic leukemia: a phase II trial of the European Organization for Research and Treat-ment of Cancer. *J Natl Cancer Inst* 1990; 82:1416–1420.
106. Urba WJ, Baseler MW, Kopp WC, et al. Deoxycoformycin-induced immunosuppression in patients with hairy cell leukemia. *Blood* 1989; 73:38–46.
107. Piro LD, Carrera CJ, Carson DA, Beutler E. Lasting remissions in hairy cell leukemia induced by a single infusion of 2-chlorodeoxyadenosine. *N Engl J Med* 1990; 322:1117–1121.
108. Juliusson G, Liliemark J. Rapid recovery from cytopenia in hairy cell leukemia after treat-ment with 2-chloro-2'-deoxyadenosine (CdA): Relation to opportunistic infections. *Blood* 1992; 79:888–894.
109. Estey EM, Kurzrock R, Kantarjian HM, et al. Treatment of hairy cell leukemia with 2-chlorodeoxyadenosine (2-CdA). *Blood* 1992; 79:882–887.
110. Tallman MS, Hakimian D, Rademaker AW, et al. Relapse of hairy cell leukemia after 2-chlorodeoxyadenosine: Long-term follow-up of the Northwestern University experience. *Blood* 1996; 88:1954–1959.
111. Hoffman MA, Janson D, Rose E, Rai KR. Treatment of hairy cell leukemia with cladribine: response, toxicity and long-term follow-up. *J Clin Oncol* 1997; 15:1138–1142.
112. Cheson BD, Vena DA, Montello MJ, et al. Treatment of hairy cell leukemia with 2-chlorodeoxyadenosine via the Group C Protocol Mechanism of the National Cancer Insti-tute: a report of 979 patients. *J Clin Oncol* 1998; 16:3007–3015.

113. Saven A, Burian C, Koziol JA, Piro LD. Long-term follow-up of patients with hairy cell leukemia after cladribine treatment. *Blood* 1998; 92:1918–1926.
114. Hakimian D, Tallman MS, Kiley C, Peterson LA. Detection of minimal residual disease by immunostaining of bone marrow biopsies after 2-chlorodeoxyadenosine for hairy cell leukemia. *Blood* 1993; 82:1798–1802.
115. Ellison DJ, Sharpe RW, Robbins BA, et al. Immunomorphologic analysis of bone marrow biopsies after treatment with 2-chlorodeoxyadenosine for hairy cell leukemia. *Blood* 1994; 84:4310–4315.
116. Kurzrock R, Strom SS, Estey E, et al. Second cancer risk in hairy cell leukemia: analysis of 350 patients. *J Clin Oncol* 1997; 15:1803–1810.
117. Au WY, Klasa RJ, Gallagher R, Le N, Gascoyne RD, Connors JM. Second malignancies in patients with hairy cell leukemia in British Columbia: a 20-year experience. *Blood* 1998; 92:1160–1164.
118. Cheson BD, Vena DA, Barrett J, Freidlin B. Second malignancies as a consequence of nucleoside analog therapy for chronic lymphoid leukemias. *J Clin Oncol* 1999;17:2454–2460.
119. Saven A, Burian C, Adusumalli J, Koziol JA. Filgrastim for cladribine-induced neutropenic fever in patients with hairy cell leukemia. *Blood* 1999; 93:2471–2477.
120. Kantarjian HM, Redman J, Keating MJ. Fludarabine phosphate therapy in other lymphoid malignancies. *Semin Oncol* 1990; 17(Suppl 8):66–70.
121. Kantarjian HM, Schachner J, Keating MJ. Fludarabine therapy in hairy cell leukemia. *Cancer* 1991; 67:1291–1293.
122. Kraut E, Chun H. Fludarabine phosphate in refractory hairy cell leukemia. *Am J Hematol* 1991; 37:59–60.
123. Golomb HM. Progress report on chlorambucil therapy in postsplenectomy patients with progressive hairy cell leukemia. *Blood* 1981; 57:464–467.
124. Lusch CJ, Ramsey HE, Katayama I. Leukemic reticuloendotheliosis: report of a case with peripheral blood remission on androgen therapy. *Cancer* 1978;41:1964–1966.
125. Blum SF. Lithium in hairy cell leukemia. *N Engl J Med* 1983; 303:464–465.
126. Lembersky BC, Ratain MJ, Golomb HM. Skeletal complications in hairy cell leukemia: diagnosis and therapy. *J Clin Oncol* 1988; 6:1280–1284.
127. Arkel YS, Lake-Lewin D, Sarapoulous AA, Berman E. Bone lesions in hairy cell leukemia. *Cancer* 1984; 53:2401.
128. Kreitman RS, Wilson WH, Robbins D, et al. Responses in refractory hairy cell leukemia to a recombinant immunotoxin. *Blood* 1999; 94:3340–3348.
129. Thomas DA, O'Brien S, Cortes J, et al. Pilot study of rituximab in refractory or relapsed hairy cell leukemia (HCL). *Blood* 2000; 94(10):705a (abstract 3116).
130. Golomb HM, Catovsky D, Golde DW. Hairy cell leukemia: a clinical review of 71 cases. *Ann Intern Med* 1978; 89:677–683.
131. Quesada JR, Gutterman J, Hersh EM. Treatment of hairy cell leukemia with alpha interferons. *Cancer* 1986; 57:1678–1680.
132. Foon KA, Maluish AE, Abrams PG, et al. Recombinant leukocyte alpha interferon therapy for advanced hairy cell leukemia. Therapeutic and immunologic results. *Am J Med* 1986; 80:351–356.
133. Rai K, Mick R, Ozer H, Silver R, Papish S, Bloomfield C. Alpha-interferon therapy in untreated active hairy cell leukemia: A Cancer and Leukemia Group B (CALGB) study. *Proc Am Soc Clin Oncol* 1987; 6:159 (abstract 624).
134. Golomb H, Fefer A, Golde D, et al. Update of a multi-institutional study of 195 patients (pts) with hairy cell leukemia (HCL) treated with interferon alfa-2b (IFN). *Proc Am Soc Clin Oncol* 1990; 6:215.
135. Kraut EH, Bouroncle BA, Grever MR. Pentostatin in the treatment of advanced hairy cell leukemia. *J Clin Oncol* 1989; 7:168–172.
136. Grem J, King S, Cheson B, Leyland-Jones B, Wittes R. Pentostatin in hairy cell leukemia: treatment by the special exception mechanism. *J Natl Cancer Inst* 1989; 81:448–453.

137. Blasinska-Morawiec RT, Blonsk J, et al. 2-chlorodeoxyadenosince (cladribine) in the treatment of hairy cell leukemia and hairy cell leukemia variant: 7-year experience in Poland. *Eur J Haematol* 1999; 62:49–56.

138. Bastie JN, Cazals-Hatem D, et al. Five years follow-up after 2-chlorodeoxyadenosine treatment in thirty patients with hairy cell leukemia: evaluation of minimal residual disease and CD4+ lymphocytopenia after treatment. *Leuk Lymphoma* 1999; 35:555–565.

4 Prolymphocytic Leukemias

Peter J. Rosen, MD and Jonathan Said, MD

INTRODUCTION

Prolymphocytic leukemias are extremely rare disease entities characterized according to their cell of origin into B- and T-cell type. Approximately 80% of the cases are of B-cell phenotype. Definitional problems exist regarding specificity of diagnosis for these unusual leukemias. The recent World Health Organization (WHO) classification recognizes the existence of these entities and attempts to delineate specific diagnostic criteria.

B-CELL PROLYMPHOCYTIC LEUKEMIA

A prolymphocytic leukemia of B-cell type was first described as a rare variant of chronic lymphocytic leukemia (CLL) by Catovsky and colleagues (1). Although not given a separate category in the REAL classification (2), it is apparent that prolymphocytic leukemia has distinctive clinical and cytologic characteristics that warrant its designation as a specific entity. Thus, the new WHO classification recognizes B-cell prolymphocytic leukemia (B-PLL) as a specific clinical/pathologic disorder (3). It is important to consider that diagnostic confusion and considerable overlap may occur with B-cell chronic lymphocytic leukemia (B-CLL) because of transitional cases, as described here.

Clinical Features

B-PLL generally presents with splenomegaly and a high white blood cell (WBC) count (usually exceeding 100,000/mm^3). More than 55% of the lymphoid cells are prolymphocytes. In contradistinction to T-PLL and B-CLL, there

From: *Current Clinical Oncology: Chronic Leukemias and Lymphomas:*
Biology, Pathophysiology, and Clinical Management
Edited by: G. J. Schiller © Humana Press Inc., Totowa, NJ

is generally no lymphadenopathy *(4)*. The spleen is often markedly enlarged, extending at least 10 cm beneath the costal margin. Characteristically, patients are anemic, with a hemoglobin less than 10 gm%, and are usually thrombocytopenic with platelet counts less that $100,000/mm^3$. Patients are generally in their late 60s or older, and there is a modest male predominance. Survival ranges between 2 and 3 yr.

Over the years, it has been recognized that a subset of patients variously termed CLL/PLL, atypical CLL or CLL-pro exist, and represent entities with a more aggressive clinical course than B-CLL. The percentage of prolymphocytes described in these cases generally ranges between 10% and 55% or 10% and 30%, depending on the series. It is presumed that many such patients have developed a prolymphocytoid transformation arising from B-CLL denoting increased resistance to traditional therapies and a very poor outcome. Other such intermediate cases appear *de novo (5)*.

Cytologic and Histologic Features

The WBC count usually exceeds $100,000/mm^3$, and at least 55% of the cells have the morphology of prolymphocytes (Fig. 1). The nuclei are round or oval, and occasionally indented. The chromatin is generally coarse or clumped, and each cell has a distinct prominent nucleolus with perinucleolar chromatin condensation. The cytoplasm is moderately basophilic, and may contain vacuoles or a few coarse azurophilic granules. In some cases, cells may have short cytoplasmic projections *(6)*. In addition, some cases have an associated monocytosis *(7)*.

Patterns of Organ Infiltration

The bone marrow is usually diffusely and extensively infiltrated, but may exhibit a nodular pattern *(8)*. In the spleen, there is involvement of both white and red pulp, with a diffuse or pseudonodular growth pattern. Pseudonodules may also been observed in the lymph nodes (Fig. 2), and consist of central cores of densely clustered prolymphocytes *(6)*.

Immunophenotype

Cells are positive for B-cell markers, including CD19 and CD20. There is also moderately strong staining for CD22 and FMC7. In contradistinction to B-CLL, CD5 and CD23 staining is usually absent. The cells are usually negative for CD11c, but may show weak expression of CD10. Flow cytometry or fluorescence microscopy reveals the presence of strong monoclonal surface immunoglobulin staining with either IgM or IgM plus IgD subtypes. This pattern differs from B-CLL, which usually has a low density of surface immunoglobulin on the cell membrane. Also, the intensity of CD20 staining is bright, as opposed to the dim staining characteristic of B-CLL. As this chapter reveals, this finding may offer unique therapeutic possibilities.

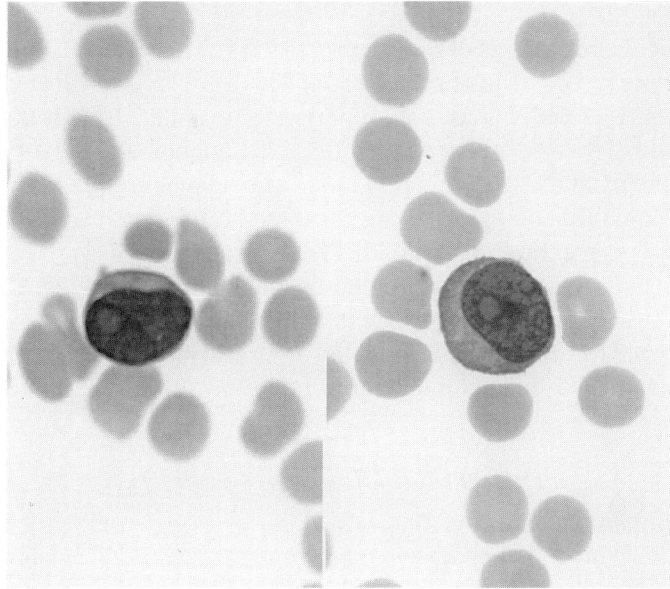

Fig. 1. Prolymphocytic leukemia, B-cell type. Cells are typical prolymphocytes with homogeneous chromatin and prominent nucleoli. (Wrights stained smear original×400.)

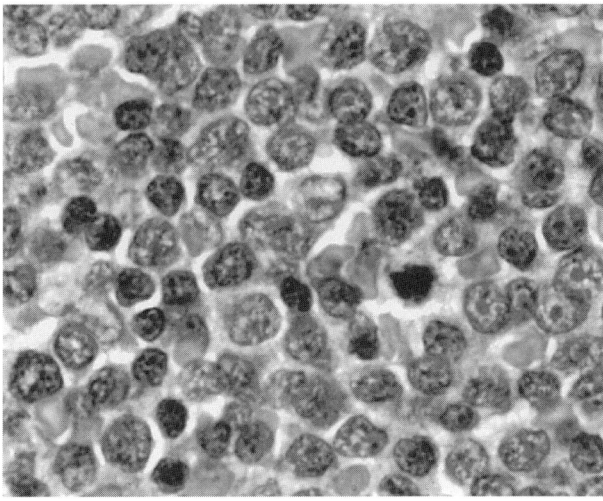

Fig. 2. Lymph-node biopsy from a patient with B-cell prolymphocytic leukemia showing replacement by prolymphocytes. (Hematoxylin and eosin, original ×400.)

Cytogenetics

The cytogenetic features of B-PLL also differ from those seen in B-CLL. For example, trisomy 12 and deletion 13 are not usually observed. However, in some series, as many as 25% of cases are reported to reveal the t(ll;14) translocation characteristically associated with mantle cell lymphoma (MCL) *(9,10)*. This translocation juxtaposes the immunoglobulin heavy-chain gene on chromosome 14 with the so-called bcl-1 gene on chromosome 11. Immunohistochemical staining for bcl-1 expression confirms this translocation on tissue sections. This observation calls into question the potential diagnostic specificity of some cases of B-PLL, suggesting that there may be considerable overlap between B-PLL and the blastoid form of MCL. This finding may also have significant therapeutic implications. In addition, point mutations involving the *p53* gene occur in about 50% of cases.

Differential Diagnosis (Table 1)

1. CLL with prolymphocytoid transformation.
   In B-CLL with prolymphocytoid transformation, the cell population is usually more heterogenous than B-PLL, with residual features of CLL by morphology and immunophenotype. Prolymphocytoid transformation is the most common form of transformation of B-CLL, and occurs in about 10% of cases after a typical chronic phase. The clinical features of CLL with prolymphocytoid transformation include increasing splenomegaly, lymphadenopathy, and poor treatment response. The peripheral blood shows a mixture of small lymphocytic and prolymphocytic cells, and prolymphocytes represent less than 55% of the lymphoid cells. The immunophenotype is usually more typical of B-CLL, retaining CD5 positivity and manifesting weak CD22 expression and weak surface immunoglobulin. CD23 is also usually evident (Table 1).

2. CLL/PLL (or CLL-Pro or atypical CLL).
   As noted previously, some patients with B-CLL present with a variant characterized by an increased proportion of prolymphocytes, often in association with other atypical morphologic findings. In these cases, the percentage of prolymphocytes is less than 55%, and according to some authors it is below 30%. Adverse cytogenetic features have been described. The course is usually more rapid than typical B-CLL.

3. Large-cell transformation of B-CLL (Richter's syndrome).
   Only rarely is there significant peripheral-blood involvement. The cells are larger than prolymphocytes and lack the characteristic phenotypic findings.

4. Hairy cell leukemia (HCL) has well-described cytologic and phenotypic features, and generally should not be confused with B-PLL. However, there is a so-called HCL variant which has morphologic features intermediate between HCL and B-PLL *(11)*. It usually presents in an age group similar to B-PLL, and has a number of clinical features at variance with HCL, including the lack of a strong male dominance, high peripheral white count, absence of monocytope-

Table 1
Differential Diagnosis Between B-CLL and B-PLL

	CLL	Prolymphocytic leukemia
Clinical features	Lymphadenopathy common	Lymphadenopathy rare
	Moderate splenomegaly	Splenomegaly often massive
	WBC count variable	WBC count high $(>100,000/mm^3)$
Cytology	Small mature lymphocytes	Large lymphocytes with fine open chromatin
	Inconspicuous nucleoli	Nucleoli prominent
Phenotype	CD5 positive	CD5 variable
	Weak surface immunoglobulin	Bright surface immunoglobulin
CD22	Weak	Strong
CD10	Negative	Variable
FMC7	Negative	Positive
CD23	Positive	Negative

nia, atypical immunophenotype, and a poor response to treatments that are usually successful in HCL.

5. Splenic lymphoma with villous lymphocytes has characteristic circulating cells with villous processes, and is negative for CD5 and CD10.

6. Acute monoblastic leukemia (M5A) blast cells may resemble prolymphocytes, but reveal diffuse cytoplasm staining for nonspecific esterase and obviously lack the immunophenotypic features of B-PLL.

7. MCL, blastoid variant.
   As previously discussed, considerable overlap may occur between B-PLL and the rare blastoid MCL. Most morphologists believe that the blastoid variant of MCL is compressed of cells resembling lymphoblasts rather than the characteristic cells of B-PLL. In addition, the cells are more uniform, and the white count is generally lower in MCL. Nevertheless, as noted, there may be a similar chromosomal translocation t(11;14), with resultant cyclin D1 expression (bcl-1) in both disorders. Review of many cases originally diagnosed as B-PLL reveal that many are likely to represent a transformed mantle cell lymphoma with t(11;14) and cyclin D1 over expression. A small proportion appear cytogenetically and immunophenotypically distinct and may represent true B-PLL (personal communication: Dr. Andrew Wotherspoon, Roya Marsden Hospital, London, UK).

Treatment and Prognosis

The therapy of B-PLL has been highly unsatisfactory. Agents utilized in B-CLL, such as chlorambucil and cyclophosphamide, generally produce suboptimal or transient responses. The older literature does contain evidence of responses to cyclophosphamide, doxorubicin, vincristine, and prednisone

(CHOP), splenic irradiation, and splenectomy. Splenectomy responses have been relatively rare, and often of short duration. Some durable responses to the CHOP regimen have been described with an occasional complete remission, but the overall response rate is probably under 30% *(12–14)*.

Newer agents employed in the management of B-PLL include the purine nucleosides and monoclonal antibodies (MAbs). Kantarjian et al. reported an initial experience with fludarabine in cases of B-PLL and prolymphocytoid transformation of B-CLL *(15)*. In their series of 17 patients, three (18%) achieved a complete response, and an additional three had a partial response. Nine patients appeared to have B-PLL at diagnosis, whereas the remaining eight developed an increasing number of prolymphocytes following a diagnosis of B-CLL. Only three had received no prior treatment. However, a disquieting note in this series is the absence of response in all five patients who had B-PLL at presentation with greater than 50% prolymphocytes. In addition, with the exception of one patient, all patients in the series showed CD5 antigen positivity on the B cells, which is generally absent in cases of typical B-PLL. Other case reports or series have demonstrated activity for fludarabine, pentostatin, and 2-chlorodeoxadenosine, suggesting that all the purine nucleosides are active *(16–19)*.

2-Chlorodeoxyadenosine is a purine analog with major activity in HCL. Saven and colleagues reported their experience in eight patients with this agent, noting five complete and three partial responses. Complete responses lasted a median of 14 mo *(18)*. The EORTC reported activity utilizing 2´-deoxycoformycin (pentostatin) in both B and T PLL. Of 14 patients treated with B-PLL, seven achieved partial remissions, with a median duration of remission of 12 mo *(19)*. In this series, no complete responses were observed.

The advent of MAb therapy for lymphomas and leukemias promises further treatment possibilities for B-PLL. Rituxan is a chimeric MAb directed against the CD20 antigen present on mature B lymphocytes and most B lymphoid malignancies. As noted, most cases of B-CLL show weak expression of CD20. The clinical experience with rituxan in B-CLL and small lymphocytic lymphoma (SLL) has been less successful than that seen in follicular lymphoma (FL). In the pivotal trial, the response rate for SLL was only 13% *(20)*. Recent studies using novel dosing schedules suggest a somewhat higher remission rate in B-CLL, exploiting dose intensity to achieve more favorable pharmacokinetics *(21)*. The higher amount of antigen density in B-PLL suggests a potentially superior role for rituxan when compared with B-CLL. O'Brien et al. have reported a series of patients with CLL and CLL variants treated in a dose-escalation trial with rituxan *(22)*. In this series of 50 patients, two with B-PLL were treated. Both patients responded, and one achieved a complete remission (CR). Further evidence for the potential activity of rituxan comes from case reports described by Tsiara et al. *(23)* and Vartholomatos et al. *(24)*. The first report described a 34-yr-old patient unresponsive to several prior programs, including CHOP and fludarabine.

After four infusions of rituxan, the patient achieved a remission that lasted at least 6 mo. The second experience involved a 31-yr-old woman with resistant PLL. In this patient, a complete remission lasted at least 8 mo.

A second MAb, CAMPATH-1H, is a humanized antibody that recognizes the CD52 antigen present on both B and T lymphocytes as well as monocytes. A recent series of seven patients included one patient with B-PLL, who achieved a complete response with this antibody. However, the response was short-lived, lasting only 3 mo, with further transformation to a large-cell lymphoma *(25)*.

Since up to 30% of patients with B-PLL manifest the t(11;14) translocation seen in mantle cell lymphoma, the possibility of employing mantle-cell regimens in this subset may be reasonable. For example, investigators at the M D Anderson Cancer Center have used a multi-agent aggressive chemotherapy regimen termed hyper-CVAD in the management of MCL, with impressive initial results *(26)*. Patients who achieved remission were then subjected to autologous stem-cell transplant. This approach may prove fruitful in B-PLL, particularly those cases with the t(ll;14) translocation. The possibility of targeting cyclin D1, the oncogene overexpressed by the bcl-1 translocation, also deserves mention.

A multifaceted approach to the treatment of B-PLL should be considered based upon the available data. One potential scenario would include combination therapy with a purine nucleoside analog plus rituxan followed by autologous stem-cell transplantation for those patients who achieved complete or near complete remissions. Because of the age of patients generally afflicted with this disease, most patients would not be candidates for traditional allogeneic transplantation. On the other hand, non-myeloablative strategies may be considered *(27)*.

T-CELL PROLYMPHOCYTIC LEUKEMIA

T-cell prolymphocytic leukemia (T-PLL) is an extremely rare and aggressive disease characterized by the proliferation of small-to-medium size prolymphocytes with a mature post-thymic T-cell phenotype. Cases previously classified as T-CLL are now subsumed within the spectrum of T-PLL *(28)*. Approximately 75% of T-PLL are characterized by typical prolymphocytes, whereas the remaining 25% consist of two variants recognized in the new WHO classification system. These variants are a small-cell form *(29)* and a variant superficially resembling the cerebriform cells of Sézary syndrome.

Clinical Features

Typically, the disease occurs in an older population, with most patients over the age of 60 at the time of diagnosis. The largest series has been published by Matutes and colleagues at the Royal Marsden Hospital in London, which described findings in 78 patients *(30)*. Although B-PLL is a syndrome typified by a very high WBC count, splenomegaly, and little or no lymphadenopathy, the

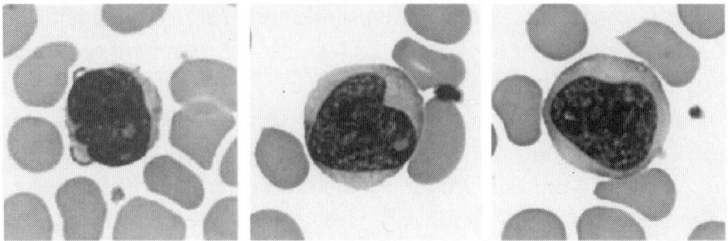

Fig. 3. T-cell prolymphocytic leukemia revealing prolymphocytes with variable nuclear irregularity and distinct nucleoli. (Wrights stained smear original ×400.)

situation is different in T-PLL. High WBC counts typically exceeding 100,000/mm^3 and enlarged spleens also are features of T-PLL, but about one-half of the patients also have lymphadenopathy. In addition, a significant minority of patients present with cutaneous lesions, which are often seen in other T-cell lymphoproliferative disorders. The skin rash has been described as maculopapular, nodular, or occasionally as a generalized erythroderma, and may be the initial manifestation of disease. Less often, patients present with pulmonary and central nervous system (CNS) or serosal involvement. While some patients may not be anemic or thrombocytopenia at presentation, hematologic deterioration usually occurs quickly.

Cytologic and Histologic Features

The characteristic cell, as recognized in peripheral blood smears, is a small-to-medium size lymphoid cell with a round or oval nucleus and a distinct nucleolus (Fig. 3). In other cases, cells have an irregular or even "knobby" nuclear outline. The cytoplasm is often sparse and basophilic without granules. Often, there may be cytoplasmic protrusions or blebs. As previously mentioned, in less than 25% of cases the cells are small without a visible nucleolus (small-cell variant), and can be confused with B-CLL. Rarely, the cells may have a cerebriform outline resembling Sézary cells. In some cases there may be overlap between the different subtypes, with both smaller and larger irregular cells present in the same patient. The cells frequently have paranuclear lysosomal inclusions that stain with acid phosphatase and nonspecific esterase *(31)* (Fig. 4).

Patterns of Organ Infiltration

The bone marrow is often diffusely infiltrated with the same cytologic features seen in the peripheral blood. As mentioned, cutaneous involvement occurs in approx 25% of patients, and may be extensive. Infiltrates often surround dermal appendages, but lack the characteristic epidermotropism of mycosis fungoides. Lymph nodes may be diffusely involved, or there may be predilection for the paracortex. Splenic involvement occurs, with infiltration of both red and white pulp.

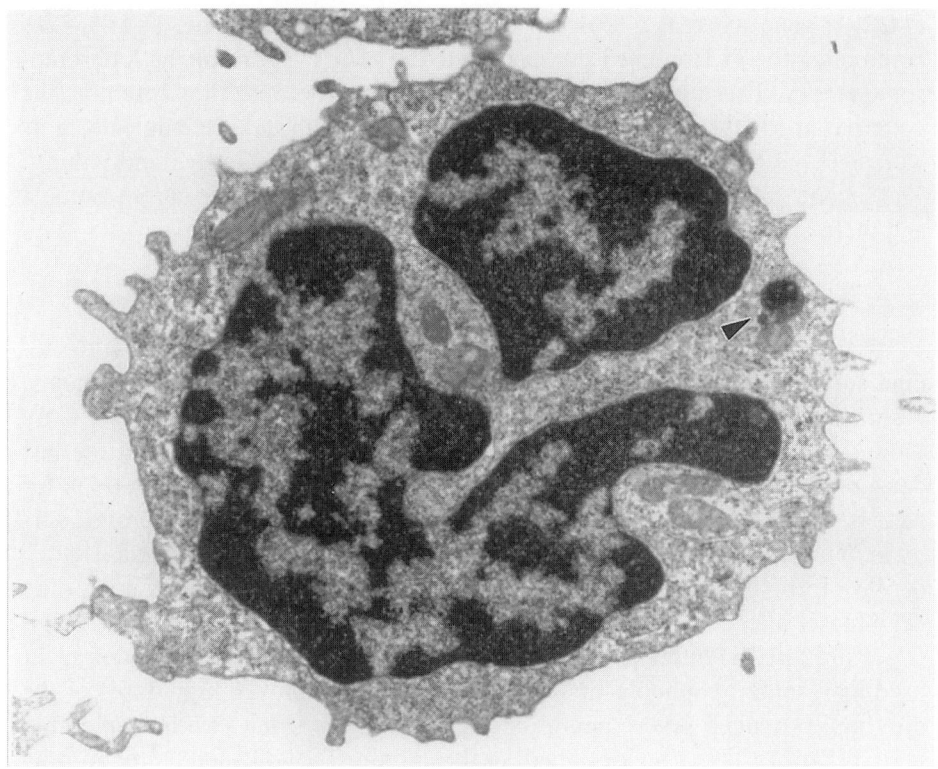

Fig. 4. Electron micrograph from a case of T-cell prolymphocytic leukemia. There is a markedly irregular or "knobby" nuclear outline, and the nucleolus is indistinct. There is a single paranuclear lysosomal granule (arrowhead). The presence of these granules explains the block-like staining for acid phosphatase or nonspecific esterase in these cases. (Uranyl acetate, lead citrate, original ×900.)

Immunophenotype

The cells in T-PLL have the phenotype of mature peripheral T-cells: negative for TdT and positive for CD2, CD3, CD5, and CD7 *(30)*. Sixty percent have a T-helper-cell phenotype (CD4+, CD8−) and about 25% reveal coexpression of CD4 and CD8. The remainder are positive for CD8 and negative for CD4. Expression of CD7 is helpful in differentiating T-PLL from Sézary syndrome, which is CD7−. The cells lack cytolytic granules staining for TIA-1 and granzyme characteristic of T-NK cells.

Cytogenetics

The most common chromosome abnormality is inversion of chromosome 14, with breakpoints on q11 and q32 *(30,32)*. qll is the site of the T-cell-receptor

(TCR) α gene whereas q32 is the site of the putative oncogene, TCL-1. Less commonly, the TCRα gene is juxtaposed to the MTCP-1 gene on the X chromosome at q28. These genetic changes are of interest because they resemble the pattern found in the T-lymphocytes seen in patients with ataxia telangiectasia, as well as in the leukemias and lymphomas that may develop in such individuals. The second most common abnormality seen in T-PLL involves chromosome 8 and includes an isochromosome 8q and/or trisomy 8 *(33)*.

Treatment and Prognosis

Historically, the prognosis associated with T-PLL has been dismal, with median survival averaging 7.5 mo. Older therapies involving alkylating agents, multiagent combinations such as CHOP, and splenectomy have benefited only a minority of patients, and usually for very brief periods of time. In the last decade, several important strides have been made in improving the outlook for patients with this disease, which hopefully will translate into an improved survival. The first agent to be extensively studied was the purine nucleoside 2´ deoxycoformycin (pentostatin). This agent is a potent inhibitor of adenosine deaminase, a key enzyme in the purine degradation pathway present in high concentrations in lymphoid tissue, particularly T-cells. Earlier trials of this agent used in T-acute lymphoblastic leukemia (T-ALL) employed high doses of the drug and produced severe neurotoxicity. Revised schedules with a favorable toxicity profile have been designed for the chronic T- and B-cell lymphoproliferative disorders. A series by Mercieca et al. in which 145 patients with T-cell malignancies were treated with pentostatin was recently reported *(34)*. Fifty-five of the 145 patients had T-PLL. Responses were observed in 25 patients (45%), and five had complete responses. The median duration of complete remission was 10 mo whereas partial responses lasted between 3 and 6 mo. Of interest, there was no significant difference in the response rate between previously treated and untreated patients. Furthermore, clinical abnormalities such as the degree of splenomegaly, lymphadenopathy, and the height of the WBC count did not adversely affect response. The median survival duration from the start of therapy was longer in responders (17.5 mo) than in non-responders (9 mo).

A second purine analog has been developed with potential activity in T-PLL. This agent, known as compound 506U is a prodrug of 9-β-D arabinofuranosylguanine (Ara-G) *(35)*. A phase I trial has been reported by Kurtzberg involving 70 patients *(36)*. The population was made up of both pediatric and adult patients with a variety of refractory hematologic malignancies. The highest degree of drug activity appeared to be in T-ALL. However, six patients with T-cell CLL, presumably T-PLL in the newer WHO classification, were included, and four achieved a partial response. This agent is associated with some neurologic toxicity, which has been dose-limiting.

Perhaps the most exciting agent introduced in the management of T-PLL has been the MAb CAMPATH-1H. As already noted, this antibody is a genetically humanized MAb directed against the CD52 antigen, and is expressed on most normal and neoplastic lymphocytes as well as monocytes and macrophages. Because it is humanized, the antibody does not evoke antimurine antibody responses, and can be given over a significant duration of time. However, as opposed to the CD20 antibody (rituxan), the broader spectrum of normal cell types depleted by the antibody leads to significant immune suppression, which may complicate management. The results obtained to date in patients with T-PLL treated with CAMPATH-1H have been extremely promising. Pawson et al. reported an initial experience in 15 patients with T-PLL, most of whom had been pretreated with pentostatin *(37)*. Nine of 15 patients (60%) achieved a complete response, and two patients (13%) showed a partial response. Treatment was administered 3× weekly at a dose of 30 mg with possible dose escalation. The duration of treatment lasted approx 6 wk, although some patients received slightly longer periods of treatment. Because of the immune suppression anticipated with the drug, prophylactic cotrimoxazole and acyclovir were administered. In this initial study, response durations were encouraging with the complete remissions lasting a median of 6 mo and some patients remained in remission for periods lasting up to 30 mo. Furthermore, patients could be retreated with the antibody following relapse with successful second complete responses observed in three relapsed patients. In addition to the potential increased risk of infections associated with the antibody, an unexpected toxicity consisted of two episodes of bone-marrow aplasia.

An expanded report of this experience was recently reported. Twenty-two patients with T-PLL have now been treated *(38)*. All patients had received prior therapy, including pentostatin in 14 patients, and all patients had progressive disease after a response or were resistant to treatment. In this series, 77% of patients responded, and 59% achieved CR. The median disease-free survival was 9 mo and survival was 13.5 mo in complete responders and 6 mo in partial responders. Four patients remain alive in remission up to 3 yr following therapy. Three patients proceeded to high-dose therapy conditioned with melphalan and total body irradiation (TBI) followed by autotransplantation. Two of these patients were autografted after relapse, and subsequently died 12 and 17 mo later, respectively. An additional patient transplanted in first remission remains alive after 16 mo. Stem-cell harvests were uncontaminated with malignant cells, as demonstrated by flow cytometry and PCR.

Further demonstration of the utility of this agent in T-PLL was reported by Cazin from France *(39)*. Nine previously treated patients were enrolled in the study and were given a higher dose of CAMPATH-1H than reported in the previous experience. Treatment was continued for 4–8 wk. Six of the nine patients achieved a CR with a median duration of 7 mo. Two of the complete responders went on to high-dose chemotherapy with an autologous stem-cell transplant, one of whom relapsed in the central nervous system. The median survival in this series was 8 mo.

These demonstrations of activity of several agents in this disease warrant cautious optimism that integration of these newer treatments followed by possible autologous stem-cell transplants or non-myeloablative allogeneic transplantation may control the disease.

REFERENCES

1. Catovsky D, Galetto J, Okos A, et al. Prolymphocytic leukaemia of B and T-cell type. *Lancet* 1973; 2:232–234.
2. Harris NL, Jaffe ES, Stein H, et al. A Revised European American Classification of Lymphoid Neoplasms: A proposal from the International Study Group. *Blood* 1994; 84:1361–1392.
3. Jaffe ES, Harris NL, Diebold J, et al. World Health Organization Classification of neoplastic diseases of the hematopoietic and lymphoid tissues. A progress report. Am *J Clin Pathol* 1999; 111(Suppl 1):S8–12.
4. Galton DAG, Goldman J, Wiltshaw E, et al. Prolymphocytic leukaemia. *Br J Haematol* 1974; 27:7–23.
5. Melo JV, Catovsky D, Galton DAG. The relationship between chronic lymphocytic leukaemia and prolymphocytic leukaemia. The patterns of evolution of "prolymphocytoid" transformation. *Br J Haematol* 1986; 64:77–86.
6. Katayama I, Aiba M, Pechet L, et al. B-lineage prolymphocytic leukemia as a distinct clinicopathologic entity. *Am J Pathol* 1980; 99:399–412.
7. Brunning RD, McKenna RW. Tumors of the bone marrow. Washington DC, Armed Forces Institute of Pathology, 1994.
8. Bearman RM, Pangalis GA, Rappaport H. Prolymphocytic leukemia: clinical, histopathological and cytochemical observations. *Cancer* 1978; 42:2360–2372.
9. Brito-Babapulle V, Pittman S, Melo JV, et al. Cytogenetic studies on prolymphocytic leukemia I: B-cell prolymphocytic leukemia. *Hematol Pathol* 1987; 1:27–33.
10. Brito-Babapulle V, Ellis J, Matutes E, et al. Translocation t (11;14) (q 13;32) in chronic lymphoid disorders. *Genes Chromosomes Cancer* 1992; 5:158–165.
11. Sainaiti L, Matutes E, Mulligan S, et al. A variant form of hairy cell leukemia resistant to α-interferon: clinical and phenotypic characteristics of 17 patients. *Blood* 1979; 76:157–162.
12. Sibbald B, Catovsky D. Complete remission in prolymphocytic leukaemia with the combination chemotherapy—CHOP. *Br J Haematol* 1979; 42:488–490.
13. Taylor HG, Butler WM, Rhoads J, et al. Prolymphocytic leukemia: treatment with combination chemotherapy to include doxorubicin. *Cancer* 1982; 49:1524–1529.
14. Swift JF, Wold HG, Gandara DR, et al. Prolymphocytic leukemia: serial responses to therapy. *Cancer* 1984; 54:978–980
15. Kantarjian HM, Childs C, O'Brien S, et al. Efficacy of fludarabine, a new adenine nucleoside analogue, in patients with prolymphocytic leukemia and the prolymphocytoid variant of chronic lymphocytic leukemia. *Am J Med* 1991; 90:223–228.
16. Sporn JR. Sustained response of refractory prolymphocytic leukemia to fludarabine. *Acta Haematol* 1991; 85:205–211.
17. Dearden C, Catovsky D. Deoxycoformycin in the treatment of mature B-cell malignancies. *Br J Cancer* 1990; 62:4–5.

18. Saven A, Lee J, Schlutz M, et al. Major activity of cladribine in patients with de novo B-cell prolymphocytic leukemia. *J Clin Oncol* 1997; 15:37–43.
19. Dohner H, Ho AD, Thaler J, et al. Pentostatin in prolymphocytic leukemia: Phase II Trial of European Organization for Research and Treatment of Cancer Leukemia Comparative Study Group. *J Natl Cancer Inst* 1993; 85:658–662.
20. McLaughlin P, Grillo-Lopez AJ, Link BK, et al. Rituximab chimeric anti CD-20 monoclonal antibody therapy for relapsed indolent lymphoma: half of patients respond to a four dose treatment program. *J Clin Oncol* 1998; 16:2825–2833.
21. Byrd JC, Grever MR, Davis B, et al. Phase I/II study of thrice weekly rituximab in chronic lymphocytic leukemia (CLL)/small cell lymphocytic lymphoma: a feasible and active regimen. *Blood* 1994; 94; abst. 314.
22. O'Brien SM, Kantarjian H, Thomas DA, et al. Rituximab dose escalation trial in chronic lymphocytic leukemia. *J Clin Oncol* 2001; 19:2165–2170.
23. Tsiara SN, Vartholomatos G, Kapsali H, et al. Monoclonal antibody rituximab for the treatment of resistant B-prolymphocytic leukemia. *Am J Oncol* 1999; 10(Suppl 3):129.
24. Vartholomatos G, Tsiara DN, Christou L, et al. Rituximab (anti-CD 20 monoclonal antibody) administration in a young patient with resistant B-prolymphocytic leukemia. *Acta Haematol* 1999; 102:94–98.
25. Bowers AL, Zongs A, Emmett E, et al. Subcutaneous CAMPATH-IH infludarabine-resistant/relapsed chronic lymphocytic and B-prolymphocytic leukaemia. *Br J Haematol* 1997; 96:617–619.
26. Khouri IF, Romaguera J, Kantarjian H, et al. Hyper-CVAD and high dose methotrexate cytarabine followed by stem cell transplantation: an active regimen for mantle cell lymphoma. *J Clin Oncol* 1998; 16:3803–3809.
27. Khouri IF, Keating M, Körbling M, et al. Transplant-lite: induction of graft versus malignancy using fludarabine-based nonablative chemotherapy and allogeneic blood progenitor-cell transplantation as treatment for lymphoid malignancies. *J Clin Oncol* 1998; 16:2817–2824.
28. Matutes E, Catovsky D. Similarities between T-cell chronic lymphocytic leukemia and the small cell variant of T-prolymphocytic leukemia. *Blood* 1996; 87:3520–3521.
29. Hoyer JD, Ross CW, Li CY, et al. True T-cell chronic lymphocytic leukemia: a morphologic and immunophenotypic study of 25 cases. *Blood* 1995; 86:1163–1169.
30. Matutes E, Brito-Babapulle V, Swansburg J, et al. Clinical and laboratory features of 78 cases of T-prolymphocytic leukemia. *Blood* 1991; 78:3269–3274.
31. Costello C, Catovsky D, O'Brien M. Cytoplasmic inclusions in a case of prolymphocytic leukemia. *Am J Clin Pathol* 1981; 76:499–501.
32. Brito-Babapulle V, Pomfret M, Matutes E, et al. Cytogenetic studies on prolymphocytic leukemia II: T cell prolymphocytic leukemia. *Blood* 1987; 70:926–931.
33. Mossafa H, Brizard A, Huret JL, et al. Trisomy 8q due to i(8q) or der(8) t(8;8) is a frequent lesion in T-prolymphocytic leukaemia: four new cases and a review of the literature. *Br J Haematol* 1994; 86:780–785.
34. Mercieca J, Matutes E, Dearden C, et al. The role of pentostatin in the treatment of T-cell malignancy: analysis of response rate in 145 patients according to disease subtype. *J Clin Oncol* 1994; 12:2588–2593.
35. Lambe CU, Averett DR, Paff MT, et al. 2-amino-6-methoxypurine arabinoside: an agent for T-cell malignancies. *Cancer Res*; 55:3352-6, 1995.
36. Kurtzberg S, Keating M, Moore JO, et al. 2-amino-9-β-arabinosyl-6-methoxy-9H-guanine (GW 506U; Compound 506U) is highly active in patients with T-cell malignancies; results of a Phase I trial in pediatric and adult patients with refractory hematological malignancies. *Blood* 1996; 88(Supp, 1):669a.

37. Pawson R, Dyer MJS, Barge R, et al. Treatment of T-cell prolymphocytic leukemia with human CD52 antibody. *J Clin Oncol* 1997; 15:2667–2672.
38. Dearden CE, Matutes E, Dyer MJS, et al. CAMPATH-1H treatment of T- prolymphocytic leukemia. *Blood* 1999; 94 (Supp 1):600a.
39. Cazin B, Wetterwald M, Ojeda M, et al. CAMPATH-1H in the treatment of T- prolymphocytic leukemia (T-PLL). *Blood* 1999; 94 (Supp 1):1259a.

5 Chronic Myeloid Leukemia

Neil P. Shah, MD, PhD
and Charles L. Sawyers, MD

CONTENTS

INTRODUCTION

Over the past twenty years, clinical and laboratory studies have led to important new insights into the biology of chronic myeloid leukemia. Basic science has defined the molecular pathogenesis of chronic myeloid leukemia (CML) as unregulated signal transduction by the Bcr-Abl tyrosine kinase. Clinical studies have demonstrated that CML can be curable through immune-mediated elimination of leukemia cells by allogeneic T lymphocytes. Recently, specific inhibition of signal transduction by the tyrosine kinase Bcr-Abl has been found to be active in managing the disease.

CLINICAL FEATURES

CML represents a proliferative clonal disorder of hematopoietic stem cells that results in expansion of not only myeloid cells, but also of erythroid cells and platelets in the peripheral blood (*see* Fig. 1). Although the median age at presen-

From: *Current Clinical Oncology: Chronic Leukemias and Lymphomas:*
Biology, Pathophysiology, and Clinical Management
Edited by: G. J. Schiller © Humana Press Inc., Totowa, NJ

tation is 53 yr, all age groups are affected, occasionally including children. Most patients also exhibit thrombocytosis, which is suggestive of the presence of a defect in a pluripotent hematopoietic stem cell. Although the most common symptoms at presentation are fatigue, anorexia, and weight loss, fully 40% of patients are entirely asymptomatic; the disease in these cases is suspected solely on the basis of an elevated white blood cell (WBC) count. Splenomegaly is the most common abnormal physical finding, and can be found in approx 50% of patients. CML typically progresses from a benign chronic phase to a rapidly fatal blast crisis after a mean duration of 3–5 yr. Often, the blast crisis phase is preceded by an accelerated phase in which increasing doses of hydroxyurea or busulfan chemotherapy are required to control the WBC count. In contrast to the complete maturation of blood cells that occurs during the chronic phase, during the blast crisis phase cells exhibit a maturation defect, and the bone marrow becomes populated predominantly by myeloblasts or lymphoblasts similar to those found in patients with acute leukemias.

MOLECULAR PATHOPHYSIOLOGY

The diagnosis of CML is based upon detection of the Philadelphia (Ph) chromosome. This abnormality was initially described in 1960 as an apparently shortened chromosome 22 *(1)*. The advent of quinacrine and Giemsa banding techniques facilitated the demonstration that the Philadelphia chromosome actually represents a balanced t(9,22) translocation *(2)*, and is present in 95% of patients with CML. Leukemic cells of the remaining 5% of CML patients frequently exhibit complex or variant translocations involving additional chromosomes that have the same molecular result—fusion of the breakpoint cluster region (Bcr) gene on chromosome 22 to the Abl (Ableson leukemia virus) gene on chromosome 9. Rarely, the ETV6 (also termed tel) gene has been found fused to Abl *(3)* in the absence of Bcr involvement. In cases of CML, the Ph chromosome is detected in cells of the myeloid, erythroid, megakaryocytic, and B lymphoid lineages, indicating that CML truly represents a disease of the hematopoietic stem-cell. Several non-random secondary chromosome changes have been observed during evolution to blast crisis, including duplication of the Ph chromosome, trisomy 8, and isochromosome 17p *(4)*. Mutations or deletions of tumor-suppressor genes such as *p16 (5)* and *p53* occur with varying frequency and are believed to contribute to the malignant phenotype of blast crisis phase *(6)*. Additionally, elevated expression of the Wilms' tumor (WT) *(7)* and EVI-1 *(8,9)* genes have also been found after progression to blast crisis.

Fig. 1. *(opposite page)* Photomicrographs of a peripheral-blood sample and bone-marrow samples from a patient with CML. (**A**) shows a peripheral-blood smear with numerous myeloid cells, including myelocytes and a basophil (center) (Wright's stain, ×40).

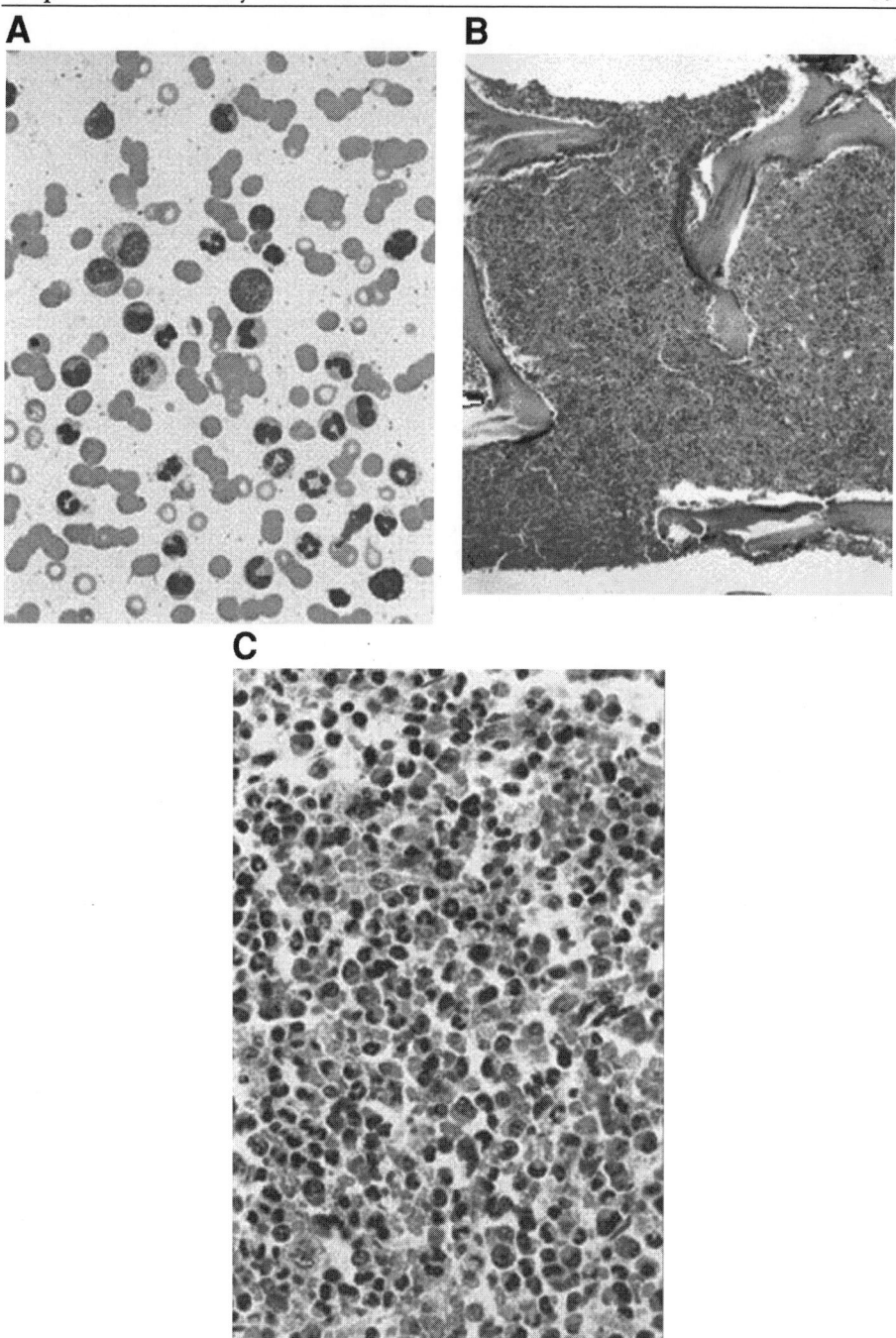

Fig. 1. *(continued)* (**B**) a bone-marrow specimen obtained with a trephine shows marked hypercellularity and virtually no fat (hematoxylin and eosin, ×40). (**C**) marked myeloid hyperplasia is evident in the bone-marrow specimen at a higher magnification (H&E, ×160).

The molecular consequence of the t(9,22) translocation is the creation of the fusion gene Bcr-Abl, whose protein product displays constitutively activated cytoplasmic tyrosine kinase activity when compared with c-Abl, its normal cellular counterpart. The fusion protein can vary in size from 185 to 230 kd, depending upon the location of the chromosomal breakpoint within the Bcr gene. The resultant fusion genes differ from each other only in the amount of Bcr coding sequence retained at the N-terminus (*see* Fig. 2). Cells from patients with typical chronic-phase CML usually harbor a 210 kd Bcr-Abl protein, whereas in cases of Ph-positive acute lymphoblastic leukemia (ALL), either a 210- or 185/190-kd Bcr-Abl protein can be detected. A larger 230-kd Bcr-Abl fusion protein is found in a subset of patients with CML who presented with a lower white-blood-cell (WBC) count, and in whom the chronic phase is prolonged *(10)*. Laboratory studies have demonstrated that the 185/190-kd Bcr-Abl protein has higher specific activity as a tyrosine kinase and is a more potent oncogene than the 210-kd isoform, suggesting that the magnitude of the tyrosine kinase signal directly affects the severity of the resultant disease phenotype *(11,12)*.

As a result of the successful cloning of the Bcr and Abl genes, highly sensitive and specific molecular probes have been developed to enable more precise detection of the Ph chromosome, thus permitting superior monitoring of disease response to therapy. Interphase fluorescence *in situ* hybridization offers a more rapid and sensitive method of detecting the Ph chromosome than standard cytogenetics *(13–16)*, but its limits of detection are not dramatically superior to classic metaphase analysis. Polymerase chain reaction (PCR) of peripheral-blood cDNA can reliably detect one Ph+ cell expressing the Bcr-Abl fusion transcript in a background of 10^5 to 10^6 normal cells *(17)*, and has resulted in reclassification of response to treatment into three groups: hematologic, cytogenetic, and molecular remissions. Hematologic remission denotes normalization of peripheral blood-cell counts and bone-marrow morphology, whereas cytogenetic and molecular remissions indicate complete disappearance of the Ph chromosome or the Bcr-Abl fusion gene, respectively. Based on the survival data of patients treated with interferon (IFN), the favorable prognostic value of hematologic and cytogenetic remissions is clear *(18)*; however, the clinical value of molecular testing has not yet been defined. Recipients of allogeneic bone-marrow transplants (AlloBMTs) who subsequently test negative by PCR clearly enjoy a favorable prognosis *(19,20)*, but positive results are difficult to interpret because of the extreme sensitivity of the PCR assay. For example, two subgroups with extremely favorable outcomes—IFN-treated patients in complete cytogenetic remission and patients who have survived for several years after bone-marrow transplantation (BMT) with no overt evidence of disease relapse—can remain PCR-positive for years *(21,22)*. Positive PCR tests in this setting are presumably a result of the persistence of scarce residual leukemic cells, although the ability of Bcr-Abl transcripts to be effectively translated into functionally active protein in this setting has not been demonstrated. Intriguingly, the presence of Bcr-Abl transcripts in healthy individuals using a two-step reverse-transcriptase polymerase chain reaction (RT-PCR) assay has been reported *(23,24)*. Newly developed quantitative PCR assays allow monitoring of the level of Bcr-Abl mRNA transcripts over time. A progressive increase in the quantity of minimal residual disease after allogeneic transplantation as measured by these assays appears to predict eventual relapse *(17)*.

MECHANISM OF LEUKEMOGENESIS

Laboratory studies have firmly established the capability of Bcr-Abl to induce leukemias in animals. Expression of the 185/190-kd Bcr-Abl gene as a transgene in mice results in acute leukemia at birth, demonstrating that the protein confers a potent oncogenic signal in hematopoietic cells *(25)*. Karyotypic studies of the leukemic cells from these mice reveal secondary chromosomal abnormalities analogous to those found in cells obtained during the blast-crisis phase in patients *(26)*. A second model of CML utilizes transfer of the Bcr-Abl gene into the hematopoietic stem cells of normal mice by recombinant retroviral infection. These animals develop a range of acute and chronic myeloid leukemias (CML) that vary in mouse strains with different genetic backgrounds *(27–29)*. These findings, in concert with the secondary chromosomal abnormalities mentioned previously, suggest that the pathogenesis of CML represents a multistep process.

Most laboratory studies of the Bcr-Abl gene have focused on defining the effects of protein overexpression on cellular proliferation and transformation. Hematopoietic cells transformed by Bcr-Abl exhibit increased proliferation, and their survival in vitro is independent of cytokines *(30,31)*. Constitutive activation of JAKs and STATs has been observed in cell lines expressing Bcr-Abl *(32)*. Bcr-Abl has also been demonstrated to constitutively phosphorylate the common beta subunit of the GM-CSF and IL-3 receptors and JAK 2 *(33)*. Additionally, Bcr-Abl is capable of protecting hematopoietic cells from programmed cell death in response to cytokine withdrawal and DNA damage induced by chemotherapy or radiation *(34,35)*. In primary CML cells, however, the effects of Bcr-Abl appear to be less dramatic, particularly with respect to apoptosis *(36,37)*. Adhesion of hematopoietic cells to extracellular matrix proteins has been seen in Bcr-Abl-expressing cells, and appears to involve an increase in integrin activity *(38)*. One molecular mechanism for this effect may involve the Bcr-Abl substrate CRKL, which, when phosphorylated, induces adhesion by allowing assembly of focal adhesion complexes *(39)*. Curiously, primary CML cells adhere poorly to bone-marrow stroma in vitro *(40)* because of defective integrin function *(41)*. Because stromal cells can regulate hematopoietic cell growth and differentiation through cytokine release and stromal cell-stem-cell content, such a defect in adhesion may allow leukemic cells to escape negative regulatory influences.

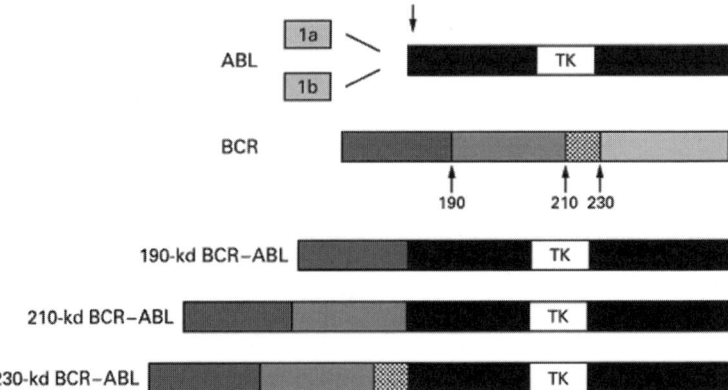

Fig. 2. Structure of BCR/ABL fusion proteins. The structure of the wild-type c-abl and c-bcr proteins are shown with the site of the breakpoints in each marked by the arrows. The sizes of the fusion proteins differ based on the contribution of different amounts of bcr sequence. The abl sequence is identical in all cases. 1a and 1b = alternative first exons of c-abl; TK = tyrosine kinase domain. Reprinted with permission from Sawyers, CL. Chronic myeolid leukemia, *N Engl J Med* 1999; 340(17):1330–1340.

Biochemical studies have demonstrated that Bcr-Abl is exclusively localized in the cytoplasm, whereas the normal cellular counterpart c-abl, which has only minimal tyrosine kinase activity because of the presence of kinase inhibitory sequences at its amino terminus (which are absent in Bcr-Abl), shuttles between the nucleus and the cytoplasm *(42–44)*. As a result of its increased kinase activity, Bcr-Abl phosphorylates several substrates, thereby activating multiple signal-transduction cascades that affect cell growth and differentiation. These substrates include Crkl *(45–47)*, p62Dok *(48,49)*, paxillin *(50)*, Cbl *(51)*, and Rin *(52)*, which are known to activate pathways involving Ras *(53)*, Raf *(54)*, phosphatidyl inositol-3 kinase *(55)*, Jun kinase *(56)*, Myc *(57)*, and Stat *(58–60)* (*see* Fig. 3). Although the precise activation of these pathways is not well understood, it is becoming increasingly apparent that Bcr-Abl activates signaling cascades normally activated by cytokines that carefully control the growth and differentiation of normal hematopoietic cells. The constitutive nature of the Bcr-Abl signal allows these cells to escape physiologic constraints on normal growth, and thereby become leukemic.

A major end point of current research is the definition of specific signal transduction events that contribute to leukemogenesis so that rational therapeutic interventions can be developed. It has become apparent that loss of Bcr-Abl tyrosine kinase activity through either mutation or by the use of pharmacologic inhibitors results in the elimination of its leukemogenic activity *(61)*. Additionally, inhibition of the Ras *(62)*, Raf, phosphatidyl inositol-3 kinase, *(55)*, Akt *(63)*, Jun kinase *(56,64)* and Myc *(57,65)* pathways blocks transformation of cells in which the Bcr-Abl tyrosine kinase is constitutively activated. Thus, it is believed that although the various signaling

Table 1
Results of Allo-BMT in Patients with CML in Chronic Phase

Study	No. of Patients	Follow-up	Survival(%)	Relapse(%)	Ref.
Matched Related Donor					
IBMTR	2231	3 yr	57	13	*(67)*
EBMT	373	8 yr	54	19	*(68)*
Seattle	351	>10 yr	70	20	*(69)*
Matched Unrelated Donor					
NMDP	779	3 yr	40	5	*(72,73)*
IBMTR	331	3 yr	38	—	*(67)*
Seattle	196	5 yr	57	—	*(75)*

IBMTR = International Bone Marrow Transplantation Registry, EBMT = European Group for Blood and Bone Marrow Transplantation, and NMDP = National Marrow Donor Program. Adapted from Sawyers, CL. Chronic myeolid leukemia, *N Engl J Med* 1999; 340(17):1330–1340.

pathways activated by Bcr-Abl exhibit great complexity, inhibition of specific pathways may attenuate the oncogenic potential of Bcr-Abl.

TREATMENT OPTIONS

During the chronic phase of CML, most patients require some form of cytoreductive therapy to avoid complications that can result from high levels of circulating neutrophils. Fortunately, CML cells are sensitive to several oral chemotherapeutic drugs. Fully 90% of patients treated with hydroxyurea or busulfan experience hematologic responses *(66)*. Hydroxyurea is preferred because both the median duration of the chronic phase and the median survival of treated patients appear to be superior to results obtained with busulfan; furthermore, its side-effect profile is more favorable *(66)*. With both agents, however, the cytogenetic response rate is minimal, and the rate of progression to blast crisis is unchanged. Therefore, these treatments must be considered palliative.

Allogeneic Bone-Marrow Transplantation (Allo-BMT)

Clearly, CML is a disease of hematopoietic stem cells. Chemotherapy doses that destroy all the leukemic cells also destroy normal bone marrow, and must therefore be supplemented with allogeneic bone-marrow or stem-cell transplantation. Longitudinal follow-up from multiple centers over several decades has confirmed that chemotherapy with busulfan and cyclophosphamide or combined chemoradiotherapy with cyclophosphamide and fractionated total body irradiation (TBI) followed by Allo-BMT is curative therapy in patients with CML in chronic phase. The International Bone Marrow Transplantation Registry (67) and European Group for Blood and Marrow Transplantation (68) have reported survival rates of 50–60% for patients in chronic phase who received chemotherapy or radiation plus chemotherapy followed by marrow cells from HLA-matched sibling donors (Table 1). The Fred Hutchinson Cancer Center in Seattle has published the largest single-institution experience, with a reported survival rate of 70% at 10 yr (69). The success rate of allogeneic transplantation is clearly influenced by the age of the recipient, and is significantly lower in patients over age 40 yr, primarily because of increased treatment-related mortality (TRM). Although age clearly constitutes a major prognostic variable, transplantation decisions in each case must be individually considered, and should take into account other variables that influence outcome, such as disease stage and the degree of donor-recipient HLA-identity.

The transplantation procedure itself has been associated with significant TRM. As a result, it may seem reasonable to delay the procedure in patients with matched related donors until the disease progresses. However, this approach is inappropriate for two reasons. First, CML patients who undergo transplantation when the disease is in the chronic phase have better survival rates than those transplanted during the accelerated or blast crisis phase (67,69). Second, patients transplanted within the first year after diagnosis have better survival rates than those who are transplanted later in the chronic phase (67,70). These findings indicate that CML cells can be capable of resisting ablative doses of chemotherapy and radiation therapy. Considering that CML invariably progresses steadily to a more malignant phenotype, and that the point in the chronic phase at which survival following transplantation begins to worsen has not been defined, allogeneic transplantation should be considered at the time of diagnosis in eligible patients with HLA-matched sibling donors.

Unfortunately, only 15–20% of CML patients are suitable candidates for allogeneic transplantation because of limiting factors such as advanced age at the time of diagnosis and the low incidence of having an HLA-identical sibling donor. Through the use of HLA-matched unrelated donors identified by bone-marrow donor registries, the number of candidates for transplantation increases to approx 30% (71). However, survival rates of transplant recipients from unrelated donors performed through the National Marrow Donor Program have generally been reported to be substantially lower than that of recipients of transplants from related donors (Table 1) (72,73), although a recent comparative review of related and unrelated transplants using serologic methods for matching at HLA-A and -B and molecular matching at DRB1 found no difference in outcome (74). Results from Seattle are more encouraging, particularly in patients less than 50 yr of age who are matched with donors at the HLA DRB1 locus using molecular studies (75). Molecular typing allows a distinction between subtypes of HLA antigens that are serologically related but immunologically distinct. Although molecular HLA typing appears to improve survival, it effectively further restricts the number of CML patients with an appropriate donor.

The Role of Graft vs Leukemia in Curing CML

Clinical transplantation research in CML has strongly implicated the role of the immune system in effecting disease cure. The first hint of this concept was a correlation between graft-vs-host disease, a potentially fatal complication of allogeneic transplantation, and the long-term success of the transplant as defined by leukemia-free survival *(76)*. The importance of this graft-vs-leukemia (GVL) effect became evident when transplants were performed using bone marrow that had been depleted of T-lymphocytes in an effort to treat graft-vs-host disease. Although these depleted allografts succeeded in reducing mortality from graft-vs-host disease, the rate of relapsed CML approached 60% *(77)*. These results implicated T-lymphocytes in the donor marrow of allogeneic transplants as critical for the induction of long-term remissions in CML patients. Formal proof of the GVL hypothesis ensued with the demonstration that donor lymphocyte infusions are capable of inducing complete remissions in the absence of any conditioning chemotherapy or radiotherapy in patients who have relapsed CML after AlloBMT *(78–80)*.

Recent efforts have focused on improving the safety of allogeneic transplantation by reducing the risk of graft-vs-host disease without sacrificing the curative GVL phenomenon. One approach involves removing and preserving T-cells from the allograft for delayed infusion. Threshold doses of T-cells that are capable of inducing a GVL, but not graft-vs-host effect when infused after engraftment, have been determined *(81)*. This reduction in graft-vs-host disease is most likely explained by delivery of T-cells at a time when target tissues such as the gut and liver have recovered from damage induced by chemotherapy or radiation, and are thus less immunogenic. A future challenge is to test this concept more widely and extend its utility to unrelated donor transplants, which harbor a much higher incidence of graft-vs-host disease.

With the goal of preserving the clinical benefits of GVL while avoiding the complications induced by graft-vs-host disease, current research in transplantation biology has addressed whether graft-vs-host disease and GVL can be separated at the cellular level. To this end, efforts to isolate leukemia-specific cytotoxic T-cell clones that might be expanded in vitro from donor T cells are underway. CML cells express the tumor-specific Bcr-Abl fusion protein; therefore, tumor-specific peptides spanning the Bcr-Abl junction could theoretically elicit a tumor-specific immune response. Such peptides have been shown to induce T-cell immune responses *(82,83)*, and recent evidence demonstrates that one such peptide could be detected on primary cells isolated from CML patients.

Table 2
Results of Clinical Trials of IFN-α and Several Drugs in Patients with CML

Trial	Treatment arm	Cytogenetic response rate[a] (%)	Survival[b] (%)	Ref.
Italian	Hydroxyurea	1	29	(86)
	IFN-α	19	50	
German	Hydroxyurea	<1	44	
	Busulfan	<1	32	(66)
	IFN-α	9.6	59	
British	Hydroxyurea/Busulfan	—	34	(88)
	IFN-α	11	52	
Japanese	Busulfan	5	32	(87)
	IFN-α	16.3	54	
French	IFN-α	24	79	(90)
	IFN + Arabonoside C	41	86	
Meta-Analysis	Chemotherapy		42	(89)
	IFN-α		57	

[a]Includes complete (no Ph[+] cells) and partial (≤33% Ph[+] cells) responses.
[b]5-yr survival except for Italian trial (6-yr survival) and French trial (3-yr survival).
Adapted from Sawyers, CL. Chronic myeolid leukemia, *N Engl J Med* 1999; 340(17):1330–1340.

Moreover, these patients mounted a cytotoxic T-lymphocyte response directed at the junction peptide that also killed autologous CML cells *(84)*.

Interferon-α

Because the majority of CML patients are not candidates for allogeneic transplantation, alternative therapies have been extensively studied. IFN-α can induce both hematologic and cytogenetic remissions in chronic-phase patients *(85)*. In several clinical trials, both cytogenetic response and overall survival rates were superior in patients treated by subcutaneous (sc) injection of 10 million U per d of IFN-α as compared to patients treated with chemotherapy *(66,86–89)* (Table 2). IFN-α therefore gained acceptance as first-line therapy in patients with CML not eligible for Allo-BMT. Twenty to thirty percent of patients treated with IFN-α achieve either a complete or partial cytogenetic response, defined as a reduction in the percentage of Ph metaphases to less than 34%. Minor responses (less than 67% Ph metaphases) occur in an additional 10% of patients. Patients who achieve complete cytogenetic remission gain the most clinical benefit from IFN-α *(18)*, but those with lesser responses also benefit, as compared with patients treated with hydroxyurea *(88)*. Only 5–10% of patients have sustained, complete disappearance of the Ph chromosome, and these patients derive the greatest benefits in survival. In an effort to improve the response rate, subsequent trials have focused on combination therapy; the most promising results have been obtained with cytarabine and IFN-α *(90)*. Interferon, however, is associated with significant side effects, which in several circumstances have led to its discontinuation despite disease response.

Little is known about the mechanism of action (MOA) of IFN-α in patients with CML. IFN-α has immune modulatory effects on tumor cells, such as increased expression of HLA class I antigens *(91)*, but it is not clear whether these play a role in its MOA in CML. In a recent study IFN-α, in combination with granulocyte-macrophage colony-stimulating factor (GM-CSF), stimulated expansion of antigen-presenting dendritic cells in vitro *(92)*. Dendritic cells from CML patients may stimulate selective killing of autologous Ph-positive but not Ph-negative cells by T-cells *(93)*, and therefore the anti-CML activity of IFN-α may be mediated through dendritic-cell activation. Recently, a strong correlation was reported between cytogenetic response to IFN-α or Allo-BMT and the presence of T-cells specific for PR1, a peptide derived from proteinase 3, strongly suggestive of a role of T-cell immunity in the elimination of the malignant clone *(94)*.

Imatinib

The search for molecular inhibitors of the tyrosine kinase activity of Bcr-Abl led to the identification of imatinib mesylate (CGP 57148B, STI571, Gleevec). Experimental studies demonstrated its ability to selectively inhibit the tyrosine kinase activity of Bcr-Abl, and through an undetermined mechanism, to cause apoptosis of cell lines established from patients with CML. The drug was approved by the FDA in May 2001 for the treatment of accelerated and blast-crisis phases, and for chronic-phase patients who had failed IFN. Phase I trial results demonstrated a hematologic response in 53 of 54 chronic-phase patients in whom IFN-α had failed. The minimum effective dose was found to be 300 mg imatinib daily *(95)*. The drug was shown to have an excellent toxicity profile, and the most common side effects were mild nausea, myalgias, edema, and diarrhea. Additionally, patients treated with imatinib have a 41% rate of complete cytogenetic response, which is superior to cytogenetic response rates obtained from historical data from IFN-α-treated patients (ref. *95a*). A randomized study comparing the activities of imatinib and INF-α in therapy-naïve patients is in progress. The efficacy of imatinib in the blast-crisis phase of CML, as well as in patients with Philadelphia chromosome-positive ALL, was also recently assessed. Fifty-five percent of patients with myeloid blast crisis CML, and 70% of patients with ALL or lymphoid blast-crisis CML responded to the drug, although responses were typically not durable *(96)*. Evaluation of leukemic cells obtained at the time of relapse revealed reactivation of Bcr-Abl in nearly all cases. Evidence for genomic amplification of the Bcr-Abl locus was found in a subset of patients at the time of relapse. Sequence analysis of the kinase domain in the remaining patients revealed a high prevalence of mutations capable of decreasing the affinity of the protein for imatinib while maintaining kinase activity *(97)*. Thus, although there have been rare reports of the deletion of Bcr-Abl resulting in loss of transcript and protein production after transformation from the chronic phase-to-blast crisis *(98)*, it appears that the leukemic cells in the most advanced stages of CML continue to express Bcr-Abl, and remain dependent upon Bcr-Abl activity for their growth and survival. Whether or not long-term administration of imatinib in chronic-phase patients will eventually select for drug-resistant disease has not yet been determined.

Clinical Decision Making: Transplantation vs Medical Therapy

Although imatinib offers an exciting new treatment alternative, its long-term efficacy relative to more established treatment modalities remains to be documented. Over the past 10 yrs, the survival of patients with CML has improved as a result of both early diagnosis through routine blood tests and the documented efficacy of transplantation and IFN-α. Although it must be emphasized that no conclusive statements can yet be made with respect to the impact of imatinib on overall survival, many experts currently recommend imatinib as first-line therapy because of its superior cytogenetic remission rate over IFN-α as well as its favorable toxicity profile. With the improved cytogenetic response rates in patients treated with imatinib, IFN-α and cytarabine, physicians counseling patients with CML eligible for Allo-BMT may face a difficult decision. The significantly improved cytogenetic response rate and safety of imatinib must be interpreted in light of inadequate long-term follow-up. Allo-BMT offers the only known cure for CML, yet is associated with substantial mortality and potentially disabling morbidity in long-term survivors. Although IFN-α is safer and has documented survival benefit, the percentage of patients who have a complete cytogenetic remission is low, and the durability of the survival benefit has not been defined in large numbers of patients. One strategy supported by decision analysis is to treat older patients or younger patients with no suitable related bone-marrow donor with IFN-α *(99)* (Table 2) or alternatively, imatinib. In those patients who achieve cytogenetic responses within 1 yr, therapy is continued and the others are treated by transplantation by using an alternate donor. With improvements in HLA matching and pre-transplant risk assessment, this algorithm will require modification. An implicit assumption of this scheme is that the success of Allo-BMT is not affected by prior IFN-α therapy, but conflicting reports have been published on this topic and the issue remains unsettled *(100–104)*. Patients who relapse after Allo-BMT can be treated successfully with infusion of donor lymphocytes *(105–107)*, withdrawal of immunosuppression, imatinib, IFN-α *(108,109)* or second allogeneic transplantation.

NOVEL TREATMENTS

Autografts

Studies of combination chemotherapy with cytarabine plus anthracylines, similar to the drugs used to treat acute myeloid leukemia, have demonstrated transient cytogenetic remissions but minimal long-term clinical benefit in patients with CML in chronic phase *(110,111)*. Many investigators have combined high-dose chemotherapy with stem-cell purification technologies to perform autologous transplants using Ph-negative stem cells. Stem cells harvested during the recovery phase after induction chemotherapy are enriched for Ph-negative stem cells, and they successfully engraft, resulting in Ph-negative hematopoiesis *(112)*. However, Ph-positive hematopoiesis inevitably recurs, usually within the first year after transplantation, and thus the patient is again in the chronic phase of the disease *(113,114)*. Relapse in this setting is probably caused by incomplete elimination of Ph-positive cells during the enrichment process. Support for this hypothesis comes from retrovirus-marking trials, which demonstrate that virus-marked harvested CML cells contribute to relapse *(115)*. This result has led to further efforts to purge stem-cell preparations of residual CML cells using anti-sense mRNA directed against Bcr-Abl *(116)* or the c-Myb gene *(117)*, in vitro culture conditions that select against Ph-positive cells *(118)*, imatinib treatment of the graft, or physical separation of Ph-negative from Ph-positive stem cells *(119)*. The clinical feasibility and safety of these strategies has been demonstrated, but their therapeutic value has not yet been proven.

Autografting alone, even when combined with effective purging strategies, is not expected to result in long-term remissions in most patients because of the lack of a GVL effect. Identical twin studies have shown a relapse rate 2–3 × higher in patients who received bone-marrow transplants from identical twins donors— an approach theoretically equivalent to the use of autografts purged of Ph-positive stem cells—when compared with patients who received HLA-matched transplants from siblings who were not syngeneic *(67,69)*. It therefore seems likely that patients who receive autografts will require some form of post-transplant therapy to remain in remission. To this end, treatment with IFN-α offers some promise because it can restore Ph-negative hematopoiesis in some patients who relapse after Allo-BMT *(120,121)*. Alternatives include imatinib and interleukin-2 (IL-2), which has activity in CML and in post-remission therapy of acute myeloid leukemia *(122)*.

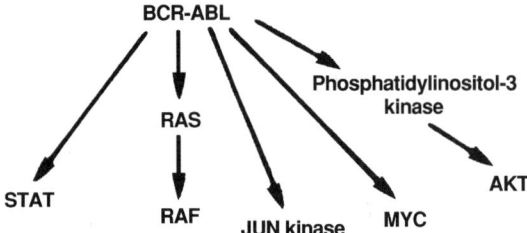

Fig. 3. Signal transduction by Bcr-Abl protein. As a result of the constitutive activation of its tyrosine kinase domain, Bcr-Abl activates several cytoplasmic and nuclear signal transduction pathways that affect growth and survival of hematopoietic cells. Reprinted with permission from Sawyers, CL. Chronic myeolid leukemia, *N Engl J Med* 1999; 340(17):1330–1340.

Non-Myeloablative Transplantation

Non-myeloablative preparative regimens have been shown to be associated with less treatment-related mortality (TRM) than traditional ablative regimens. Several investigators have recently enrolled CML patients who were believed to be unacceptable candidates for standard allogeneic transplantation (because of high risk for TRM) in clinical trials designed to assess the efficacy of non-myeloablative transplantation. In an early report, molecular remission was reported in each of three patients who underwent infusion of HLA-identical stem cells following a non-myeloablative conditioning regimen consisting of cyclo-phosphamide and fludarabine *(123)*. Preliminary reports from Seattle indicate 100% donor engraftment in patients conditioned with low-dose fludarabine and 2 gy of total body irradiation (TBI). Eight of the first 12 patients achieved molecular remission. The transplant-related mortality was reported to be less than 5% (*see* ref. *123a*). By appearing to preserve the GVL effect of allogeneic transplantation while reducing transplant-related mortality, non-myeloablative transplants may represent another effective means of managing CML for a sub-group of patients. However, most results to date have been obtained from patients who received stem cells from an HLA-identical sibling, and the number of patients who may thus qualify for non-myeloablative transplantation may be limited.

Molecular Therapy

Recent success in defining the molecular basis for many types of cancer has shifted drug discovery efforts toward identifying compounds such as imatinib that specifically antagonize proteins involved in specific signal transduction pathways by cancer cells. Knowledge about the specific pathways that are critical for the leukemogenic activity of Bcr-Abl provides a number of potential targets for drug therapy. One promising target is the Ras pathway, which is required for the anti-apoptotic as well as the transforming activity of Bcr-Abl *(62,124)*. A series of candidate anti-Ras drugs known as farnesyl transferase inhibitors, which block a lipid modification required for Ras to function as a signaling molecule *(125)*, are currently being studied in clinical trials in patients with other cancers. The identification of imatinib-resistant kinase domain mutations in the blast-crisis phase of CML demonstrates the necessity to continue the search for effective therapies.

CONCLUSION

Allo-BMT is firmly established as the treatment of choice for patients with CML, but only a small percentage of patients benefit from this curative procedure because of limitations imposed by donor availability and recipient age. IFN-α—alone or in combination with other drugs—is suitable for most patients, but fails to induce long-term cytogenetic remissions in the majority of patients, and is associated with substantial toxicity. Imatinib clearly has activity in the treatment of chronic-phase CML which has progressed despite IFN-α, but its impact on improving overall survival has not yet been defined. Laboratory and clinical research in CML has defined the critical roles of both the Bcr-Abl fusion protein in the pathogenesis of the disease, as well as the immune system in curing patients who have undergone transplantation. Based on these insights, new treatment strategies are currently under investigation using other pharmacologic inhibitors of the Bcr-Abl signal transduction pathway and peptides or cell-based immunotherapy to activate a leukemia-specific immune response.

REFERENCES

1. Nowell PC, Hungerford DA. A minute chromosome in human chronic granulocytic leukemia. *Science* 1960; 132:1497.
2. Rowley JD. A new consistent chromosomal abnormality in chronic myelogenous leukemia identified by quinacrine fluorescence and Giemsa banding. *Nature* 1973; 243:290–291.
3. Andreasson P, Johansson B, Carlsson M, Jarlsfelt I, Fioretos T, Mitelman F, et al. BCR/ABL-negative chronic myeloid leukemia with ETV6/ABL fusion. *Genes Chromosomes Cancer* JID - 9007329 1997; 20:299–304.
4. Bernstein R. Cytogenetics of chronic myelogenous leukemia. *Semin Hematol* 1988; 25:20–34.
5. Sill H, Goldman JM, Cross NC. Homozygous deletions of the p16 tumor-suppressor gene are associated with lymphoid transformation of chronic myeloid leukemia. *Blood* 1995; 85: 2013–2016.
6. Ahuja H, Bar-Eli M, Arlin Z, Advani S, Allen SL, Goldman J, et al. The spectrum of molecular alterations in the evolution of chronic myelocytic leukemia. *J Clin Investig* 1991; 87:2042–2047.
7. Menssen HD, Renkl HJ, Rodeck U, Maurer J, Notter M, Schwartz S, et al. Presence of Wilms' tumor gene (wt1) transcripts and the WT1 nuclear protein in the majority of human acute leukemias. *Leukemia* 1995; 9:1060–1067.

8. Mitani K, Ogawa S, Tanaka T, Miyoshi H, Kurokawa M, Mano H, et al. Generation of the AML1-EVI-1 fusion gene in the t(3;21)(q26;q22) causes blastic crisis in chronic myelo-cytic leukemia. *EMBO J* JID - 8208664 1994; 13:504–510.

9. Carapeti M, Goldman JM, Cross NC. Overexpression of EVI-1 in blast crisis of chronic myeloid leukemia. *Leukemia* JID - 8704895 1996; 10:1561.

10. Pane F, Frigeri F, Sindona M, Luciano L, Ferrara F, Cimino R, et al. Neutrophilic-chronic myeloid leukemia: a distinct disease with a specific molecular marker (BCR/ABL with C3/A2 junction). *Blood* 1996; 88:2410–2414.

11. Lugo TG, Pendergast A, Muller AJ, Witte ON. Tyrosine kinase activity and transformation potency of Bcr-Abl oncogene products. *Science* 1990; 247:1079–1082.

12. Voncken JW, Kaartinen V, Pattengale PK, Germeraad WT, Groffen J, Heisterkamp N. BCR/ABL p210 and p190 cause distinct leukemia in transgenic mice. *Blood* 1995; 86:4603–4611.

13. Cox MC, Maffei L, Buffolino S, Del Poeta G, Venditti A, Cantonetti M, et al. A compara-tive analysis of FISH, RT-PCR, and cytogenetics for the diagnosis of Bcr-Abl-positive leukemias. *Am J Clin Pathol* JID - 0370470 1998; 109:24–31.

14. Sinclair PB, Green AR, Grace C, Nacheva EP. Improved sensitivity of BCR-ABL detec-tion: a triple-probe three-color fluorescence in situ hybridization system. *Blood* JID-7603509 1997; 90:1395–1402.

15. Acar H, Stewart J, Boyd E, Connor MJ. Identification of variant translocations in chronic myeloid leukemia by fluorescence in situ hybridization. *Cancer Genet Cytogenet* JID-7909240 1997; 93:115–118.

16. Yanagi M, Shinjo K, Takeshita A, Tobita T, Yano K, Kobayashi M, et al. Simple and reliably sensitive diagnosis and monitoring of Philadelphia chromosome-positive cells in chronic myeloid leukemia by interphase fluorescence in situ hybridization of peripheral blood cells. *Leukemia* JID - 8704895 1999; 13:542–552.

17. Cross NC, Feng L, Chase A, Bungey J, Hughes TP, Goldman JM. Competitive polymerase chain reaction to estimate the number of BCR-ABL transcripts of chronic myeloid leuke-mia patients after bone marrow transplantation. *Blood* 1993; 82:1929–1936.

18. Kantarjian HM, Smith TL, O'Brien S, Beran M, Pierce S, Talpaz M, et al. Prolonged survival in chronic myelogenous leukemia after cytogenetic response to interferon-α therapy. *Ann Intern Med* 1995; 122:254–261.

19. Hughes TP, Morgan GJ, Martiat P, Goldman JM. Detection of residual leukemia after bone marrow transplant for chronic myeloid leukemia: role of polymerase chain reaction in predicting relapse. *Blood* 1991; 77:874–878.

20. Radich JP, Gehly G, Gooley T, Bryant E, Clift RA, Collins S, et al. Polymerase chain reaction detection of the BCR-ABL fusion transcript after allogeneic marrow transplanta-tion for chronic myeloid leukemia: results and implications in 346 patients. *Blood* 1995; 85:2632–2638.

21. Hochhaus A, Lin F, Reiter A, Skladny H, van Rhee F, Shepherd PC, et al. Variable numbers of BCR-ABL transcripts persist in CML patients who achieve complete cytogenetic remis-sion with interferon-alpha. *Br J Haematol* 1995; 91:126–131.

22. Miyamura K, Tahara T, Tanimoto M, Morishita Y, Kawashima K, Morishima Y, et al. Long persistent Bcr-Abl positive transcript detected by polymerase chain reaction after marrow transplant for chronic myelogenous leukemia without clinical relapse: a study of 64 patients. *Blood* 1993; 81:1089–1093.

23. Bose S, Deininger M, Gora-Tybor J, Goldman JM, Melo JV. The presence of typical and atypical BCR-ABL fusion genes in leukocytes of normal individuals: biologic significance and implications for the assessment of minimal residual disease. *Blood* JID-7603509 1998; 92:3362–3367.

24. Biernaux C, Loos M, Sels A, Huez G, Stryckmans P. Detection of major Bcr-Abl gene expression at a very low level in blood cells of some healthy individuals. *Blood* JID-7603509 1995; 86:3118–3122.

25. Heisterkamp N, Jenster G, ten Hoeve J, Zovich D, Pattengale PK, Groffen J. Acute leukemia in bcr/abl gene transgenic mice. *Nature* 1990; 344:251–253.

26. Voncken JW, Morris C, Pattengale P, Dennert G, Kikly C, Groffen J, et al. Clonal development and karyotype evolution during leukemogenesis of BCR/ABL transgenic mice. *Blood* 1992; 79:1029–1036.

27. Daley GQ, van Etten RA, Baltimore D. Induction of chronic myelogenous leukemia in mice by the P210bcr/abl gene of the Philadelphia chromosome. *Science* 1990; 247:824–830.

28. Kelliher MA, McLaughlin J, Witte ON, Rosenberg N. Induction of a chronic myelogenous leukemia syndrome in mice with v-abl and BCR/ABL. *Proc Natl Acad Sci USA* 1990; 87: 6649–6665.

29. Elefanty AG, Hariharan IK, Cory S. Bcr-Abl, the hallmark of chronic myeloid leukaemia in man, induces multiple haematopoietic neoplasms in mice. *EMBO J* 1990; 9:1069–1078.

30. McLaughlin J, Chianese E, Witte O. In vitro transformation of immature hematopoietic cells by the P210 BCR/ABL oncogene product of the Philadelphia chromosome. *Proc Natl Acad Sci USA* 1987; 84:6558–6562.

31. Gishizky ML, Witte ON. Initiation of deregulated growth of multipotent progenitor cells by Bcr-Abl in vitro. *Science* 1992; 256:836–839.

32. Chai SK, Nichols GL, Rothman P. Constitutive activation of JAKs and STATs in Bcr-Abl-expressing cell lines and peripheral blood cells derived from leukemic patients. *J Immunol* JID - 2985117R 1997; 159:4720–4728.

33. Wilson-Rawls J, Liu J, Laneuville P, Arlinghaus RB. P210 Bcr-Abl interacts with the interleukin-3 beta c subunit and constitutively activates Jak2. *Leukemia* JID-8704895 1997; 11(Suppl 3):428–431.

34. Nishii K, Kabarowski JH, Gibbons DL, Griffiths SD, Titley I, Wiedemann LM, et al. ts BCR-ABL kinase activation confers increased resistance to genotoxic damage via cell cycle block. *Oncogene* 1996; 13:2225–2234.

35. Evans CA, Owen-Lynch PJ, Whetton AD, Dive C. Activation of the Abelson tyrosine kinase activity is associated with suppression of apoptosis in hemopoietic cells. *Cancer Res* 1993; 53:1735–1738.

36. Amos TA, Lewis JL, Grand FH, Gooding RP, Goldman JM, Gordon MY. Apoptosis in chronic myeloid leukaemia: normal responses by progenitor cells to growth factor deprivation, X-irradiation and glucocorticoids. *Br J Haematol* 1995; 91:387–393.

37. Albrecht T, Schwab R, Renkes M, Peschel C, Huber C, Aulitzky WE. Primary proliferating immature myeloid cells from CML patients are not resistant to induction of apoptosis by DNA damage and growth factor withdrawal. *Br J Haematol* 1996; 95:501–507.

38. Bazzoni G, Carlesso N, Griffin JD, Hemler ME. Bcr/Abl expression stimulates integrin function in hematopoietic cell lines. *J Clin Investig* 1996; 98:521–528.

39. Senechal K, Heany C, Druker B, Sawyers CL. Structural requirements for function of the Crkl adaptor protein in fibroblasts and hematopoietic cells. *Mol Cell Biol* 1998; 18: 5082–5090.

40. Gordon MY, Dowding CR, Riley GP, Goldman JM, Greaves MF. Altered adhesive interactions with marrow stroma of haematopoietic progenitor cells in chronic myeloid leukaemia. *Nature* 1987; 328:342–344.

41. Bhatia R, McCarthy JB, Verfaillie CM. Interferon-alpha restores normal beta 1 integrin-mediated inhibition of hematopoietic progenitor proliferation by the marrow microenvironment in chronic myelogenous leukemia. *Blood* 1996; 87:3883–3891.

42. van Etten RA, Jackson P, Baltimore D. The mouse type IV c-abl gene product is a nuclear protein, and activation of transforming ability is associated with cytoplasmic localization. *Cell* 1989; 58:669–678.

43. Lewis JM, Baskaran R, Taagepera S, Schwartz MA, Wang JYJ. Integrin regulation of c-Abl tyrosine kinase activity and cytoplasmic-nuclear transport. *Proc Natl Acad Sci USA* 1996; 93:15,174–15,179.

44. Pluk H, Dorey K, Superti-Furga G. Autoinhibition of c-Abl. *Cell* 2002; 108:247–259.

45. Nichols GL, Raines MA, Vera JC, Lacomis L, Tempst P, Golde DW. Identification of CRKL as the constitutively phosphorylated 39-kD tyrosine phosphoprotein in chronic myelogenous leukemia cells. *Blood* 1994; 84:2912–2918.

46. ten Hoeve J, Arlinghaus RB, Guo JQ, Heisterkamp N, Groffen J. Tyrosine phosphorylation of CRKL in Philadelphia[+] leukemia. *Blood* 1994; 84:1731–1736.

47. Oda T, Heaney C, Hagopian JR, Okuda K, Griffin JD, Druker BJ. Crkl is the major tyrosine-phosphorylated protein in neutrophils from patients with chronic myelogenous leukemia. *J Biol Chem* 1994; 269:22,925–22,928.

48. Carpino N, Wisniewski D, Strife A, Marshak D, Kobayashi R, Stillman B, et al. p62dok: A constitutively tyrosine-phosphorylated, GAP-associated protein in chronic myelogenous leukemia progenitor cells. *Cell* 1997; 88:197–204.

49. Yamanashi Y, Baltimore D. Identification of the Abl- and rasGAP-associated 62 kDa protein as a docking protein, Dok. *Cell* 1997; 88:205–211.

50. Salgia R, Uemura N, Okuda K, Li JL, Pisick E, Sattler M, et al. CRKL links p210BCR/ABL with paxillin in chronic myelogenous leukemia cells. *J Biol Chem* 1995; 270:29,145–29,150.

51. de Jong R, ten Hoeve J, Heisterkamp N, Groffen J. Crkl is complexed with tyrosine-phosphorylated Cbl in Ph-positive leukemia. *J Biol Chem* 1995; 270:21,468–21,471.

52. Afar DE, Han L, McLaughlin J, Wong S, Dhaka A, Parmar K, et al. Regulation of the oncogenic activity of BCR-ABL by a tightly bound substrate protein RIN1. *Immunity* 1997; 6:773–782.

53. Mandanas RA, Leibowitz DS, Gharenbaghi K, Tauchi T, Burgess GS, Miyazawa K, et al. Role of p21 Ras in p210 Bcr-Abl transformation of murine myeloid cells. *Blood* 1993; 82:1838–1847.

54. Okuda K, Matulonis U, Salgia R, Kanakura Y, Druker B, Griffin JD. Factor independence of human myeloid leukemia cell lines is associated with increased phosphorylation of the proto-oncogene Raf-1. *Exp Hematol* 1994; 22:1111–1117.

55. Skorski T, Kanakaraj P, Nieborowska-Skorska M, Ratajczak MZ, Wen SC, Zon G, et al. Phosphatidylinositol-3 kinase activity is regulated by BCR/ABL and is required for the growth of Philadelphia chromosome-positive cells. *Blood* 1995; 86:726–736.

56. Raitano AB, Halpern JR, Hambuch TM, Sawyers CL. The Bcr-Abl leukemia oncogene activates Jun Kinase and requires Jun for transformation. *Proc Natl Acad Sci USA* 1995; 92:11,746–11,750.

57. Sawyers CL, Callahan W, Witte ON. Dominant negative myc blocks transformation by ABL oncogenes. *Cell* 1992; 70:901–910.

58. Shuai K, Halpern J, ten Hoeve J, Rao X, Sawyers CL. Constitutive activation of STAT5 by the BCR-ABL oncogene in chronic myelogenous leukemia. *Oncogene* 1996; 13:247–254.

59. Carlesso N, Frank DA, Griffin JD. Tyrosyl phosphorylation and DNA binding activity of signal transducers and activators of transcription (STAT) proteins in hematopoietic cell lines transformed by Bcr/Abl. *J Exp Med* 1996; 183:811–820.

60. Ilaria RL, van Etten RA. P210 and P190 BCR/ABL induce the tyrosine phosphorylation and DNA binding activity of multiple specific STAT family members. *J Biol Chem* 1996; 271:31,704–31,710.

61. Druker BJ, Tamura S, Buchdunger E, Ohno S, Segal GM, Fanning S, et al. Effects of a selective inhibitor of the Abl tyrosine kinase on the growth of Bcr-Abl positive cells. *Nat Med* 1996; 2:561–566.

62. Sawyers CL, McLaughlin J, Witte ON. Genetic requirement for Ras in the transformation of fibroblasts and hematopoietic cells by the Bcr-Abl oncogene. *J Exp Med* 1995; 181:307–313.
63. Skorski T, Bellacosa A, Nieborowska-Skorska M, Martinez R, Choi JK, Trotta R, et al. Transformation of hematopoietic cells by BCR/ABL requires activation of a P1-3k/Akt-dependent pathway. *EMBO J* 1997; 16:6151–6161.
64. Dickens M, Rogers JS, Cavanagh J, Raitano A, Xia Z, Halpern J, et al. A cytoplasmic inhibitor of the JNK signal transduction pathway. *Science* 1997; 277:693–696.
65. Afar DEH, Goga A, McLaughlin J, Witte O, Sawyers CL. Differential complementation of Bcr-Abl point mutants with c-Myc. *Science* 1994; 264:424–426.
66. Hehlmann R, Heimpel H, Hasford J, Kolb HJ, Pralle H, Hossfeld DK, et al. Randomized comparison of interferon-α with busulfan and hydrozyurea in chronic myelogenous leukemia. *Blood* 1994; 84:4064–4077.
67. Horowitz MM, Rowlings PA, Passweg JR. Allogeneic bone marrow transplantation for CML: a report from the International Bone Marrow Transplant Registry. *Bone Marrow Transplant* 1996; 17:S5–S6
68. van Rhee F, Szydlo RM, Hermans J, Devergie A, Frassoni F, Arcese W, et al. Long-term results after allogeneic bone marrow transplantation for chronic myelogenous leukemia in chronic phase. *Bone Marrow Transplant* 1997; 20:553–560.
69. Clift RA, Anasetti C. Allografting for chronic myeloid leukaemia. *Bailliere's Clin Haematol* 1997; 10:319–336.
70. Thomas ED, Clift RA, Fefer A, Appelbaum FR, Beatty P, Bensinger WI, et al. Marrow transplantation for the treatment of chronic myelogenous leukemia. *Ann Intern Med* 1986; 104:155–163.
71. O'Brien SG. Autografting for chornic myeloid leukaemia. *Bailliere's Clin Haematol* 1997; 10:369–388.
72. McGlave P, Bartsch G, Anasetti C, Ash R, Beatty P, Gajewski J, et al. Unrelated donor marrow transplantation therapy for chronic myelogenous leukemia: initial experience of the national marrow donor program. *Blood* 1993; 81:543–550.
73. McGlave P, Shu XO, Wen W, Anasetti C, Nademanee A, Champlin R, Antin JH, Kerna NA, King R, Weisdorf DJ. Unrelated donor marrow transplantation for chronic myelogenous leukemia: 9 years' experience of the national marrow donor program. *Blood* 2000;95:2219–2225.
74. Davies SM, DeFor TE, McGlave PB, Miller JS, Verfaillie CM, Wagner JE, et al. Equivalent outcomes in patients with chronic myelogenous leukemia after early transplantation of phenotypically matched bone marrow from related or unrelated donors. *Am J Med* JID - 0267200 2001; 110:339–346.
75. Hansen JA, Gooley TA, Martin PJ, Applebaum F, Chauncey TR, Clift RA, et al. Bone marrow transplants from unrelated donors for patients with chronic myeloid leukemia. *N Engl J Med* 1998; 338:962–68.
76. Weiden PL, Sullivan KM, Flournoy N, Storb R, Thomas ED. Antileukemic effect of chronic graft-versus-host disease: contribution to improved survival after allogeneic marrow transplantation. *N Engl J Med* 1981; 304:1529–1533.
77. Goldman JM, Gale RP, Horowitz MM, Biggs JC, Champlin RE, Gluckman E, et al. Bone marrow transplantation for chronic myelogenous leukemia in chronic phase. Increased risk for relapse associated with T-cell depletion. *Ann Intern Med* 1988; 108:806–814.
78. Kolb HJ, Mittermuller J, Clemm C, Holler E, Ledderose G, Brehm G, et al. Donor leukocyte transfusions for treatment of recurrent chronic myelogenous leukemia in marrow transplant patients. *Blood* 1990; 76:2462–2465.
79. Drobyski WR, Keever CA, Roth MS, Koethe S, Hanson G, McFadden P, et al. Salvage immunotherapy using donor leukocyte infusions as treatment for relapsed chronic myelogenous leukemia after allogeneic bone marrow transplantation: efficacy and toxicity of a defined T-cell dose. *Blood* 1993; 82:2310–2318.

80. Porter DL, Roth MS, McGarigle C, et al. Induction of graft-versus-host disease as immunotherapy for relapsed chronic myeloid leukemia. *N Engl J Med* 1994; 330:100–106.
81. Mackinnon S, Papadopoulos EB, Carabasi MH, Reich L, Collins NH, Boulad F, et al. Adoptive immunotherapy evaluating escalating doses of donor leukocytes for relapse of chronic myeloid leukemia after bone marrow transplantation: separation of graft-versus-leukemia responses from graft-versus-host disease. *Blood* 1995; 86:1261–1268.
82. Bocchia M, Korontsvit T, Xu Q, Mackinnon S, Yang SY, Sette A, et al. Specific human cellular immunity to Bcr-Abl oncogene-derived peptides. *Blood* 1996; 87:3587–3592.
83. Nieda M, Nicol A, Kikuchi A, Kashiwase K, Taylor K, Suzuki K, et al. Dendritic cells stimulate the expansion of Bcr-Abl specific CD8$^+$ T cells with cytotoxic activity against leukemic cells from patients with chronic myeloid leukemia. *Blood* 1998; 91:977–983.
84. Clark RE, Dodi IA, Hill SC, Lill JR, Aubert G, Macintyre AR, et al. Direct evidence that leukemic cells present HLA-associated immunogenic peptides derived from the BCR-ABL b3a2 fusion protein. *Blood* JID - 7603509 2001; 98:2887–2893.
85. Talpaz M, McCredie KB, Mavligit GM, Gutterman JU. Leukocyte interferon-induced myeloid cytoreduction in chronic myelogenous leukemia. *Blood* 1983; 62:689–692.
86. The Italian Cooperative Study Group on Chronic Myeloid Leukemia. Interferon alfa-2 as compared with conventional chemotherapy for the treatment of chronic myeloid leukemia. *N Engl J Med* 1994; 330:820–825.
87. Ohnishi K, Ohno R, Tomonaga M, Kamada N, Onozawa K, Kuramoto A, et al. A randomized trial comparing interferon-α with busulfan for newly diagnosed chronic myelogenous leukemia in chronic phase. *Blood* 1995; 86:906–916.
88. Allan NC, Richards SM, Shepherd PC. UK medical research council randomised, multicentre trial of interferon-alpha n1 for chronic myeloid leukaemia: improved survival irrespective of cytogenetic response. *Lancet* 1995; 345:1392–1397.
89. Chronic Myeloid Leukemia Trialists' Collaborative Group. Interferon alpha versus chemotherapy for chronic myeloid leukemia: a meta-analysis of seven randomized trials. *J Natl Cancer Inst* 1997; 89:1616–1620.
90. Guilhot F, Chastang C, Michallet M, Guerci A, Harousseau J-L, Maloisel F, et al. Interferon alpha-2b combined with cytarabine versus interferon alone in chronic myelogenous leukemia. *N Engl J Med* 1997; 337:223–229.
91. Friedman RL, Stark GR. alpha-Interferon-induced transcription of HLA and metallothionein genes containing homologous upstream sequences. *Nature* 1985; 314:637–639.
92. Lardon F, Snoeck HW, Berneman ZN, Van Tendeloo VF, Nijs G, Lenjou M, et al. Generation of dendritic cells from bone marrow progenitors using GM-CSF, TNF-alpha, and additional cytokines: antagonistic effects of IL-4 and IFN-gamma and selective involvement of TNA-alpha receptor-1. *Immunology* 1997; 91:553–559.
93. Choudhury A, Gajewski JL, Liang JC, Popat U, Claxton DF, Kliche KO, et al. Use of leukemic dendritic cells for the generation of antileukemic cellular cytotoxicity against Philadelphia chromosome-positive chronic myelogenous leukemia. *Blood* 1997; 89:1133–1142.
94. Molldrem JJ, Lee PP, Wang C, Felio K, Kantarjian HM, Champlin RE, et al. Evidence that specific T lymphocytes may participate in the elimination of chronic myelogenous leukemia. *Nat Med* JID - 9502015 2000; 6:1018–1023.
95. Druker BJ, Talpaz M, Resta DJ, Peng B, Buchdunger E, Ford JM, et al. Efficacy and safety of a specific inhibitor of the BCR-ABL tyrosine kinase in chronic myeloid leukemia. *N Engl J Med* JID - 0255562 2001; 344:1031–1037.
95a. Kantarjian H, Sawyers C, Hachhaus A, et al. Hematologi and cytogenetic responses to imatinib mesylate in chronic myelogenous leukemia. *N Engl J Med* 2003;346:645–652.
96. Druker BJ, Sawyers CL, Kantarjian H, Resta DJ, Reese SF, Ford JM, et al. Activity of a specific inhibitor of the BCR-ABL tyrosine kinase in the blast crisis of chronic myeloid leukemia and acute lymphoblastic leukemia with the Philadelphia chromosome. *N Engl J Med* JID - 0255562 2001; 344:1038–1042.

97. Gorre ME, Mohammed M, Ellwood K, Hsu N, Paquette R, Rao PN, et al. Clinical resistance to STI-571 cancer therapy caused by BCR-ABL gene mutation or amplification. *Science* JID-0404511 2001; 293:876–880.

98. Bartram CR, Janssen JW, Becher R, de Klein A, Grosveld G. Persistence of chronic myelocytic leukemia despite deletion of rearranged bcr/c-abl sequences in blast crisis. *J Exp Med* JID-2985109R 1986; 164:1389–1396.

99. Lee SJ, Kuntz KM, Horowitz MM, McGlave PB, Goldman JM, Sobocinski KA, et al. Unrelated donor bone marrow transplantation for chronic myelogenous leukemia: a decision analysis. *Ann Intern Med* 1997; 127:1080–1088.

100. Beelen DW, Graeven U, Elmaagacli AH, Niederle N, Kloke O, Opalka B, et al. Prolonged administration of interferon-alpha in patients with chronic-phase Philadelphia chromosome-positive chronic myelogenous leukemia before allogeneic bone marrow transplantation may adversely affect transplant outcome. *Blood* 1995; 85:2981–2990.

101. Giralt SA, Kantarjian HM, Talpaz M, Rios MB, Del Giglio A, Andersson BS, et al. Effect of prior interferon alpha therapy on the outcome of allogeneic bone marrow transplantation for chronic myelogenous leukemia. *J Clin Oncol* 1993; 11:1055–1061.

102. Zuffa E, Bandini G, Santucci MA, Martinelli G, Rosti G, Testoni N, et al. Prior treatment with alpha-interferon does not adversely affect the outcome of allogeneic BMT in chronic phase chronic myeloid leukemia. *Haematologica* 1998; 83:321–326.

103. Hehlmann R, Hochhaus A, Kolb HJ, Hasford J, Gratwohl A, Heimpel H, et al. Interferon-alpha before allogeneic bone marrow transplantation in chronic myelogenous leukemia does not affect outcome adversely, provided it is discontinued at least 90 days before the procedure. *Blood* JID-7603509 1999; 94:3668–3677.

104. Giralt S, Szydlo R, Goldman JM, Veum-Stone J, Biggs JC, Herzig RH, et al. Effect of short-term interferon therapy on the outcome of subsequent HLA-identical sibling bone marrow transplantation for chronic myelogenous leukemia: an analysis from the international bone marrow transplant registry. *Blood* JID-7603509 2000; 95:410–415.

105. Kolb HJ, Mittermuller J, Clemm C, Holler E, Ledderose G, Brehm G, et al. Donor leukocyte transfusions for treatment of recurrent chronic myelogenous leukemia in marrow transplant patients. *Blood* JID-7603509 1990; 76:2462–2465.

106. Drobyski WR, Keever CA, Roth MS, Koethe S, Hanson G, McFadden P, et al. Salvage immunotherapy using donor leukocyte infusions as treatment for relapsed chronic myelogenous leukemia after allogeneic bone marrow transplantation: efficacy and toxicity of a defined T-cell dose. *Blood* JID-7603509 1993; 82:2310–2318.

107. Porter DL, Roth MS, McGarigle C, Ferrara JL, Antin JH. Induction of graft-versus-host disease as immunotherapy for relapsed chronic myeloid leukemia. *N Engl J Med* JID-0255562 1994; 330:100–106.

108. Higano CS, Chielens D, Raskind W, Bryant E, Flowers ME, Radich J, et al. Use of alpha-2a-interferon to treat cytogenetic relapse of chronic myeloid leukemia after marrow transplantation. *Blood* JID-7603509 1997; 90:2549–2554.

109. Arcese W, Goldman JM, D'Arcangelo E, Schattenberg A, Nardi A, Apperley JF, et al. Outcome for patients who relapse after allogeneic bone marrow transplantation for chronic myeloid leukemia. Chronic Leukemia Working Party. European Bone Marrow Transplantation Group. *Blood* JID-7603509 1993; 82:3211–3219.

110. Sharp JC, Joyner MV, Wayne AW, Kemp J, Crofts M, Birch AD, et al. Karyotypic conversion in Ph1-positive chronic myeloid leukaemia with combination chemotherapy. *Lancet* 1979; 1:1370–1372.

111. Smalley RV, Vogel J, Huguley CM Jr, Miller D. Chronic granulocytic leukemia: cytogenetic conversion of the bone marrow with cycle-specific chemotherapy. *Blood* 1977; 50:107–113.

112. Carella AM, Chimirri F, Podesta M, Pitto A, Piaggio G, Dejana A, et al. High-dose chemoradiotherapy followed by autologous Philadelphia chromosome-negative blood progenitor

cell transplantation in patients with chronic myelogenous leukemia. *Bone Marrow Transplant* 1996; 17:201–205.

113. McGlave PB, De Fabritiis P, Deisseroth A, Goldman J, Barnett M, Reiffers J, et al. Autologous transplants for chronic myelogenous leukaemia: results from eight transplant groups. *Lancet* 1994; 343:1486–1488.

114. Reiffers J, Goldman J, Meloni G, Cahn JY, Gratwohl A. Autologous stem cell transplantation in chronic myelogenous leukemia: a retrospective analysis of the European Group for Bone Marrow Transplantation. *Bone Marrow Transplant* 1994; 14:407–410.

115. Deisseroth AB, Zu Z, Claxton D, Hanania EG, Fu S, Ellerson D, et al. Genetic marking shows that Ph+ cells present in autologous transplants of chronic myelogenous leukemia (CML) contribute to relapse after autologous bone marrow in CML. *Blood* 1994; 83:3068–3076.

116. de Fabritis P, Amadori S, Petti MC, Mancini M, Montefusco E, Picardi A, et al. In vitro purging with BCR-ABL antisense oligodeoxynucleotides does not prevent haematologic reconstitution after autologous bone marrow transplantation. *Leukemia* 1995; 9:662–664.

117. Gewirtz AM. Treatment of chronic myelogenous leukemia (CML) with c-myb antisense oligodeoxynucleotides. *Bone Marrow Transplant* 1994; 14:57–61.

118. Barnett MJ, Eaves CJ, Phillips GL, Gascoyne RD, Hogge DE, Horsman DE, et al. Autografting with cultured marrow in chronic myeloid leukemia: results of a pilot study. *Blood* 1994; 84:724–732.

119. Verfaillie CM, Bhatia R, Miller W, Mortari F, Roy V, Burger S, et al. BCR/ABL-negative primitive progenitors suitable for transplantation can be selected from the marrow of most early-chronic phase but not accelerated-phase chronic myelogenous leukemia patients. *Blood* 1996; 87:4770–4779.

120. Higano CS, Chielens D, Raskind W, Bryant E, Flowers ME, Radich J, et al. Use of alpha-2a-interferon to treat cytogenetic relapse of chronic myeloid leukemia after marrow transplantation. *Blood* 1997; 90:2549–2554.

121. Arcese W, Goldman JM, D'Arcangelo E, Schattenberg A, Nardi A, Apperley JF, et al. Outcome for patients who relapse after allogeneic bone marrow transplantation for chronic myeloid leukemia. *Blood* 1993; 82:3211–3219.

122. Toren A, Ackerstein A, Slavin S, Nagler A. Role of interleukin-2 in human hematological malignancies. *Med Oncol* 1995; 12:177–186.

123. Childs R, Epperson D, Bahceci E, Clave E, Barrett J. Molecular remission of chronic myeloid leukaemia following a non-myeloablative allogeneic peripheral blood stem cell transplant: in vivo and in vitro evidence for a graft-versus-leukaemia effect. *Br J Haematol* JID - 0372544 1999; 107:396–400.

123a. Applebaum FR. Perspectives on the future of chronic myeloid leukemia treatment. *Seminars in Hematology* 2001;38(3)Suppl 8:35–42.

124. Cortez D, Stoica G, Pierce JH, Pendergast AM. The BCR-ABL tyrosine kinase inhibits apoptosis by activating a Ras-dependent signaling pathway. *Oncogene* 1996; 13:2589–2594.

125. Gibbs JB, Oliff A, Kohl NE. Farnesyltransferase inhibitors: ras research yields a potential cancer therapeutic. *Cell* 1994; 77:175–178.

6 Sézary Syndrome

The Redefinition of a Clinico-Pathologic Entity and Its Implication for Staging, Prognosis, and Treatment

Lauren C. Pinter-Brown, MD

CONTENTS

HISTORY

Sézary syndrome (SS) is widely believed to be a distinctive leukemic and erythrodermic variant of mycosis fungoides (MF). In 1938, Sézary and Bouvrain *(1)* wrote of a patient who presented with complaints of intense pruritus, who was found to have erythroderma, lymphadenopathy, and abnormal "monster" hyper-

From: *Current Clinical Oncology: Chronic Leukemias and Lymphomas:*
Biology, Pathophysiology, and Clinical Management
Edited by: G. J. Schiller © Humana Press Inc., Totowa, NJ

convoluted mononuclear cells circulating in the peripheral blood. Twenty-three years later, the Sézary syndrome was recognized in the American medical literature by Taswell and Winkelmann *(2)*.

With the advent of immunologic techniques enabling the identification of T-lymphocytes, the term cutaneous T-cell lymphoma (CTCL) was proposed as a term that would encompass MF, SS, and any other T-cell lymphoma with primary manifestations in the skin. In 1978, an international workshop sponsored by the National Cancer Institute (NCI) and the Mycosis Fungoides Cooperative Group (MFCG) accepted this concept and proposed a staging classification based on the TNM (tumor, node, metastasis) scheme *(3)*.

EPIDEMIOLOGY

SS is rare, representing approx 5% of all newly reported cases of CTCL *(4)*. Although population-based registries may fail to completely capture all new diagnoses of patients with malignancies such as CTCL that are frequently diagnosed in a clinic setting, analysis of Surveillance, Epidemiology, and End Results (SEER) and National Center of Health Statistics data show that in the period of 1973–1992, the incidence of CTCL in the United States was 0.36/10 person-years, or about 1000 new cases per yr. The age-adjusted incidence rate ratio for Afro-Americans/Caucasians was 1.7 and for Asians/Caucasians, 0.6 *(5,6)*.

Both the incidence and mortality data demonstrate a greater frequency of CTCL among men than women (approx 1.5:1), with an increasing incidence with advancing age (median age 63 yr), although the diagnosis has been made in much younger patients, and rarely in children *(6)*.

ETIOLOGY

The risk factors for the development of CTCL are unclear. Much speculation has focused on exposures to physical and chemical agents, to retroviruses, and to other forms of chronic antigenic stimulation, but rigorous epidemiologic data demonstrating these hypothesized associations are lacking *(6)*. There has been a particular interest in the connection between the production of Staphlycoccal enterotoxins during bacterial colonization of the skin and SS *(7–9)*.

Immunosuppression or incompetence may also be risk factors for CTCL. Reports of cases in which the diagnosis of CTCL has been made after organ transplantation, and in the setting of HIV infection, have been published *(6)*.

CLINICAL ASPECTS

In one of the largest series describing the clinical aspects of SS, generalized erythroderma, edema, and intense pruritus were seen in the vast majority of patients. These symptoms and signs were accompanied by palpable lymphadenopathy (57%), alopecia (32%), onychodystrophy (32%), and keratoderma of the palms and soles (29%) *(10)*. Ectropion of the eyelids with possible ocular irritation, hyperkeratosis of the palms and soles causing painful fissures, exfoliation (sometimes causing decreased hearing secondary to occlusion of the external auditory canal by scale), hyperpigmentation, and "leonine facies" (the accentuation of normal facial skin folds) can also occur *(11,12)*.

PATHOLOGIC ASPECTS

No clinical feature seen in CTCL or SS is pathognomonic. Thus, histologic diagnoses of tissue or blood, supplemented with immunophenotypic, cytogenetic, and/or gene rearrangement studies, are necessary to establish this diagnosis.

Like MF, hematoxylin-and-eosin (H&E) stained biopsy specimens of skin may show a subepidermal band-like infiltrate of atypical lymphocytes, characterized by cerebriform nuclei. Epidermotropism, the infiltration of these atypical lymphoid cells into the epidermis, is often seen. Single cells or clusters of cells found in the epidermis and surrounded by a clear halo are known as Pautrier's microabscesses.

In series reporting the pathologic findings of skin biopsies taken from patients with SS, 17–33% had findings indicative only of chronic dermatitis *(13,14)*, and 27% lacked any light-microscopic finding of CTCL *(14)*. In one series *(13)* examining 18 specimens from 10 patients, the skin biopsies of only two patients showed consistent findings of cerebriform cells, demonstrating the need for taking multiple and/or serial skin biopsies from patients in whom there is a strong suspicion of CTCL. Such biopsies should be taken from skin that has not been treated with steroids or other agents, as these may influence the histologic findings.

In the case of erythrodermic patients in whom the diagnosis of SS is suspected, tissues other than skin—such as lymph nodes or blood—may contribute to the physician's ability to make a diagnosis. Examination of the blood should reveal the Sézary cell, a lymphocyte with a hyperconvoluted or cerebriform nuclear contour, a high nuclear/cytoplasmic ratio, and condensed chromatin at the nuclear membrane. Electron microscopy of the buffy coat can confirm the presence of cells that have deep and narrow—almost serpiginous nuclear indentations *(11,15)* (*see* Fig. 1).

Examination of excisional lymph-node specimens of palpable nodes may also confirm the diagnosis of CTCL. One study of seven SS patients shows a significant correlation between cytology obtained by fine-needle aspiration and histologic evidence of lymphomatous involvement *(16)*.

IMMUNOPHENOTYPING

Although the finding of Sézary cells in the blood is the hallmark of SS, morphologically identical cells can often be found in the blood of patients with

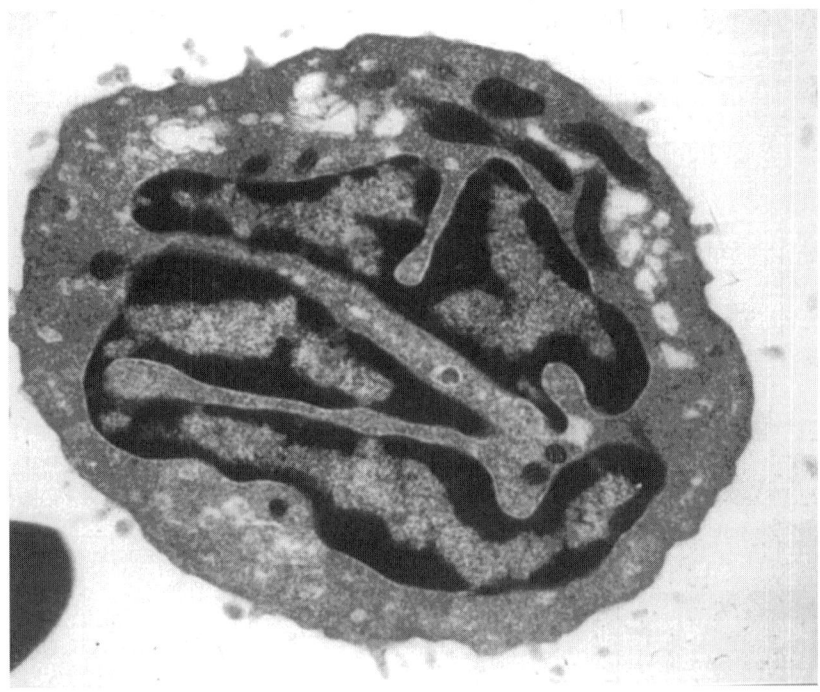

Fig. 1. Detection microgreph of Sézary's cell.

benign skin conditions *(17)* and even in the blood of healthy subjects *(18)*, and not always in smaller numbers. Then, flow immunophenotyping, or immunophenotyping of fixed tissue specimens can contribute to diagnostic specificity. Most cases of SS are clonal expansions of cells that are CD2,3,4,5 positive and CD 8-negative, mature T-helper lymphocytes. Cases of SS with expression of CD8 rather than CD4, or lack of CD 2,3, or 5 have been described. Approximately two-thirds of cases lack CD7 expression, an antigen found on most mature T-cells *(19)*. Indeed, the loss of normal T-cell antigens such as CD 2, 3, 5, or 7 is much more commonly seen in the blood of patients with SS compared to normals *(20)*.

More recently, several groups have noted the expansion of a CD4-positive CD26-negative clone in the blood of patients with CTCL, and have suggested that the finding of an expanded population of such cells may be more specific to the diagnosis *(21–23)*. Bernengo et al. suggest that the finding of more than 30% CD4-positive CD26-negative lymphocytes in peripheral blood will correctly identify blood involvement with CTCL *(22)*.

CYTOGENETICS

Although no specific chromosomal abnormality has been associated with CTCL, random numerical and structural abnormalities are often encountered, and may help to define a malignant clone *(19,24–27)*.

MOLECULAR GENETICS

Evidence of clonality in peripheral blood and skin can be demonstrated more frequently by a number of molecular techniques such as Southern blot testing for TCR rearrangments, a less sensitive method than PCR-based assays that detect rearrangements in the TCR gene *(30)*. Numerous methods are currently available to analyze PCR products, including electrophoresis on denaturing gradient gel or heteroduplex temperature-gradient gel, and single-strand conformational polymorphism analysis. A comparison of these techniques in specimens from those diagnosed with CTCL has not been undertaken *(19)*.

Despite decreased sensitivity, Southern blot techniques are capable of detecting an expanded clone in both the blood *(28,29)*, skin, and nodes *(29)* in nearly all specimens from patients with SS. False-positive results can occur, however *(28)*, mandating the use of other confirmatory data before establishing a diagnosis of malignancy.

Using the more sensitive PCR-based assays, even patients with early-stage MF can be found to have circulating clonal T-cells *(31)*. Data from Delfau-Larve et al. suggest that the finding of identical clones in both skin and blood may be additional criteria for the diagnosis of CTCL in histologically uncertain cases. The finding of a dominant T-cell clone in the blood alone is of unknown significance, being found with the same frequency in cases of CTCL and those without CTCL, but more frequently in both groups with increasing age *(32)*.

PROPOSED TERMINOLOGY AND DIAGNOSTIC CRITERIA FOR ERYTHRODERMIC CTCL (E-CTCL) AND SS

The International Society for Cutaneous Lymphomas (ISCL) was founded in 1992 to enhance interaction among regional and international cutaneous lymphoma groups, enabling consensus on such areas as definition, terminology, and staging criteria. To this end, the ISCL organized two conferences on E-CTCL and SS *(19)*.

The group proposed that E-CTCL should be considered to be a variant of CTCL characterized by chronic erythroderma, a diffuse, generalized erythema involving more than 90% of the skin surface. E-CTCL can be further divided into three clinical groups.

The first group is erythrodermic MF (E-MF), E-CTCL that lacks the blood findings of SS, and develops during the course of otherwise typical MF (involvement of the skin in patches, plaques, and tumors).

The second is SS, a distinctive form of leukemic E-CTCL characterized by the finding of Sézary cells in skin, blood, and other tissues, typically with evidence of T-cell clonality. The manifestations of SS typically develop de novo, but may be preceded by a prodrome of pruritus or nonspecific dermatitis. In rare cases in which clinical and pathologic features of SS are preceded by MF, the term "SS preceded by MF" should be used to distinguish this condition from the more typical presentation of SS.

Cases of SS must fulfill at least one criteria of "leukemic" involvement. These include:

1. An absolute Sézary count of ≥1000 cells per mm3.*
2. An increase in CD4-positive cells with a CD4/CD8 ratio ≥10 by flow cytometry.*
3. An increase in CD3-positive or CD4-positive cells with evidence of circulating cells that exhibit aberrant loss or expression of T-cell markers (CD2,3,4,5) by flow cytometry. Deficient CD7 (CD4-positive, CD7-negative expression in ≥40% lymphocytes) represents a tentative criterion.
4. Relative or absolute lymphocytosis with evidence of a T-cell clone in the blood by Southern blot or PCR technique.*
5. A chromosomally abnormal T-cell clone.

The third E-CTCL group is designated E-CTCL, not otherwise specified, a group that would include cases of E-CTCL that fail to fulfill the criteria for either E-MF or SS.

Two additional diagnostic categories included Adult T-Cell Leukemia (ATLL) with features of Sézary syndrome, and pseudo-CTCL erythroderma. The first acknowledges the existence of cases of ATLL that mimic the findings of SS, but have evidence of incorporation of human T- lymphotropic viral type 1 DNA into the tumor-cell genome. The latter includes cases of benign inflammatory erythrodermas often caused by drugs that mimic the findings of E-CTCL. When such cases mimic the findings of SS, with Sézary cells ≥1000 per m3 or with CD4/CD8 ratio ≥10, such cases would be designated as pseudo-SS. This situation has been described during treatment with anticonvulsants, particularly phenytoin.

---

* If the diagnosis of CTCL in not substantiated by skin or node studies, additional evidence of malignancy is required, such as evidence of T cells with aberrant expression of T-cell markers, or demonstration of the identical T-cell clone in the skin and blood by Southern blot or PCR-based methods.

PATHOPHYSIOLOGY

Although patch or plaque MF may persist for years in patients in the absence of obvious lymph-node or blood involvement, it would be incorrect to view this condition as a lymphoma solely confined to the skin.

MF/SS arises from a distinctive subset of T-lymphocytes that normally patrol and home to the skin—the activated/memory-helper T-lymphocyte. Naïve helper T-lymphocytes recirculate from the peripheral blood to the nodes. When their T-cell-receptor is activated by a specific antigen that is presented by cutaneous dentritic cells in regional draining nodes, these naïve helper T-lymphocytes undergo a transition to memory T-lymphocytes, thereafter displaying the memory T-cell phenotype, CD45RO. During this transition, these T-cells acquire new molecular keys, allowing them to exit the blood vessels and enter extranodal tissue. One such molecule is the cutaneous lymphoid antigen (CLA), an adhesion molecule that mediates lymphocyte tethering to endothelial cells in cutaneous post-capillary venules through interaction with E-selectin. Then, the specific memory-helper T-lymphocytes expressing this antigen become skin-homing cells that may cycle between three compartments: the blood, lymph nodes, and skin. The same cell population has been implicated in the pathogenesis of such "benign" disorders as cutaneous graft vs host disease, psoriasis, and allergic and atopic dermatitis, but the demonstration of a clone of such cells distinguishes MF/SS from nonmalignant states *(33)*.

Additionally, the malignant cell population of MF/SS has been shown to exhibit abnormalities in cytokine production that may account for many of the observed immune alterations seen in the disease, such as elevations in IgE and increased eosinophils in skin and blood. Studies of peripheral-blood mononuclear cells from patients with SS show these cells to produce IL4, IL5, and possibly IL10, with decreased production of IL2, IL12, and interferon (IFN), a cytokine profile similar to the murine subset of helper T-lymphocytes, Th2 *(34–36)*. It has also been noted that early skin lesions of MF contain ample CD8-positive cyto-toxic T-lymphocytes making IFN. IL12 from macrophages may further augment the cytotoxic T-lymphocyte population's production of IFN, but may itself be decreased by IL10 made by the malignant population. IL4 made by the malignant population and IFN made by the cytotoxic T-lymphocyte population can each antagonize the biologic effects of the other cytokine, and can inhibit the produc-tion of the other. As the disease progresses, nonmalignant cytotoxic T-lympho-cytes disappear from the skin and from the blood *(35)*.

In the early stages of CTCL, when the density of malignant cells is low, IFN produced by responding cytotoxic T-lymphocytes may counteract the biologic effects of the IL-4 produced by the malignant cells and inhibit IL4-driven expan-sion of the abnormal Th2 cell population. As the malignant population expands and increases IL4 production, the biologic activity and production of IFN will

Table 1
Skin, Lymph Node, and Visceral Staging System

T-Stage	Adenopathy	Lymph node class on biopsy	Visceral
T_1: Limited plaque (<10% of body surface area)	Ad+: Palpable adenopathy	LN1: Reactive node	V+: Positive visceral biopsy V−: Negative visceral biopsy
T_2: Generalized plaque (≥10% of body surface area)	Ad−: No palpable adenopathy	LN_2: Dermatopathic node, small clusters of convoluted cells	
T_3: Cutaneous tumor		LN_3: Dermatopathic node, large clusters of convoluted cells (>6 per cluster)	
T_4: Erythroderma		LN_4: Lymph-node effacement	

Modified from Sausville et al. *(40)*.

Table 2
Staging System for CTCL

IA	T_1; Ad−; LN_1, LN_2; V−
IB	T_2; Ad−; LN_1; LN_2; V−
IIA	T_1, T_2; Ad+; LN_1, LN_2; V−
IIB	T_3; Ad±; LN_1, LN_2; V−
III	T_4; Ad±; LN_1, LN_2; V−
IVA	T_{1-4}; Ad±; LN_3 or LN_4; V−
IVB	T_{1-4}; Ad±; $LN_1 - LN_4$; V+

Modified from Sausville et al. *(40)*.

decrease, accelerating the escape from immune surveillance that has been only partially effective at best *(35)*.

Another IFN-dependent function is the expression of intercellular adhesion molecule 1 (ICAM1) by keratinocytes. Increased keratinocyte expression of ICAM1 is a common finding in early CTCL, perhaps explaining the lymphocyte's predilection for the epidermis through binding of their LFA 1 (lymphocyte function-associated protein) to ICAM 1. Rook and Heald hypothesized that decreased production of IFN in the later stages of CTCL may in turn cause the loss of ICAM 1 expression on keratinocytes, thus allowing the cells to move away from the epidermis *(35)*. The predilection of malignant cells for skin in the early stages of MF may explain the success of topical treatments, which would treat the bulk of the malignant cells, yet later stages of MF/SS in which the T-cells have lost their strict dependence on the skin require systemic therapies.

Further studies of peripheral-blood mononuclear cells from patients with SS suggest that IL7, as produced by keratinocytes in normal skin, may induce significant proliferation of the malignant cell population (37,38).

STAGING

In 1979, the NCI/MFCG adopted a TNM classification for CTCL, which came to include both a clinical evaluation of the skin and nodes and the histopathologic evaluation of nodes and visceral tissue. A designation of B0 was given to patients with <5% atypical circulating cells, and B1 to patients with ≥5% atypical circulating cells, although these designations did not affect the patients' stage (39). This classification was modified in 1988 by Sausville (40) with the addition of a lymph-node grading system to further delineate histopathologic lymph-node findings. Tables 1 and 2 demonstrate this staging system for CTCL. Using this staging system, patients with SS will be designated as either stage III or IV.

The more recent ISCL recommendations include a further designation of B2 for blood that fulfills the proposed diagnostic criteria for SS, and the proposal that a B2 designation should be considered a component of stage IVA. The B1 designation would be retained for patients with ≥5% per 100 lymphocytes plus PCR or other evidence of a T-cell clone in the blood. If only Sézary counts are available, then ≥20% abnormal lymphocytes should be used as the criterion for minimal blood involvement (19).

When assessing a patient diagnosed with CTCL for stage of disease, the analysis should focus on those areas of the body trafficked by T-cells: the skin, nodes, blood, and viscera especially the liver, lung, and marrow. The physical examination should focus on the type and extent of skin involvement, regions and dimensions of palpable lymphadenopathy, and the presence of organomegaly. Blood evaluation should include a complete blood count with white-blood-cell differential, and liver-function testing including lactate dehydrogenase (LDH). Pathologic evaluation of the blood may include an examination of the buffy coat, flow cytometry, and/or T-cell gene rearrangement studies. Any palpable lymph node should be biopsied, and a chest radiograph should be performed.

The role of routine body CT scanning to detect adenopathy in patients with MF/SS has been addressed by Bass et al. (41). In this study, the results of body CT scanning did not change either the stage or management of any patient with stage I CTCL, and therefore cannot be recommended for all patients with CTCL. However, the authors concluded that body CT scanning could be clinically useful to patients with CTCL who had clinical stage II and greater, not only to clarify stage and optimize treatment planning, but also for accurate baseline assessment and for subsequent assessment of disease progression.

A standardized assessment for visceral involvement has not yet been established in MF/SS (42). In a study of prospective staging evaluation of patients with

CTCL, peripheral-blood involvement and advanced lymph-node histopathologic class (LN3 or 4) were found to correlate with visceral involvement *(43)*. Foss and Sausville have suggested that it would be reasonable to use nodal and blood involvement as surrogate markers for visceral involvement. In the case of abnormal visceral function or appearance, such as the findings of chest radiograph abnormalities or hepatomegaly and/or liver function abnormalities, it may be reasonable to consider biopsy of those organs to delineate the cause of such abnormalities and to further optimize management of the patient *(42)*.

With respect to the routine examination of bone-marrow, a study of marrow examinations from 60 patients with CTCL showed that approx 22% of bone-marrow examinations were positive for atypical cerebriform cells in either an infiltrative or nodular pattern. The majority of positive marrow examinations were found in patients with advanced disease (stage III or IV) or with peripheral-blood involvement *(44)*.

In addition to the staging procedures that would be recommended for all patients diagnosed with CTCL, patients diagnosed with SS should complete staging evaluations with body CT scanning, bone-marrow evaluation, and visceral biopsy as directed by physical, laboratory, and radiographic examination.

PROGNOSTIC FACTORS

In addition to the clinical stage of the patient, others have searched for additional clinical or laboratory parameters that may aid in prognostication. Kim et al. *(45)* performed a retrospective cohort study of 106 patients with either erythrodermic MF or SS. Independent prognostic factors including age $\geq$65 yr at presentation, stage IV, and the presence of circulating Sézary cells >5% in the peripheral blood were adverse prognostic features in multivariate analysis. Given these three prognostic factors, the Stanford Group found that three distinct groups could be described. The favorable group who had no poor prognostic features enjoyed a median survival of 10.2 yr, and the unfavorable group, who had two or three poor prognostic features, had a median survival of only 1.5 yr. An intermediate group with one poor prognostic feature had a median survival of 3.7 yr.

Others have focused on the measurement of the soluble alpha receptor for IL2 (sIL-2R) as both a means to follow a patient's clinical course and to help with prognostication. In his study of 101 patients with MF/SS, Wasik found that sIL-2R correlated with stage, Sézary count, and LDH. The median value of sIL-2R was 3× higher for erythrodermic compared to other patients with CTCL. In 40 patients studied with erythroderma, including 23 with SS, most erythrodermic patients had values greater than 1000 U/mL. In a multivariate analysis, sIL-2R was found to correlate with survival of erythrodermic patients, and to be a better predictor of prognosis than stage, Sézary cell count or LDH *(46)*. Bernengo's study of 17 patients with SS confirms that sIL-2R values correlate with the clinical course of disease, and with LDH and Sézary cell count *(47)*.

COMPLICATIONS

The major cause of death in patients with SS, and CTCL in general, is infection. Infections contribute to 27–60% of deaths. In a retrospective study of 356 patients with MF/SS, the most common infections causing morbidity in this patient group were acquired bacterial skin infections, most often with staph species and beta streptococcus. Cutaneous bacterial infections were usually treated in an outpatient setting. The second most common infections were cutaneous herpes simplex and herpes zoster infections. Twenty-seven percent of these infections were disseminated in the skin, usually in patients with stage III and IV disease (48). This proclivity for herpes simplex virus (HSV) to disseminate in skin may be explained by the known decrease in cytotoxic T-cells in skin and blood of patients with advancing CTCL. Kaposi's variceliform eruption, the dissemination of herpes simplex in skin with a pre-existing dermatosis, presents as evanescent umbilicated vesiculopapules with formation of punched-out skin lesions, and is well-described in patients with CTCL.

Bacteremias and bacterial pneumonia were observed in 88% of patients who died of infection. In this series, Gram-negative infection was most common in patients with stage III and IV disease (48). In another study of 60 patients with CTCL in which sepsis occurred in 23% of patients, the most common organism was Gram-positive cocci (49). In both studies, advanced stage was the most important risk factor for infection (48,49).

Another complication of CTCL is transformation to large T-cell lymphoma. In series studying pathologic specimens from patients with CTCL, between 8% and 45% of patients have evidence of cytologic transformation, variably defined as the presence of large cells greater than 4× the size of a small lymphocyte in more than 25% of the cellular infiltrate, or large cells forming microscopic nodules (50–53). Patients with stage IIB or greater appeared to have a higher incidence of transformation (50,53) with 31% of patients stage IIB–IV vs 14% of patients stage I-IIA (50). The median time from diagnosis to transformation is from 12–21.5 mo (50,52,53). Patients are also diagnosed with cytologic evidence of transformation at initial presentation 10–40% of the time (51,52). Cytologic transformation significantly shortens the patient's life as compared to patients diagnosed with CTCL who do not have cytologic evidence of transformation (51,52) with median survival after transformation from 2–22 mo (50,53,54). Two series found that patients whose disease transformed in cutaneous sites fared significantly better than patients whose disease transformed in extracutaneous sites (51,52). In Vergier's study (54) of a French population of 45 patients diagnosed with CTCL in transformation, extracutaneous transformation and age over 60 yr were associated with a worse prognosis in a multivariate analysis. Diamandidou et al. noted that early transformation (less than 2 yr from diagnosis) and stage IIB–IV disease were associated with inferior survival. Their study population included only 2 stage III patients of a total study population of 26, and may not be wholly applicable to this discussion of patients with SS. Additionally, it was believed that the combination of elevated 2-microglobulin and LDH predicted the possibility of transformation *(50)*.

A third complication of CTCL is secondary or associated malignancies. Perhaps first described by Abel *(55)*, this patient population has been noted to develop non-melanoma skin cancers, unusual in the formation in non-sunexposed areas and sometimes metastatic behavior. In a review of 71 patients with CTCL, 10% were noted to have developed cutaneous neoplasms with an average follow-up of 8 yr. Of the patients who developed cutaneous neoplasms, the majority had received either electron-beam radiation or PUVA treatment *(56)*. A more recent study performed in the United Kingdom by Scarisbrick *(57)* evaluated 71 patients with SS followed for 6.8 yr. A total of 23% of patients developed other malignancies: eight squamous-cell carcinoma of the skin, two squamous-cell carcinoma of the oral mucosa, and nine other internal malignancies. The incidence of squamous-cell carcinoma of the skin was 42× that observed in a study of age-matched controls. The mean time from the diagnosis of SS to the diagnosis of the secondary malignancy was 7 yr. Notably, there was no difference in treatment modalities between the entire SS group and those who developed cancer, suggesting that the increase in skin cancer may be inherent to the disease itself, perhaps related to increasing immunoincompetence with stage.

In the United States, Olsen *(58)* found that in 63 patients with CTCL followed at Duke University for 15 yr, the secondary malignancies occur at a rate 2.4× greater than expected. In a SEER population-based study of the period from 1973–1983, Kantor *(59)* found the rate of secondary cancers in 544 patients diagnosed with CTCL to be 6%, with a risk ratio of 1.7. Among patients diagnosed with SS, the rate of secondary malignancy was 12%. Of note in the group as a whole, the incidence of non-Hodgkin's lymphoma, lung, and colon cancer were particularly increased. Finally, in a recent study of 319 patients with CTCL in Finland, Valeva *(60)* found an increased incidence of cancer (standardized incidence ratio of 1.4) with a particular increase in lung cancer (standardized incidence ratio 2.7), especially small-cell carcinoma (standardized incidence ratio 8.5), and other lymphomas, including Hodgkin's disease (standardized incidence ratio 7.0).

GENERAL TREATMENT CONSIDERATIONS

A multitude of treatment options currently exist for patients with SS. All are offered with palliative intent; no treatment to date has been proven to increase long-term or median survival of treated patients. Considering the often intense symptoms and alterations in appearance that SS engenders, treatments that offer good palliation are welcomed. As the patient with SS may experience a decrease in survival because of concomitant infection in association with declining immunocompetence, the most desirable treatments allow for palliation and at the same time, preservation of immune function.

To allow an evaluation of treatment options, series in the English-language literature have been identified that report treatment of subjects with CTCL or SS. If patients with SS were not specifically discussed, the data from all patients with erythrodermic CTCL (stage III or T4) were examined. Few studies, in fact, have specifically mentioned patients with SS. In evaluating studies in this manner, I hope to update an excellent review of treatment options for patients with SS published over 10 yr ago by Wieselthier and Koh *(11)*.

The discussion of treatment options is divided into topical treatments, including light treatment, topical chemotherapy, and radiation therapy, and systemic therapies including retinoids, interferon (IFN), extracorporeal photopheresis, and treatment with either single-agent or combination chemotherapy. New treatment options are discussed, including treatment with rexinoids and fusion toxins, and experimental treatment options are also included. Treatment utilizing combinations of multiple modalities are also mentioned.

PUVA

PUVA therapy, the combination of the oral ingestion of 8-methoxypsoralen (8-MOPP), a compound naturally found in a variety of fruits and vegetables that can be photoactivated, followed by UVA exposure to the patient's skin, was first described as a treatment for CTCL by Gilchrest in 1976 *(61)*. Since that time, many series have confirmed its efficacy in the treatment of patients with early-stage (stage I) MF. Within these series, few patients with SS were included, mostly those who had been previously treated with other modalities *(11)*. Only Abel *(62)* reported on a series that included patients with SS and erythroderma who were treated primarily with PUVA therapy. In this study, although 7 of 10 patients with erythroderma experienced a clinical complete remission in skin, no patients with SS experienced a complete response in all sites of disease. Despite less frequent maintenance treatments, relapses occurred in patients with a median of 10.5 mo, implying the need for long-term maintenance PUVA, perhaps with higher frequency. The observation that erythrodermic patients initiated treatment with less UVA exposure ($0.1–0.2 \ J/cm^2$/treatment) because of extreme photosensitivity is germane.

There have been no further published studies dealing with the use of PUVA therapy in patients with CTCL since Wieselthier and Koh made the observation that PUVA therapy for patients with SS—many of whom had been previously treated with other modalities—resulted in a complete remission (CR) about 25% of the time, and that remission durations were usually short. PUVA therapy was also not associated with a decrease in Sézary cell count in those studies in which this measurement was recorded *(11)*. As circulating Sézary cells are known to be in equilibrium with the skin, this result is not surprising, and PUVA therapy alone as a primary therapy modality for patients with SS cannot be recommended.

More recently, Kuzel et al. *(63)* reported the long-term follow-up of 39 patients with stage IB and greater CTCL who participated in phase I and phase II trials examining the combination of interferon-2a (IFN-2a) and PUVA therapy. In this study, most patients had received previous treatment with other modalities. Treatment consisted of IFN-2a given subcutaneously or intramuscularly escalated in 3-mU increments over a 6–8 wk period with a target dose of 12 mU 3× weekly. Treatment was continued for 2 yr. This was combined with PUVA therapy, which was maintained indefinitely at less frequency than induction. Of eight stage III patients, five experienced a CR and two a partial remission (PR), similar to the CR rate of 62% and overall response rate (RR) of 90% observed in the entire group of patients. All CRs were pathologically confirmed. With a median follow-up of 28 mo, the median response duration of the entire group was 28 mo. Again, the observation that photosensitization occurs with the combination of IFN-2a and PUVA, particularly in erythrodermic patients, mandates careful initiation and gradual increases of UVA exposure in this patient group. Here, the combination of PUVA with IFN appears to result in a RR higher than that seen with either modality alone in stage III patients with CTCL.

Topical Chemotherapy

The most common chemotherapeutic agent used topically for patients with CTCL is nitrogen mustard (mechlorethamine hydrochloride), used by the patient in either an aqueous or ointment form. The largest series reported is a retrospective review by Vonderheid *(64)* of 331 patients with CTCL treated between 1968 and 1982. The patients were treated with the aqueous form of topical nitrogen mustard daily until clear, and then continued treatment daily or every other day for 3 yr. Twenty-nine patients with SS were included in the group of treated patients. Although 60% of the stage III patients experienced a clinical and often a pathologic CR, and approx 30% of these had a sustained CR (≥4 yr), only two patients with SS experienced a sustained CR. The results from other series summarized by Wieselthier and Koh *(11)* also support the conclusion that although the use of topical nitrogen mustard can be very effective, and perhaps curative when used to treat patients with early-stage (stage I) CTCL, the results in patients with SS are not as compelling, primarily because of the shorter duration of remission.

Zackheim *(65)* also reported on the use of topical BCNU (100 mg BCNU/50 cc 95% alcohol). Although patients with limited CTCL had a higher response rate, of nine patients with stage III CTCL, there was a CR of 22% and PR of 22%.

Radiation Therapy

At Stanford University, a depth-limited method for giving total skin radiation therapy to patients diagnosed with CTCL was initiated in 1958. Total skin electron-beam therapy (TSEBT) using a classical six-field technique was introduced in the early 1960s. 2.5–9 meV electrons were used, depending on the depth of the skin lesions, and a total dose of 3600 cGy with 400 cGy in four fractions per wk was achieved. A 10-d split midway through treatment allowed resolution of skin toxicity. The feet, perineum, and other shaded areas received electron patches (2000 cGy in 20 fractions).

A similar technique was employed in Hamilton, Ontario from 1969, allowing a compilation of the data from both institutions in a review by Jones *(66)*. In all, the responses of 992 patients with CTCL are described—42 at Stanford and 20 at Hamilton were stage III. Overall, 3–5% of patients had B1 involvement, but the results of these patients were not commented upon separately.

Examination of the data showed that 26% of stage III patients at Stanford and 50% of stage III patients treated at Hamilton achieved CR. Response rates appeared to be higher in erythrodermic patients who received a higher total radiation dose and/or higher-energy electrons. Comparatively, CR rates were much higher in patients with stage IA disease—96% at Stanford and 84% at Hamilton.

Long-term relapse-free survivals were markedly different when comparing patients with stage IA disease to patients with stage III disease. At Stanford, the 20-yr relapse-free survival for patients with stage IA disease was 46%, and the 15-yr relapse-free survival at Hamilton was 33%. Although some would consider these patients to be cured of their disease, the 2.5–5 yr relapse-free survival for patients with stage III disease was 10% at Stanford and 23% at Hamilton.

A summary of worldwide data, excluding Stanford and Hamilton, yielded similar results *(66)*. Then, with updated information, the conclusions of Wieselthier and Koh *(11)* are still unchallenged—that with a relatively low CR rate and short remission period, TSEBT of patients with SS cannot be recommended as primary therapy.

Recently, two authors have focused on the use of radiation therapy for treatment of erythrodermic patients with CTCL, particularly those without demonstrable involvement on buffy-coat smears. Jones *(67)* retrospectively reviewed the combined data of Hamilton and Yale University. A total of 45 patients with erythrodermic CTCL were treated between 1970 and 1996. Of all patients, 21 had B1 involvement, and 15 patients had TSEBT as their first therapy after diagnosis. Of the 28 patients classified as stage III, 19 of these had no blood involvement by examination of buffy-coat smears, 13 had been previously treated with other modalities, and eight ultimately received more intense doses of radiation therapy (between 32 and 40 gy with 4–6 meV electrons). Of the stage III patients without B1 involvement, 63% achieved at CR, pathologically confirmed. The 5-yr progression-free survival was 69%. It may be possible to select a group of erythrodermic patients who may fare better with TSEBT. These results remain unconfirmed by other institutions.

Wilson *(68)* retrospectively examined the results obtained when erythrodermic patients with CTCL were treated with TSEBT at Hamilton and Yale University from 1974 to 1997. Of the 44 such patients described, 21 who were treated at Yale University additionally received extracorporeal photopheresis (EP) in a nonrandomized fashion in either a neoadjuvant, concomitant, or adjuvant fashion 2 d per mo for a median of 6 mo. Of all patients, 73% had received prior treatment modalities, and 59% had blood involvement. Median follow-up after completion of radiation therapy was 2 yr. Overall, CR was achieved in 73% of patients after radiation, with a disease-free survival at 3 yr of 63%. Examining the results with respect to use or non-use of EP, 3-yr disease-free survival was 49% for those who received radiation alone and 81% for those who received radiation+EP, achieving statistical significance at a 0.024 level. A prospective randomized trial of TBEBT therapy with or without the use of EP in erythrodermic CTCL patients would be warranted, given these results.

Interferons

The use of IFN for the treatment of patients with CTCL was first reported by Bunn et al. in 1984 *(69)*. The maximally tolerated dose was determined from phase I trials, and patients with CTCL participating in this NCI trial were treated with 50 mU/m2 IFN-2a 3× a wk indefinitely in responding patients. Twenty patients with advanced CTCL were treated, and all had received treatment with other modalities. Although they had failed other treatments, the RR in this patient group was 45%, with a CR rate of 15%.

Since this report, over 200 patients with CTCL who have received treatment with IFN have been reported in the international medical literature. Patients were treated with all stages of CTCL, both as the primary treatment and as salvage treatment after another treatment modality. Although there are two types of recombinant alpha IFN, and recombinant gamma IFN is commercially available, most studies utilized IFN-2a given either subcutaneously or intramuscularly. Target dose, method of dose escalation, dose frequency, and length of treatment vary widely among the studies; however, many conclusions can be drawn. The reader is referred to a detailed review of the use of IFN for treatment of patients with CTCL by Olsen *(70)*.

Olsen's review of all the published series using IFN in the treatment of CTCL revealed an overall RR was 54%, with a CR of 17%. She further concluded after examination of her data *(70,71)* that the lowest dose with efficacy and tolerability was 3 mU daily, and that there appeared to be a dose-response correlation because patients who did not respond to a lower dose could have a response induced by dose escalation. Whether efficacy can be seen with alternate-day dosing, as in other tumors, is unclear. Papa's study *(72)* showed that although an objective response could generally be seen by 3–5 mo, the achievement of maximal response may take much longer *(70)*. Additionally, although patients with all stages

Table 3
Studies of IFN Treatment in SS

Investigator	Type IFN	Dose	SS/ Total patients	Response CR	PR	Duration	Pre-treatment
Bunn (69)	IFNα2a	50 mu/m^2 TIW indefinitely	5/20 (T$_4$)	–	2/5 all patients	Median 5 mo	Yes
Tura (74)	IFNα2a	3 mu ×3 d 9 mu ×3 d 18 mu ×3 mo until 3 mo after CR	2/15 (SS)	–	2/2	–	12/15 yes
Nicholas (75)	IFNα2a	6 mu QD × 1 mo	1/6 (SS)	–	1/1	4 mo	No
Olsen (71)	IFNα2a	3 mu QD × 10 wk vs 36 mu QD (3 mu QD × 3, 18 mu QD × 3, 36 mu) TIW maintenance	2/22 (SS)	–	–	–	Yes
Kohn (73)	IFNα2a	10 mu/m^2 D1 50 mu/D$_2$-5 Q3 wk × 4 if CR	6/24 (T$_4$) 5/24 (B$_1$)	–	–	Median 8 mo all patients	Yes
Papa (72)	IFNα2a	3 mu with increase by 3 mu Q3D 18 mu ×12 wk maintenance TIW	6/43 (SS)	–	2/2	–	4—no 2—yes
Jumbou (76)	IFNα2a	6 mu QD × 1 mo decrease to 3 mu QD maintenance TIW indefinitely	11/51 (SS)	2/11	1/11	Mean period response 31 mo	35—no 21—yes
Kaplan (77)	IFN	0.25 mg/m^2/d ×1 wk 0.5 mg/m^2/d ×8 wk	3/16 (Stage III)	–	1/3	19 mo	Yes

Table 4
Studies of IFN and Retinoid Treatment in SS

Investigator	Type IFN	Dose	SS/ Total patients	Response		Duration	Pretreatment
				CR	PR		
Thestrup-Pederson (78)	IFN 2a + etretinate	3 mu ×3 d, then Q4D increase 9, 18, then 36 mu ×3 mo then TIW + etretinate 0.7 mg/kg	2/7 (T$_4$)	–	–	–	Yes
Dreno (79)	IFN 2a + etretinate	6–9 mu QD ×3 mo if NR, add etretinate 0.5 mg/kg/d	13/45 (SS)	–	2 combo 3 IFN	–	Most yes
Altomare (80)	IFN 2b + etretinate	1 mu/m^2/d ×3 d then 2.5, then 5 mu/m^2 on d7 ×12 wk + etretinate 0.75 mg/kg/d	2/13 (stage III)	1		10 mo	1 Yes

of CTCL showed responses, patients with visceral disease were unlikely to respond *(70,73)*.

Table 3 tabulates the data published in the English medical literature that is specifically related to the treatment of patients with SS. In keeping with the data for published studies of patients with all stages of CTCL treated with IFN, the overall RR was 48%, with a CR of 9%.

Kaplan *(77)* studied the utility of treatment with another IFN, treating 16 patients with stage IB to IVB CTCL with IFN-γ for 8 wk. The overall RR was 31%. All responses seen were PRs. A similar RR was achieved in the small group of patients with stage III CTCL.

Several investigators have also attempted to use IFN in combination with retinoids in the treatment of patients with CTCL. Table 4 tabulates series that specifically mention treatment of patients with SS *(78–80)*. In these series, both types of IFN have been used in combination with etretinate, a pan-retinoid. Although the information about RRs in patients with SS is limited, after tabulation of all series utilizing IFN and retinoid combinations, Olsen (70) concluded that the responses achieved with the combination were the same as the responses achieved with IFN as a single agent.

Extracorporeal Photopheresis

In 1974, Edelson—and later, other groups *(11)*—showed that SS could be palliated by the use of aggressive leukapheresis *(81)*. The treatment of the erythrodermic form of CTCL with EP, a more efficient type of leukapheresis was first described by the same author in 1987 *(81)*. In this multicenter trial, the photopheresis instrument was introduced, a device that integrates an initial discontinuous leukapheresis procedure with the subsequent exposure of the buffy-coat product to UVA light in a single device. The photopheresis procedure utilized in this study involved ingestion of 8-MOPP by the subjects. One to two hours later, the subjects had an intravenous (iv) needle placed, and their leukocytes were separated from the erythrocytes by centrifugation of the blood in the photopheresis instrument. Then, 240 cc of methoxsalen containing leukocytes were exposed to UVA (2J/cm2) by passage through a 1-mm pathway in a sterile disposable cassette contained within the machine. This was followed by a return of the treated cells through the same iv needle to the patient. In this study, the procedure was performed on two consecutive days at 4-wk intervals.

Thirty-three patients with the erythrodermic form of CTCL—all of whom had been previously treated with some other modality, most commonly systemic chemotherapy—entered the study. A skin score was tabulated as the sum of the products of severity and surface-area percentage to allow a determination of these patients' response. On the basis of these skin scores, 24 of 29 patients who were evaluable for response (83%) had a documented response, some with a prolonged duration. Of all the patients treated, 27 of 37 patients responded, with an average 64% decrease in cutaneous involvement after 22 ± 10 wk. Complications of treatment were minimal *(82)*.

Given these encouraging results, multiple single-institution experiences with EP in the treatment of CTCL have been published, many of them retrospective. Considering the results of the initial trial, the majority of the patients described in the literature have had the erythrodermic form of CTCL In some instances, patients may have been treated with an accelerated treatment program, with treatments given every 1–2 wk. Additionally, after the maintenance of a response for 6 mo, a tapering schedule was generally used. In a review of the largest series of patients with CTCL treated with EP, Zic *(83)* notes that in the 136 patients with erythrodermic CTCL described, a RR of 55% was observed, with CR of 16%. It is unclear whether treatment with EP can prolong patient survival *(85)*.

Ideal candidates for EP have included patients with circulating Sézary cells, normal or modestly elevated leukocyte counts (<15,000), and preservation of CD8 counts (>15%). Patients with bulky lymphadenopathy and/or visceral disease are unlikely to respond to EP alone *(84)*. The occurrence of nausea, which sometimes follows the ingestion of 8-MOPP, should be diminished by newer machines that allow liquid 8-MOPP to be injected directly into the extracorporeal system, eliminating the need for oral ingestion by the patient.

The mechanism through which response is achieved with EP is not clear. When cells are exposed simultaneously to 8-MOPP and UVA, covalently linked DNA strands result. Edelson certainly demonstrated that the treated and reinfused cells have such decreased viability *(82)*, but as the majority of tumor cells are not being treated, other mechanisms must exist. The most commonly accepted mechanism invokes the increased quantities of antigen peptides that have been demonstrated on the surface of 8-MOP-treated cells. The reinfusion of these cells would then engender an enhanced cytotoxic response against similar neoplastic cells *(83,85)*.

Many studies have utilized adjunctive treatments to EP such as IFN *(83,85)* or retinoids *(87)*, but these studies have involved small numbers of patients and have not been performed in a systematic fashion. Then, although the use of EP in the treatment of patients with SS is a safe, viable, and fairly well-studied option, the advisability of the use of adjunctive treatments with EP is unclear, and is dependent on the clinical situation.

Retinoids

Retinoids are vitamin A analogs that include natural derivatives of vitamin A (retinoic acid) and synthetic derivatives. They are known to affect neoplastic cells through the inhibition of cell proliferation, by the induction of apoptosis, and the promotion of cell differentiation *(88)*. These biologic effects are mediated through specific nuclear receptors in cells. The two major types of nuclear retinoic acid receptors are retinoic acid receptors (RAR) and retinoic x receptors (RXR).

Since Wieselthier and Koh's *(11)* review of panretinoids (affecting both types of RARs) in the treatment of patients with SS, little new material has been published regarding the use of panretinoids. In general, it appears that the panretinoids may produce a higher RR and CR rate in patients with earlier stages of CTCL *(88)* compared with patients with erythrodermic CTCL. It also appears that patients with erythrodermic CTCL may be particularly sensitive to the known mucocutaneous side effects of panretinoids, experiencing increased exfoliation, and erythema in the first 1–2 mo on the retinoids, often necessitating discontinuation of treatment *(89)*.

Kuzel et al. *(90)* reported on the use of a RAR-specific retinoid, all trans retinoic acid (ATRA), in the treatment of MF, in a study of 29 patients who had failed at least one previous therapy. Patients were treated with 45 mg/m2 in two daily doses. The median number of previous therapies experienced by these patients was three. The overall RR was 17%, with a median duration of remission of 4.5 mo.

More recently, Duvic et al. *(91)* reported the results of a multi-institution phase II trial of a new synthetic RXR specific drug known as bexarotene. This rexinoid was recently approved by the Food and Drug Administration (FDA) in the United States for the treatment of the cutaneous manifestations of patients with CTCL who are refractory to one prior treatment. The study involved 94 patients with stage IIB-IVB CTCL who had proven refractory to at least one prior systemic treatment. A total of 56 patients were treated with the approved dose of 300 mg/m2/day orally; the remainder was treated with greater doses. A median of five therapies preceded the participation of these patients' in the study. Of the patients who received a 300 mg/m2 dose, 32% had stage III disease, and 27% of patients had known circulation of Sézary cells. Rigid response criteria were used in this trial, consisting of a Physicians Global Assessment of Clinical Condition score and a Composite Assessment of Index Lesions Disease Severity score. A Primary Endpoint Classification, the highest confirmed response on either response criteria determined the final response designation.

Utilizing these response measures, 24% of patients with SS showed a response to treatment manifested by decreased erythema and scaling within 8 wk. Some patients had a temporary reduction in their CD4 + CD7 − circulating cells. Improvement in secondary end points, such as the size of lymphadenopathy and a decrease in the patients' perception of pruritus, were also seen.

A RR of 45% (CR 2%) was seen in the entire study group who received 300 mg/m2/d with a median duration of response of 299 d, and a median time to response of 180 d. A suggestion of a dose-response effect was seen when the group of 38 patients receiving a dose higher than 300 mg/m2/d was examined. This group of patients experienced a RR of 55% with a CR of 13% (pathologically documented).

Side effects were not rare, but were manageable. The most common side effects seen were hypertriglyceridemia (occasionally associated with pancreatitis) and elevated cholesterol. The majority of patients required the addition of anti-lipid-lowering agents. A central but reversible hypothyroidism was also seen, sometimes requiring thyroid replacement. Headaches were occasionally noted. It should be remembered that all retinoids are potent teratogens, and that a proper method of contraception should be offered to all patients of child-bearing age.

Interestingly, 28 patients on the study had received prior treatment with other retinoids, and 54% of these patients experienced a response to bexarotene, with a 14% CR. Notably, this trial is unique among trials examining retinoids, as rigid, objective response criteria were utilized in a multi- institution setting. The study population was also heavily pretreated, and was documented as such. It remains difficult to compare this data to older trials utilizing other retinoid preparations, who were found to have a 30% RR for patients with SS in the conglomerate *(11)*.

Fusion Toxins

Denileukin diftitox (DAB389IL-2, ONTAK) is a novel recombinant fusion protein consisting of peptide sequences for the enzymatically active and membrane translocatory domains of diphtheria toxin and human interleukin (IL)-2. This single-polypeptide chain is then capable of binding to the surface of cells expressing the IL-2 receptor (IL2-R) and inhibiting their protein synthesis, thereby causing the cell's death *(92)*.

The human IL2R consists of three subunits, the (p55, CD25), (p75, CD122), and (p65, CD132) subunits. The CD122 and CD 132 proteins together define an intermediate-affinity IL2- R; CD25 protein defines a low-affinity receptor; all three define the high-affinity receptor. Although DAB389IL2 will bind to all three forms of the IL2R, only cells that have the intermediate or high-affinity receptor will internalize the toxin. Expression of the high-affinity IL2R is normally limited to activated T- or B-lymphocytes or macrophages; however, expression of one or more IL2R subunits can be seen in neoplasms of lymphoid origin, including CTCL.

DAB389IL2 (ONTAK) has been approved by the FDA for the treatment of patients with CTCL who are refractory to other treatments, and whose tumor cells can be demonstrated by immunohistochemical means to express CD25 in ≥20% of cells. Olsen et al. *(92)* reported the results of a phase III, multi-institution trial that randomized patients with refractory CTCL stage IB-IVA to two dose levels of DAB389IL2.

To be eligible for participation, patients were to have biopsy-proven CTCL, with ≥20% of their tumor cells expressing CD25. Patients were required to have recurrent or persistent disease after at least four prior treatments, or if stage IVA, failed at least one prior treatment regimen. Patients were randomized to treatment with one of two dose levels, 9 or 18gm/kg/d of DAB389IL2 given intravenously over 15 min-1 h on five consecutive days every 21 d. Acetaminophen and antihistamines were allowed for premedication, but no steroids could be used.

A rigorous analysis of response was undertaken to assess total tumor burden, which used a severity-weighted assessment tool (including an erythroderma scale) to assess skin, flow cytometry to assess blood, and examination of nodes by physical examination and CT scanning. An independent panel of physicians verified all responses.

A group of 71 patients were randomly assigned and treated. Overall, 63% of patients had stage IIB or greater disease. The patients had received a median of five previous therapies. Overall, 30% of the patients had an objective response, with 10% CR. The difference in RR between the two dose levels was not statistically significant. However, a trend toward improved RR with the higher dose in patients with more advanced disease ($\geq$stage IIB) was seen. This is exemplified by the responses of patients who were classified as stage III. The lower dose group without response (0 of 5) and the higher dose group with a RR of 33% (2 of 6).

The median time to first response was 6 wk, and the median duration of response was 6.9 mo. Documented objective responses were paralleled by a statistically significant improvement in quality of life as measured by patient responses to a FACT-G. Quality of life was not adversely affected in non-responders.

Most side effects were seen within the first two courses of treatment. The most common toxicities included constitutional symptoms and symptoms related to hypersensitivity, which occurred during infusion. These may be ameliorated in the future with steroid pretreatment, which could not be given during the trial. Reversible abnormalities in liver function tests were also seen, largely resolving by the beginning of the second cycle of treatment.

A vascular capillary leak syndrome (VLS) was seen and retrospectively defined as the simultaneous occurrence of hypoalbuminemia ($\leq$2.8 g/dL), edema, and/or hypotension. This syndrome occurred within 14 d of treatment. It was usually self-limited, but when treatment was required, it consisted of treatment for the primary clinical problem—mild diuretics for fluid overload, and/or hydration for patients who experience hypotension. Thirteen patients who experienced VLS were retreated, the majority with no ill effect. Those who developed VLS on rechallenge had albumen $\leq$2.8 mg/dL at the start of the course in which the second episode of VLS occurred. An albumen <3 g/dL at the start of treatment and/or preexisting edema seemed to predict for the occurrence of VLS, and may predispose to the syndrome.

Then, DAB389IL2 (ONTAK) is a novel genetically engineered agent with substantial activity in patients diagnosed with CTCL, whose disease is refractory to other agents. Like the preceding treatment options, myelosuppression and/or immunosuppression do not occur with this treatment, making it an attractive tool in the treatment of the highly symptomatic patient with CTCL. In general, clinical benefit was seen during the first two cycles of treatment, allowing the clinician to make treatment decisions for their patients with a short trial of the drug.

The question remains whether screening for the presence of CD 25 is an adequate method of screening for likelihood of response to DAB389IL2. During the trial, results from multiple biopsies taken from different anatomic sites on different days from the same patient yielded variable results. In 44% of the patients examined, there were conflicting results regarding the level of CD25 expression. Whether this variable is biologic and caused by the relative insensitivity of the test is unknown. It is also unclear whether patients whose neoplastic cells have a level of CD25 expression below this threshold will benefit from treatment with the drug. A study designed to answer this question is in progress.

Additionally, evidence from Foss *(93)* suggests that retinoids, such as ATRA, may upregulate the expression of CD25 on mycosis fungoides (MF) cell lines, perhaps allowing the cells to be more sensitive to treatment with agents such as DAB389IL2. Such sequencing of treatment in patients may provide a productive avenue for future research trials.

Single-Agent Chemotherapy

Results with treatment of small numbers of patients with MF/SS using single-agent chemotherapy such as prednisone, cisplatin, velban, bleomycin, etoposide, or VM-26 have been published in the English medical literature *(94,95)*. Although it is unclear whether one agent is clearly superior to the other, most information focuses on the treatment of patients with SS with the so-called Winkelmann regimen—chlorambucil and prednisone—and its variants, and with the use of methotrexate.

At least three series recount results in patients with SS who have been treated with chlorambucil and prednisone. The usual dose of chlorambucil used has been 4 mg orally daily combined with prednisone 20 mg orally given daily. In three studies *(96–98)* that were mostly retrospective, a total of 59 patients with SS were described. Most patients were believed to have a response to this regimen, with CR of 15% reported. Most recently, Coors *(99)* has reported on a variation of this regimen employing chlorambucil 10–12 mg oral daily for 3 d with fluocortolone 75 mg orally the first day, and tapering by 25 mg each subsequent day with treatments every 2 wk. In a study involving 13 erythrodermic patients with CTCL who were previously untreated, 11 with circulating cells, 54% of patients were believed to have a clinical CR, and the remainder to have partial responses. The mean duration of remission was 16.5 mo. Most responses were seen after three cycles. Oral daily cytoxan has also been used with some efficacy (personal experience). These regimens are simple and appear to be efficacious in the palliation of symptoms; however, the leukemogenic potential of the alkylating agents may dampen enthusiasm for their use as primary treatments.

Table 5
Studies of Purine Analogs in the Treatment of SS

Investigator	Treatment	SS/Total	Response		Duration response	Pretreated
			CR	PR		
Mercleca (101)	Deoxycoformycin 4 mg/m²/wk × 4 then Q2 wk	$\frac{16\ SS}{145}$	3	7	CR up to 7 yr PR 3–12 mo	67% pretreated
Greiner (102)	4.5 mg/m² Q 1–4 wk	$\frac{3}{18}$ (stage III)	1	–	Disease-free survival 76 mo	Some
Ho For EORTC (103)	4 mg/m² Q wk × 3, then Q 2 wk × 6, then Q 4 wk × 6 mo	$\frac{21\ SS}{76}$	1	6	Disease-free survival 24.9 wk	81% ≤1 prior regimen 19% ≥2
Kurzrock (104)	3.75–5 mg/m² iv ×3 d Q3 wk	$\frac{14\ SS}{28}$	4	6	Median response duration 3.5 mo	Yes
Foss (105)	4 mg/m² iv d1–3 + IFN α2a 10 mu/m² im d 22, then 50 mu/m² d 23–26	$\frac{18\ T}{41}$	2	–	Median progression-free survival 13.1 mo	6/41 naïve
Saven (106)	2 chlordeoxyadenosine 0.1 mg/kg/d × 7d Q 28 d	$\frac{3\ SS}{15}$	–	1	5 mo	Yes
Kong (107)	Some patients had 5d, by continuous infusion or 2-h infusion	$\frac{7}{25}$ (stage III)	1	1	Median duration CR 4.5 mo; PR 2 mo	Yes
Foss (108)	Fludarabine 25 mg/m² d1–5 q 28 D + IFNα 5 mu TIW	$\frac{13\ T}{35}$	3	6	Median progression-free survival 5.9 mo	Yes: 21/35
Scarisbrick (109)	18 mg/m² × 3 d + cytoxan 250 mg/m² + GCSF × 3d	$\frac{8\ SS}{12}$ 5 evaluable	1	4	Median duration response 10 mo	Yes

The use of methotrexate in this patient population was described in a retrospective review by Zackheim *(99)*. Seventeen patients with SS were treated with methotrexate doses ranging from 10–15 mg orally every week to 50 mg intravenously. CR was observed to be 41% and overall RR to be 76%, with a concomitant decrease in circulating Sézary cells with skin improvement. Improvement was usually seen in the first 2 mo of therapy. Duration of these responses ranged from 9–63 mo. Such simple and relatively nontoxic therapy remains attractive, despite the advent of newer chemotherapeutic agents.

Many studies have focused on the use of purine analogs such as deoxycoformycin, fludarabine, and chlorodeoxyadenosine because of the theoretic vulnerability of T-lymphocytes to agents whose mechanism of action involves adenosine deaminase. Table 5 includes all studies in the English literature that have examined these purine analogs in patients with SS.

Overall, with respect to the use of deoxycoformycin, perhaps the most heavily studied agent, the RR is 40% and CR is 15%, very similar to the rates determined by Foss *(110)* in her review of the use of purine analogs in CTCL. Mercieca *(101)* and Kurzrock's *(104)* data are notable for the demonstration of a particularly high rate of response in patients with SS compared to patients with classical MF. For instance, in Mercieca's study, the RR for patients with SS was 62%, compared with an overall RR for patients with classical MF of 30% *(101)*. Despite these dramatic response rates, the duration of responses is short, and few patients experience long-term remissions.

Ho *(103)* noted that most responses were rapid, with one-third of patients in that study experiencing responses in the first 3 wk. Kurzrock *(104)* also noted that some patients experience a "flare" in their erythroderma upon initiation of treatment. Finally, there appears to be no augmentation of the response rate with the addition of IFN to deoxycoformycin (105).

It is important to note that all of the purine analogs are associated with a sometimes sustained decrease in CD4 positive lymphocytes. In these studies, the rate of infection, particularly with herpesvirus, was high—ranging from 19% HSV infections *(104)* to 17% herpes zoster sometimes disseminated *(105)*. This is particularly troubling in this patient population, where immunoincompetence is frequently documented, as are infections with herpes viruses.

Similar response rates are documented with the use of 2´chlorodeoxyadenosine; however, with relatively high rates of myelosuppression, which can be prolonged and insidious *(107)*. When the drug was administered by continuous infusion requiring indwelling catheter placement, a significant amount of catheter-related, bacteremias were seen *(107)*.

Despite the disappointing RR of 19% noted in the Southwest Oncology Group study of fludarabine in CTCL *(111)*, combinations of this drug with IFN- and with cytoxan have been studied *(108,109)*. The prolonged and frequent myelosuppression demonstrated in each of these studies and the accompanying opportunistic infections make these regimens undesirable in this palliative setting.

Table 6
Studies of Combined Chemotherapy in the Treatment of SS

Investigator	Treatment	SS/Total	Response CR	Response PR	Duration response	Pretreated
Tirelli (116)	CVP	2/9	–	–	— / Overall RR 66% CR 44%	Some yes Comment:
Sentis (117)	CVP	2/17	–	1	—	No
Zakem (118)	BAMM	4/10 T$_4$	2	–	4–36 + mo	Yes
Doberauer (119)	VP16, bleomycin, methotrexate	4/11 T$_4$	–	1	3 mo	Yes
Schappell (120)	Methotrexate 5 FU, leukovorin	2 SS/10	"excellent"		26–78 mo duration response	Yes
Fierro (121)	VICOP-B 12 wk idarubicin, cytoxan, VP16, vincristine, bleomycin	2/25	No responses		— / 32% grade IV neutropenia	10/25 yes Comment: overall RR 84% median duration 8.7 mo
Fierro (122)	CVP, CHOP	13/35	–	1	5.9 mo / Overall RR 30%	Yes Comment:
Foss (123)	EPOCH + GCSF	6/15	2	–	Median progression-free survival 8 mo	Yes Comment: 61% grade III, IV hematologic toxicity 40% staph bacteremia

Newer agents, which have not been studied specifically in patients with SS, have shown efficacy in the palliative treatment of patients with CTCL, and show promise. Zinzanc *(112)* described the treatment of 30 patients with tumor or erythrodermic-phase CTCL with gemcitabine. Gemcitabine was given every wk for 3 wk with 1-wk rest at a dose of 1200 mg/m2 intravenously each day for a total of three courses. CR were observed in 10% of patients, with an overall RR of 70%. The median duration of all responses was 15 mo. No grade III or IV hematologic toxicity was seen.

Adriamycin was described as an effective agent in the treatment of patients with CTCL in 1977 *(113)*; however, the specter of cardiotoxicity and alopecia have made this drug less desirable in this palliative setting. Recently, the newer pegalated anthracyclines have been studied *(114)*. Treating 10 patients with various stages of recalcitrant or relapsing CTCL (none in stage III) with peg-doxorubicin at a dose of 20 mg/m2 monthly, a CR of 55%, and overall RR of 80% was reported. The median response duration was 15.7 mo. Only one patient experienced a grade IV hematologic toxicity (anemia). In a phase I study of temazolomide *(115)*, responses in patients with CTCL were observed when the drug was given 150 mg/m2 orally for 5 d monthly. Clearly, these new agents merit further study in this patient population.

Combination Chemotherapy

Table 6 tabulates series utilizing combination chemotherapies in the treatment of patients with SS. Most regimens combine the drugs cytoxan, adriamycin, vincristine, and prednisone with permutations of bleomycin and methotrexate. The overall RR of these patients is 34%, lower than the RR of 81% when Bunn *(88)* evaluated trials studied all stages of CTCL. Response durations are short. Particularly in studies utilizing indwelling catheters *(123)*, the risk of bacteremia is high.

Although a number of single-agent and combination chemotherapy regimens have demonstrated efficacy, the goal of therapy at this time for patients with SS is palliative. As such, the increased toxicity and risk of myelosuppression seen with combination regimens must be carefully weighed against the possible benefit to the patient.

The value of high-dose therapy is unclear. Bigler *(124)* reported on the use of autologous transplantation in six patients with advanced CTCL (stage IIB and IV) in which various preparative regimens were used. Although five of the six patients experienced at CR, three of the patients who experienced complete responses had relapsed by 100 d.

To date, there is only one case report of a patient with refractory SS who was successfully treated with an allogeneic—in this case unrelated—donor bone-marrow transplant *(125)*. Studies of so-called mini allogeneic transplants are underway in this patient population.

Combined Modality Therapy

The first prospective randomized trial examining treatment options for patients with CTCL was performed at the NCI and was reported in 1989 *(126)*. In this trial, 103 patients with various stages of CTCL were randomized to receive sequential palliative single-modality/agent therapy (topical nitrogen mustard, PUVA, TSEBT, and finally, oral methotrexate) vs combination chemotherapy with cytoxan, doxorubicin, etoposide, and vincristine for 8 courses combined with TSEBT. Despite a statistically significant increase in RR for the combined modality therapy at the expense of increased toxicity, the disease-free survival in both groups was unchanged. Subsequent single-institution trials have yielded similar results *(127–129)*. This approach would be most appropriate in the setting of rapidly progressive advanced disease, or perhaps transformed disease where an increased response rate may outweigh increased toxicity.

Miscellaneous Treatments

Cytokine therapy has been utilized in small numbers of patient with CTCL. The use of IL-2 therapy has been described by two groups. Gisselbrecht *(130)* used 20 mU/m2/d of IL-2 by continuous infusion for 5 d wk 1, for 3 d wk 4, and for 3 d wk 5 in 61 patients with lymphoma. Among the patient groups were two patients with SS and two patients with MF who experienced PR. Marolleau*(131)* also described the use of high-dose IL-2 in a similar schedule, including three patients with SS in the study group. One patient experienced a PR. These responses were achieved with significant cardiovascular toxicity. There have been no reports in the literature of the use of lower doses of IL-2, which may be attainable in an outpatient setting with less toxicity.

The use of IL-12 in a phase I trial was reported by Rook *(132)*. Of 10 patients with refractory CTCL, two patients with SS were treated with one PR, and toxicity was tolerable.

Cyclosporine has been utilized as an agent that may palliate the pruritus and erythema of SS, despite continuing concerns about the resultant immunosuppression. Four single case reports, utilizing doses of 12–17.5 mg orally, suggest that response durations of 4–14+ mo can be achieved with this therapy *(11)*. A series of five patients, including two with SS *(133)* also demonstrated a favorable response in some patients.

Finally, agents such as campath 1 H, a human anti-CD 52 monoclonal antibody (MAb) that affects both B- and T-lymphocytes, may prove to be efficacious for the treatment of patients with CTCL. In a multicenter Phase II trial of campath treatment in advanced, low-grade non-Hodgkin's lymphomas *(134)*, previously treated patients received 30 mg of campath in a 2-h infusion 3× weekly for a maximum of 12 wk. Four of eight patients with MF treated in this way responded to treatment, including two CRs. Median time to progression was 10 mo.

It should be noted, however, that in the entire group, seven patients were diagnosed with opportunistic infections including HSV reactivation, thrush, Pneumocystis, CMV pneumonitis, aspergillus infection, and disseminated tuberculosis. Of 50 total patients, three patients died of infection. Perhaps with more experience in the use of this drug and in the prophylaxis against the opportunistic infections that it engenders, this agent will prove promising in the treatment of patients with CTCL.

CONCLUSION

In summary, SS should be considered a distinct clinicopathologic entity in which palliative systemic therapy is most useful. Studies of novel therapeutic modalities such as mini allogeneic bone-marrow transplantation may ultimately yield a curative approach to this devastating syndrome.

REFERENCES

1. Sézary A, Bouvrain Y. Erythrodermie avec presence de cellules monstreuses dans le derme et dans le sang circulant. *Bull Soc Fr Dermatol Syphiligr* 1938; 45:254–260.
2. Taswell HF, Winkelmann BK. Sézary syndrome—a malignant reticulemic erythroderma. *J Am Med Assoc* 1961; 117:465–472.
3. Lamberg SI, Bunn PA Jr. Cutaneous T-cell lymphomas. Summary of the Mycosis Fungoides Cooperative Group-National Cancer Institute Workshop. *Arch Dermatol* 1979; Sep;115(9): 1103–1105.
4. Weinstock MA, Horm JW. Population-based estimate of survival and determinants of prognosis in patients with mycosis fungoides. *Cancer* 1988; 62(8):1658–1661.
5. Weinstock MA, Gardstein B. Twenty-year trends in the reported incidence of mycosis fungoides and associated mortality. *Am J Public Health* 1999; (8):1240–1244.
6. Koh HK, Charif M, Weinstock MA. Epidemiology and clinical manifestations of cutaneous T-cell lymphoma. *Hematol Oncol Clin N Am* 1995; (5):943–960.
7. Tokura Y, Heald PW, Yan SL, Edelson RL. Stimulation of cutaneous T-cell lymphoma cells with superantigenic staphylococcal toxins. *J Invest Dermatol* 1992; 98(1):33–37.
8. Tokura Y, Yagi H, Ohshima A, Kurokawa S, Wakita H, Yokote R, et al. Cutaneous colonization with staphylococci influences the disease activity of Sezary syndrome: a potential role for bacterial superantigens. *Br J Dermatol* 1995; 133(1):6–12.
9. Jackow CM, Cather JC, Hearne V, Asano AT, Musser JM, Duvic M. Association of erythrodermic cutaneous T-cell lymphoma, superantigen-positive Staphylococcus aureus, and oligoclonal T-cell receptor V beta gene expansion. *Blood* 1997; 89(1):32–40.
10. Winkelmann RK. Clinical studies of T-cell erythroderma in the Sezary syndrome. *Mayo Clin Proc* 1974; 49(8):519–525.
11. Wieselthier JS, Koh HK. Sezary syndrome: diagnosis, prognosis, and critical review of treatment options. *J Am Acad Dermatol* 1990; 22(3):381–401.
12. Schein PS, Macdonald JS, Edelson R. Cutaneous T-cell lymphoma. *Cancer* 1976; 38(4): 1859–1861.
13. Buechner SA, Winkelmann RK. Sezary syndrome. A clinicopathologic study of 39 cases. *Arch Dermatol* 1983; 119(12):979–986.

14. Trotter MJ, Whittaker SJ, Orchard GE, Smith NP. Cutaneous histopathology of Sezary syndrome: a study of 41 cases with a proven circulating T-cell clone. *J Cutan Pathol* 1997; 24(5):286–291.
15. Weinberg JM, Jaworsky C, Benoit BM, Telegan B, Rook AH, Lessin SR. The clonal nature of circulating Sezary cells. *Blood* 1995; 86(11):4257–4262.
16. Galindo LM, Garcia FU, Hanau CA, Lessin SR, Jhala N, Bigler RD, et al. Fine-needle aspiration biopsy in the evaluation of lymphadenopathy associated with cutaneous T-cell lymphoma (mycosis fungoides/Sezary syndrome). *Am J Clin Pathol* 2000; 113(6): 865–871.
17. Duncan SC, Winkelmann RK. Circulating Sezary cells in hospitalized dermatology patients. *Br J Dermatol* 1978; 99(2):171–178.
18. Meyer CJ, van Leeuwen AW, van der Loo EM, van de Putte LB, van Vloten WA. Cerebriform (Sezary like) mononuclear cells in healthy individuals: a morphologically distinct population of T cells. Relationship with mycosis fungoides and Sezary's syndrome. *Virchows Arch B Cell Pathol* 1977; 25(2):95–104.
19. Vonderheid EC, Bernengo MG, Burg G, Duvic M, Heald P, Laroche L, et al. Update on erythrodermic cutaneous t cell lymphoma: report of the International Society for Cutaneous Lymphomas. Submitted.
20. Harmon CB, Witzig TE, Katzmann JA, Pittelkow MR. Detection of circulating T cells with CD4+CD7− immunophenotype in patients with benign and malignant lymphoproliferative dermatoses. *J Am Acad Dermatol* 1996; 35(3 Pt 1):404–410.
21. Scala E, Russo G, Cadoni S, Narducci MG, Girardelli CR, De Pita O, et al. Skewed expression of activation, differentiation and homing-related antigens in circulating cells from patients with cutaneous T cell lymphoma associated with CD7-T helper lymphocytes expansion. *J Invest Dermatol* 1999, 113(4):622–627.
22. Bernengo MG, Novelli M, Quaglino P, Lisa F, De Matteis A, Savoia P, et al. The relevance of the CD4+ CD26− subset in the identification of circulating Sezary cells. *Br J Dermatol* 2001; 144(1):125–135.
23. Jones D, Dang NH, Duvic M, Washington LT, Huh YO. Absence of CD26 expression is a useful marker for diagnosis of T-cell lymphoma in peripheral blood. *Am J Clin Pathol* 2001; 115(6):885–892.
24. Johnson GA, Dewald GW, Strand WR, Winkelmann RK. Chromosome studies in 17 patients with the Sezary syndrome. *Cancer* 1985; 55(10):2426–2433.
25. Nowell PC, Vonderheid EC, Besa E, Hoxie JA, Moreau L, Finan JB. The most common chromosome change in 86 chronic B cell or T cell tumors: a 14q32 translocation. *Cancer Genet Cytogenet* 1986; 19(3–4):219–227.
26. Karenko L, Hyytinen E, Sarna S, Ranki A. Chromosomal abnormalities in cutaneous T-cell lymphoma and in its premalignant conditions as detected by G-banding and interphase cytogenetic methods. *J Invest Dermatol* 1997; 108(1):22–29.
27. Thangavelu M, Finn WG, Yelavarthi KK, Roenigk HH Jr, Samuelson E, Peterson L, et al. Recurring structural chromosome abnormalities in peripheral blood lymphocytes of patients with mycosis fungoides/Sezary syndrome. *Blood* 1997; 89(9):3371–3377.
28. Bakels V, van Oostveen JW, Gordijn RL, Walboomers JM, Meijer CJ, Willemze R. Diagnostic value of T-cell receptor beta gene rearrangement analysis on peripheral blood lymphocytes of patients with erythroderma. *J Invest Dermatol* 1991; 97(5):782–786.
29. Dommann SN, Dommann-Scherrer CC, Dours-Zimmermann MT, Zimmermann DR, Kural-Serbes B, Burg G. Clonal disease in extracutaneous compartments in cutaneous T-cell lymphomas. A comparative study between cutaneous T-cell lymphomas and pseudo lymphomas. *Arch Dermatol Res* 1996; 288(4):163–167.

30. Fraser-Andrews EA, Woolford AJ, Russell-Jones R, Seed PT, Whittaker SJ. Detection of a peripheral blood T cell clone is an independent prognostic marker in mycosis fungoides. *J Invest Dermatol* 2000; 114(1):117–121.

31. Muche JM, Lukowsky A, Asadullah K, Gellrich S, Sterry W. Demonstration of frequent occurrence of clonal T cells in the peripheral blood of patients with primary cutaneous T-cell lymphoma. *Blood* 1997; 90(4):1636–1642.

32. Delfau-Larue MH, Laroche L, Wechsler J, Lepage E, Lahet C, Asso-Bonnet M, et al. Diagnostic value of dominant T-cell clones in peripheral blood in 363 patients presenting consecutively with a clinical suspicion of cutaneous lymphoma. *Blood* 2000; 96(9):2987–2992.

33. Robert C, Kupper TS. Inflammatory skin diseases, T cells, and immune surveillance. *N Engl J Med* 1999; 341(24):1817–1828.

34. Vowels BR, Cassin M, Vonderheid EC, Rook AH. Aberrant cytokine production by Sezary syndrome patients: cytokine secretion pattern resembles murine Th2 cells. *J Invest Dermatol* 1992; 99(1):90–94.

35. Rook AH, Heald P. The immunopathogenesis of cutaneous T-cell lymphoma. *Hematol Oncol Clin N Am* 1995; 9(5):997–1010.

36. Rook AH, Kubin M, Cassin M, Vonderheid EC, Vowels BR, Wolfe JT, et al. IL-12 reverses cytokine and immune abnormalities in Sezary syndrome. *J Immunol* 1995; 154(3):1491–1498.

37. Dalloul A, Laroche L, Bagot M, Mossalayi MD, Fourcade C, Thacker DJ, et al. Interleukin-7 is a growth factor for Sezary lymphoma cells. *J Clin Invest* 1992; 90(3):1054–1060.

38. Foss FM, Koc Y, Stetler-Stevenson MA, Nguyen DT, O'Brien MC, Turner R, et al. Costimulation of cutaneous T-cell lymphoma cells by interleukin-7 and interleukin-2: potential autocrine or paracrine effectors in the Sezary syndrome. *J Clin Oncol* 1994; 12(2):326–335.

39. Bunn PA Jr, Lamberg SI. Report of the Committee on Staging and Classification of Cutaneous T-Cell Lymphomas. *Cancer Treat Rep* 1979; 63(4):725–728.

40. Sausville EA, Eddy JL, Makuch RW, Fischmann AB, Schechter GP, Matthews M, et al. Histopathologic staging at initial diagnosis of mycosis fungoides and the Sezary syndrome. Definition of three distinctive prognostic groups. *Ann Intern Med* 1988; 109(5):372–382.

41. Bass JC, Korobkin MT, Cooper KD, Kane NM, Platt JF. Cutaneous T-cell lymphoma: CT in evaluation and staging. *Radiology* 1993; 186(1):273–278.

42. Foss FM, Sausville EA. Prognosis and staging of cutaneous T-cell lymphoma. *Hematol Oncol Clin N Am* 1995; 9(5):1011–1019.

43. Bunn PA Jr, Huberman MS, Whang-Peng J, Schechter GP, Guccion JG, Matthews MJ, et al. Prospective staging evaluation of patients with cutaneous T-cell lymphomas. Demonstration of a high frequency of extracutaneous dissemination. *Ann Intern Med* 1980; 93(2):223–230.

44. Salhany KE, Greer JP, Cousar JB, Collins RD. Marrow involvement in cutaneous T-cell lymphoma. A clinicopathologic study of 60 cases. *Am J Clin Pathol* 1989; 92(6):747–754.

45. Kim YH, Bishop K, Varghese A, Hoppe RT. Prognostic factors in erythrodermic mycosis fungoides and the Sezary syndrome. *Arch Dermatol* 1995; 131(9):1003–1008.

46. Wasik MA, Vonderheid EC, Bigler RD, Marti R, Lessin SR, Polansky M, et al. Increased serum concentration of the soluble interleukin-2 receptor in cutaneous T-cell lymphoma. Clinical and prognostic implications. *Arch Dermatol* 1996; 132(1):42–47.

47. Bernengo MG, Fierro MT, Novelli M, Lisa F, Appino A. Soluble interleukin-2 receptor in Sezary syndrome: its origin and clinical application. *Br J Dermatol* 1993; 128(2):124–129.

48. Axelrod PI, Lorber B, Vonderheid EC. Infections complicating mycosis fungoides and Sezary syndrome. *J Am Med Assoc* 1992; 267(10):1354–1358.

49. Posner LE, Fossieck BE Jr, Eddy JL, Bunn PA Jr. Septicemic complications of the cutaneous T-cell lymphomas. *Am J Med* 1981; 71(2):210–216.

50. Diamandidou E, Colome-Grimmer M, Fayad L, Duvic M, Kurzrock R. Transformation of mycosis fungoides/Sezary syndrome: clinical characteristics and prognosis. *Blood* 1998; 92(4):1150–1159.

51. Salhany KE, Cousar JB, Greer JP, Casey TT, Fields JP, Collins RD. Transformation of cutaneous T cell lymphoma to large cell lymphoma. A clinicopathologic and immunologic study. *Am J Pathol* 1988; 132(2):265–277.

52. Greer JP, Salhany KE, Cousar JB, Fields JP, King LE, Graber SE, et al. Clinical features associated with transformation of cerebriform T-cell lymphoma to a large cell process. *Hematol Oncol* 1990; 8(4):215–227.

53. Dmitrovsky E, Matthews MJ, Bunn PA, Schechter GP, Makuch RW, Winkler CF, et al. Cytologic transformation in cutaneous T cell lymphoma: a clinicopathologic entity associated with poor prognosis. *J Clin Oncol* 1987; 5(2):208–215.

54. Vergier B, de Muret A, Beylot-Barry M, Vaillant L, Ekouevi D, Chene G, et al. Transformation of mycosis fungoides: clinicopathological and prognostic features of 45 cases. French Study Group of Cutaneious Lymphomas. *Blood* 2000; 95(7):2212–2218.

55. Abel EA, Sendagorta E, Hoppe RT. Cutaneous malignancies and metastatic squamous cell carcinoma following topical therapies for mycosis fungoides. *J Am Acad Dermatol* 1986; 14(6):1029–1038.

56. Smoller BR, Marcus R. Risk of secondary cutaneous malignancies in patients with long-standing mycosis fungoides. *J Am Acad Dermatol* 1994; 30(2 Pt 1):201–204.

57. Scarisbrick JJ, Child FJ, Evans AV, Fraser-Andrews EA, Spittle M, Russell-Jones R. Secondary malignant neoplasms in 71 patients with Sezary syndrome. *Arch Dermatol* 1999; 135(11):1381–1385.

58. Olsen EA, Delzell E, Jegasothy BV. Second malignancies in cutaneous T cell lymphoma. *J Am Acad Dermatol* 1984; 10(2 Pt 1):197–204.

59. Kantor AF, Curtis RE, Vonderheid EC, van Scott EJ, Fraumeni JF Jr. Risk of second malignancy after cutaneous T-cell lymphoma. *Cancer* 1989; 63(8):1612–1615.

60. Vakeva L, Pukkala E, Ranki A. Increased risk of secondary cancers in patients with primary cutaneous T cell lymphoma. *J Invest Dermatol* 2000; 115(1):62–65.

61. Gilchrest BA, Parrish JA, Tanenbaum L, Haynes HA, Fitzpatrick TB. Oral methoxsalen photochemotherapy of mycosis fungoides. *Cancer* 1976; 38(2):683–689.

62. Abel EA, Sendagorta E, Hoppe RT, Hu CH. PUVA treatment of erythrodermic and plaque-type mycosis fungoides. Ten-year follow-up study. *Arch Dermatol* 1987; 123(7):897–901.

63. Kuzel TM, Roenigk HH Jr, Samuelson E, Herrmann JJ, Hurria A, Rademaker AW, et al. Effectiveness of interferon alfa-2a combined with phototherapy for mycosis fungoides and the Sézary syndrome. *J Clin Oncol* 1995; 13(1):257–263.

64. Vonderheid EC, Tan ET, Kantor AF, Shrager L, Micaily B, Van Scott EJ. Long-term efficacy, curative potential, and carcinogenicity of topical mechlorethamine chemotherapy in cutaneous T cell lymphoma. *J Am Acad Dermatol* 1989; 20(3):416–428.

65. Zackheim HS, Epstein EH Jr, McNutt NS, Grekin DA, Crain WR. Topical carmustine (BCNU) for mycosis fungoides and related disorders: a 10-year experience. *J Am Acad Dermatol* 1983; 9(3):363–374.

66. Jones GW, Hoppe RT, Glatstein E. Electron beam treatment for cutaneous T-cell lymphoma. *Hematol Oncol Clin N Am* 1995; 9(5):1057–1076.

67. Jones GW, Rosenthal D, Wilson LD. Total skin electron radiation for patients with erythrodermic cutaneous T-cell lymphoma (mycosis fungoides and the Sezary syndrome). *Cancer* 1999; 85(9):1985–1995.

68. Wilson LD, Jones GW, Kim D, Rosenthal D, Christensen IR, Edelson RL et al. Experience with total skin electron beam therapy in combination with extracorporeal photopheresis in

the management of patients with erythrodermic (T4) mycosis fungoides. *J Am Acad Dermatol* 2000; 43(1 Pt 1):54–60.

69. Bunn PA Jr, Foon KA, Ihde DC, Longo DL, Eddy J, Winkler CF, et al. Recombinant leukocyte A interferon: an active agent in advanced cutaneous T-cell lymphomas. *Ann Intern Med* 1984; 101(4):484–487.

70. Olsen EA, Bunn PA. Interferon in the treatment of cutaneous T-cell lymphoma. *Hematol Oncol Clin North Am* 1995; 9(5):1089–1107.

71. Olsen EA, Rosen ST, Vollmer RT, Variakojis D, Roenigk HH Jr, Diab N, et al. Interferon alfa-2a in the treatment of cutaneous T cell lymphoma. *J Am Acad Dermatol* 1989; 20(3):395–407.

72. Papa G, Tura S, Mandelli F, Vegna ML, Defazio D, Mazza P, et al. Is interferon alpha in cutaneous T-cell lymphoma a treatment of choice? *Br J Haematol* 1991; 79(Suppl 1):48–51.

73. Kohn EC, Steis RG, Sausville EA, Veach SR, Stocker JL, Phelps R, et al. Phase II trial of intermittent high-dose recombinant interferon alfa-2a in mycosis fungoides and the Sezary syndrome. *J Clin Oncol* 1990; 8(1):155–160.

74. Tura S, Mazza P, Zinzani PL, Ghetti PL, Poletti G, Gherlinzoni F, et al. Alpha recombinant interferon in the treatment of mycosis fungoides (MF). *Haematologica* 1987; 72(4):337–340.

75. Nicolas JF, Balblanc JC, Frappaz A, Chouvet B, Delcombel M, Thivolet J. Treatment of cutaneous T cell lymphoma with intermediate doses of interferon alpha 2a. *Dermatologica* 1989; 179(1):34–37.

76. Jumbou O, N'Guyen JM, Tessier MH, Legoux B, Dreno B. Long-term follow-up in 51 patients with mycosis fungoides and Sezary syndrome treated by interferon-alfa. *Br J Dermatol* 1999; 140(3):427–431.

77. Kaplan EH, Rosen ST, Norris DB, Roenigk HH Jr, Saks SR, Bunn PA Jr. Phase II study of recombinant human interferon gamma for treatment of cutaneous T-cell lymphoma. *J Natl Cancer Inst* 1990; 82(3):208–212.

78. Thestrup-Pedersen K, Hammer R, Kaltoft K, Sogaard H, Zachariae H. Treatment of mycosis fungoides with recombinant interferon-alpha 2a2 alone and in combination with etretinate. *Br J Dermatol* 1988; 118(6):811–818.

79. Dreno B, Celerier P, Litoux P. Roferon-A in combination with Tigason in cutaneous T-cell lymphomas. *Acta Haematol* 1993; (89 Suppl 1):28–32.

80. Altomare GF, Capella GL, Pigatto PD, Finzi AF. Intramuscular low dose alpha-2B interferon and etretinate for treatment of mycosis fungoides. *Int J Dermatol* 1993; 32(2):138–141.

81. Edelson R, Facktor M, Andrews A, Lutzner M, Schein P. Successful management of the Sezary syndrome. Mobilization and removal of extravascular neoplastic T cells by leukapheresis. *N Engl J Med* 1974; 291(6):293–294.

82. Edelson R, Berger C, Gasparro F, Jegasothy B, Heald P, Wintroub B, Vonderheid E, Knobler R, Wolff K, Plewig G, et al. Treatment of cutaneous T-cell lymphoma by extracorporeal photochemotherapy. Preliminary results. *N Engl J Med* 1987; 316(6):297–303.

83. Zic JA, Miller JL, Stricklin GP, King LE Jr. The North American experience with photopheresis. *Ther Apher* 1999; 3(1):50–62.

84. Gottlieb SL, Wolfe JT, Fox FE, DeNardo BJ, Macey WH, Bromley PG, et al. Treatment of cutaneous T-cell lymphoma with extracorporeal photopheresis monotherapy and in combination with recombinant interferon alfa: a 10-year experience at a single institution. *J Am Acad Dermatol* 1996; 35(6):946–957.

85. Russell-Jones R. Extracorporeal photopheresis in cutaneous T-cell lymphoma. Inconsistent data underline the need for randomized studies. *Br J Dermatol* 2000; 142(1):16–21.

86. Vonderheid EC, Bigler RD, Greenberg AS, Neukum SJ, Micaily B. Extracorporeal photopheresis and recombinant interferon alfa 2b in Sézary syndrome. Use of dual marker labeling to monitor therapeutic response. *Am J Clin Oncol* 1994; 17(3):255–63.

87. Lim HW, Harris HR. Etretinate as an effective adjunctive therapy for recalcitrant palmar/
     plantar hyperkeratosis in patients with erythrodermic cutaneous T cell lymphoma undergo-
     ing photopheresis. *Dermatol Surg* 1995; 21(7):597–599.
88. Bunn PA Jr, Hoffman SJ, Norris D, Golitz LE, Aeling JL. Systemic therapy of cutaneous
     T-cell lymphomas (mycosis fungoides and the Sezary syndrome). *Ann Intern Med* 1994;
     121(8):592–602.
89. Thomsen K, Molin L, Volden G, Lange Wantzin G, Hellbe L. 13-cis-retinoic acid effective
     in mycosis fungoides. A report from the Scandinavian Mycosis Fungoides Group. *Acta Derm
     Venereol* 1984; 64(6):563–566.
90. Siegel RS, Martone B, Guitart J, Samuelson E, Rosen ST, Kuzel TM. Phase II trial of all-trans
     retinoic acid (ATRA) in the treatment of relapsed/refractory mycosis fungoides/Sezary syn-
     drome (MF/SS). *Blood* 1999; 94(10 Suppl 1):97a.
91. Duvic M, Hymes K, Heald P, Breneman D, Martin AG, Myskowski P, et al. Bexarotene is
     effective and safe for treatment of refractory advanced-stage cutaneous T-cell lymphoma:
     multinational phase II-III trial results. *J Clin Oncol* 2001; 19(9):2456–2471.
92. Olsen E, Duvic M, Frankel A, Kim Y, Martin A, Vonderheid E, et al. Pivotal phase III trial
     of two dose levels of denileukin diftitox for the treatment of cutaneous T-cell lymphoma. *J
     Clin Oncol* 2001; 19(2):376–388.
93. Gurgun G, Urbano A, Foss F. Enhanced cytotoxicity to DAB389IL2 (ONTAK) in human
     T-cell lines by retinoic acid. *Blood* 1999; 94(10 Suppl 1):281a.
94. Rosen ST, Foss FM. Chemotherapy for mycosis fungoides and the Sezary syndrome. *Hematol
     Oncol Clin N Am* 1995; 9(5):1109–1116.
95. Sorio R, Tirelli U, Zagonel V, Carbone A, Monfardini S. Phase II study of teniposide (VM26)
     in cutaneous T-cell lymphomas. *Am J Clin Oncol* 1990; 13(1):14–16.
96. Hamminga L, Hartgrink-Groeneveld CA, van Vloten WA. Sézary's syndrome: a clinical
     evaluation of eight patients. *Br J Dermatol* 1979; 100(3):291–296.
97. Winkelmann RK, Diaz-Perez JL, Buechner SA. The treatment of Sezary syndrome. *J Am
     Acad Dermatol* 1984; 10(6):1000–1004.
98. McEvoy MT, Zelickson BD, Pineda AA, Winkelmann RK. Intermittent leukapheresis: an ad-
     junct to low-dose chemotherapy for Sezary syndrome. *Acta Derm Venereol* 1989; 69(1):73–76.
99. Coors EA, von den Driesch P. Treatment of erythrodermic cutaneous T-cell lymphoma with
     intermittent chlorambucil and fluocortolone therapy. *Br J Dermatol* 2000; 143(1):127–131.
100. Zackheim HS, Epstein EH Jr. Low-dose methotrexate for the Sezary syndrome. *J Am Acad
     Dermatol* 1989; 21(4 Pt 1):757–762.
101. Mercieca J, Matutes E, Dearden C, MacLennan K, Catovsky D. The role of pentostatin in the
     treatment of T-cell malignancies: analysis of response rate in 145 patients according to
     disease subtype. *J Clin Oncol* 1994; 12(12):2588–2593.
102. Greiner D, Olsen EA, Petroni G. Pentostatin (2'-deoxycoformycin) in the treatment of cuta-
     neous T-cell lymphoma. *J Am Acad Dermatol* 1997; 36(6 Pt 1):950–955.
103. Ho AD, Suciu S, Stryckmans P, De Cataldo F, Willemze R, Thaler J, et al. Pentostatin in
     T-cell malignancies—a phase II trial of the EORTC. Leukemia Cooperative Group. *Ann
     Oncol* 1999; 10(12):1493–1498.
104. Kurzrock R, Pilat S, Duvic M. Pentostatin therapy of T-cell lymphomas with cutaneous
     manifestations. *J Clin Oncol* 1999; 17(10):3117–3121.
105. Foss FM, Ihde DC, Breneman DL, Phelps RM, Fischmann AB, Schechter GP, et al. Phase
     II study of pentostatin and intermittent high-dose recombinant interferon alfa-2a in advanced
     mycosis fungoides/Sezary syndrome. *J Clin Oncol* 1992; 10(12):1907–1913.
106. Saven A, Carrera CJ, Carson DA, Beutler E, Piro LD. 2-Chlorodeoxyadenosine: an active
     agent in the treatment of cutaneous T-cell lymphoma. *Blood* 1992 80(3):587–592.

107. Kong LR, Samuelson E, Rosen ST, Roenigk HH Jr, Tallman MS, Rademaker AW, et al. 2-Chlorodeoxyadenosine in cutaneous T-cell lymphoproliferative disorders. *Leuk Lymphoma* 1997; 26(1-2):89–97.
108. Foss FM, Ihde DC, Linnoila IR, Fischmann AB, Schechter GP, Cotelingam JD, et al. Phase II trial of fludarabine phosphate and interferon alfa-2a in advanced mycosis fungoides/Sezary syndrome. *J Clin Oncol* 1994; 12(10):2051–2059.
109. Scarisbrick JJ, Child FJ, Clift A, Sabroe R, Whittaker SJ, Spittle M, et al. A trial of fludarabine and cyclophosphamide combination chemotherapy in the treatment of advanced refractory primary cutaneous T-cell lymphoma. *Br J Dermatol* 2001; 144(5):1010–1015.
110. Foss FM. Activity of pentostatin (Nipent) in cutaneous T-cell lymphoma: single-agent and combination studies. *Semin Oncol* 2000; 27(2 Suppl 5):58–63.
111. Von Hoff DD, Dahlberg S, Hartstock RJ, Eyre HJ. Activity of fludarabine monophosphate in patients with advanced mycosis fungoides: a Southwest Oncology Group study. *J Natl Cancer Inst* 1990; 82(16):1353–1355.
112. Zinzani PL, Baliva G, Magagnoli M, Bendandi M, Modugno G, Gherlinzoni F, et al. Gemcitabine treatment in pretreated cutaneous T-cell lymphoma: experience in 44 patients. *J Clin Oncol* 2000; 18(13):2603–2606.
113. Levi JA, Diggs CH, Wiernik PH. Adriamycin therapy in advanced mycosis fungoides. *Cancer* 1977; 39(5):1967–1970.
114. Wollina U, Graefe T, Kaatz M. Pegylated doxorubicin for primary cutaneous T-cell lymphoma: a report on ten patients with follow-up. *J Cancer Res Clin Oncol* 2001; 127(2):128–134.
115. O'Reilly SM, Newlands ES, Stevens MF, Smith DB, Brampton MH, Slack JA, et al. Temozolomide has activity against primary brain tumors, melanoma and mycosis fungoides. *Br J Cancer* 1992; 65(Suppl 16):13.
116. Tirelli U, Carbone A, Veronesi A, Galligioni E, Trovo MG, Tumolo S, et al. Combination chemotherapy with cyclophosphamide, vincristine, and prednisone (CVP) in TNM-classified stage IV mycosis fungoides. *Cancer Treat Rep* 1982; 66(1):167–169.
117. Sentis HJ, Willemze R, Van Vloten WA. Systemic polychemotherapy in patients with mycosis fungoides and lymph node involvement: a follow-up study of 17 patients. *Acta Derm Venereol* 1985; 65(2):179–183.
118. Zakem MH, Davis BR, Adelstein DJ, Hines JD. Treatment of advanced stage mycosis fungoides with bleomycin, doxorubicin, and methotrexate with topical nitrogen mustard (BAM-M). *Cancer* 1986; 58(12):2611–2616.
119. Doberauer C, Ohl S. Advanced mycosis fungoides: chemotherapy with etoposide, methotrexate, bleomycin, and prednimustine. *Acta Derm Venereol* 1989; 69(6):538–540.
120. Schappell DL, Alper JC, McDonald CJ. Treatment of advanced mycosis fungoides and Sezary syndrome with continuous infusions of methotrexate followed by fluorouracil and leucovorin rescue. *Arch Dermatol* 1995; 131(3):307–313.
121. Fierro MT, Doveil GC, Quaglino P, Savoia P, Verrone A, Bernengo MG. Combination of etoposide, idarubicin, cyclophosphamide, vincristine, prednisone and bleomycin (VICOP-B) in the treatment of advanced cutaneous T-cell lymphoma. *Dermatology* 1997; 194(3):268–272.
122. Fierro MT, Quaglino P, Savoia P, Verrone A, Bernengo MG. Systemic polychemotherapy in the treatment of primary cutaneous lymphomas: a clinical follow-up study of 81 patients treated with COP or CHOP. *Leuk Lymphoma* 1998; 31(5-6):583–588.
123. Akpek G, Koh HK, Bogen S, O'Hara C, Foss FM. Chemotherapy with etoposide, vincristine, doxorubicin, bolus cyclophosphamide, and oral prednisone in patients with refractory cutaneous T-cell lymphoma. *Cancer* 1999; 86(7):1368–1376.

124. Bigler RD, Crilley P, Micaily B, Brady LW, Topolsky D, Bulova S, et al. Autologous bone marrow transplantation for advanced stage mycosis fungoides. *Bone Marrow Transplant* 1991; 7(2):133–137.
125. Molina A, Nademanee A, Arber DA, Forman SJ. Remission of refractory Sezary syndrome after bone marrow transplantation from a matched unrelated donor. *Biol Blood Marrow Transplant* 1999; 5(6):400–404.
126. Kaye FJ, Bunn PA Jr, Steinberg SM, Stocker JL, Ihde DC, Fischmann AB, et al. A randomized trial comparing combination electron-beam radiation and chemotherapy with topical therapy in the initial treatment of mycosis fungoides. *N Engl J Med* 1989; 321(26):1784–1790.
127. Winkler CF, Sausville EA, Ihde DC, Fischmann AB, Schechter GP, Kumar PP, et al. Combined modality treatment of cutaneous T cell lymphoma: results of a 6-year follow-up. *J Clin Oncol* 1986; 4(7):1094–1100.
128. Duvic M, Lemak NA, Redman JR, Eifel PJ, Tucker SL, Cabanillas FF, et al. Combined modality therapy for cutaneous T-cell lymphoma. *J Am Acad Dermatol* 1996; 34(6):1022–1029.
129. Wilson LD, Licata AL, Braverman IM, Edelson RL, Heald PW, Feldman AM, et al. Systemic chemotherapy and extracorporeal photochemotherapy for T3 and T4 cutaneous T-cell lymphoma patients who have achieved a complete response to total skin electron beam therapy. *Int J Radiat Oncol Biol Phys* 1995; 32(4):987–995.
130. Gisselbrecht C, Maraninchi D, Pico JL, Milpied N, Coiffier B, Divine M, et al. Interleukin-2 treatment in lymphoma: a phase II multicenter study. *Blood* 1994; 83(8):2081–2085.
131. Marolleau JP, Baccard M, Flageul B, Rybojad M, Laroche L, Verola O, et al. High-dose recombinant interleukin-2 in advanced cutaneous T-cell lymphoma. *Arch Dermatol* 1995; 131(5):574–579.
132. Rook AH, Wood GS, Yoo EK, Elenitsas R, Kao DM, Sherman ML, et al. Interleukin-12 therapy of cutaneous T-cell lymphoma induces lesion regression and cytotoxic T-cell responses. *Blood* 1999; 94(3):902–908.
133. Street ML, Muller SA, Pittelkow MR. Cyclosporine in the treatment of cutaneous T cell lymphoma. *J Am Acad Dermatol* 1990; 23(6 Pt 1):1084–1089.
134. Lundin J, Osterborg A, Brittinger G, Crowther D, Dombret H, Engert A, et al. CAMPATH-1H monoclonal antibody in therapy for previously treated low-grade non-Hodgkin's lymphomas: a phase II multicenter study. European Study Group of CAMPATH-1H Treatment in Low-Grade Non-Hodgkin's Lymphoma. *J Clin Oncol* 1998; 16(10):3257–3263.

7 Large Granular Lymphocyte Proliferative Diseases

Mustafa Benekli, MD and Maria R. Baer, MD

INTRODUCTION

Large granular lymphocytes (LGL) represent 10–15% of peripheral-blood mononuclear cells in healthy people. They are a morphologically unique subset of lymphocytes, with an eccentrically located nucleus and abundant, pale blue cytoplasm with numerous discrete azurophilic granules; the latter are the basis for the name LGL *(1,2)*. LGL include cells of two lineages, distinguished by their immunophenotypes. T-cell LGL (T-LGL) express CD3, and natural killer-cell LGL (NK-LGL) are CD3-negative *(2–4)*. T-LGL are responsible for antibody-dependent cellular cytotoxicity and NK-LGL for natural killer cell (NK) activity *(1)*. T-LGL likely represent in vivo-activated cytotoxic T-lymphocytes, which display non-major histocompatibility complex (MHC)-restricted cytotoxicity in vitro, and have clonal T-cell-receptor (TCR) gene rearrangements. NK-LGL also mediate non-MHC restricted cytotoxicity, but do not have TCR gene rearrangements.

Both T-LGL and NK-LGL may undergo malignant transformation, giving rise to two distinct malignancies. T-cell large granular lymphoproliferative disease (T-LGLD) is a distinct clonal chronic T-cell disorder. T-LGLD is a rela-

From: *Current Clinical Oncology: Chronic Leukemias and Lymphomas:*
Biology, Pathophysiology, and Clinical Management
Edited by: G. J. Schiller © Humana Press Inc., Totowa, NJ

Table 1
Terminology

Term	Refs.
T-cell CLL	(6,8)
Chronic T-cell lymphocytosis with neutropenia	(9)
T-gamma proliferations	(10)
T8 CLL	(11)
NK and suppressor T-cell CLL	(12)
Neutropenia with T lymphocytosis	(13)
T-gamma lymphoproliferative disease	(14)
T-suppressor-cell CLL	(15)
Granulated T-cell lymphocytosis with neutropenia	(16)
T-gamma lymphocytosis	(17)
LGL leukemia	(18)
T8 hyperlymphocytosis	(19)
Lymphoproliferative disease of granular lymphocytes	(20,21)
Granular lymphocyte proliferative disorder	(22)
T-cell and NK-cell LGL leukemia	(2)

tively common condition; its frequency appears to be underreported in the literature *(5)*. The disease is clinically indolent. Patients often present with recurrent infections related to neutropenia; other manifestations may include anemia and associated rheumatoid arthritis (RA) and other autoimmune phenomena. In contrast, NK-cell LGLD usually runs a more aggressive course, with frequent visceral organ involvement. Severe anemia and thrombocytopenia are more common than in T-LGLD, but neutropenia is less common, and immunologic abnormalities are rarely observed. Clonality remains unproven in most NK-LGL cases.

HISTORICAL PERSPECTIVE

Terminology

T-LGLD was first described in the 1970s. It was initially classified as a subtype of chronic lymphocytic leukemia (CLL), and only later accepted as a distinct clinicopathological entity. In 1975, Brouet et al. reported 11 patients with T-cell CLL *(6)*; at least six of these had abnormal lymphocytes morphologically identical to LGL. McKenna et al. provided the first description of the syndrome of circulating LGL with chronic neutropenia in 1977 *(7)*. A variety of terms have been proposed for this distinct syndrome over the following years (Table 1). These include T-cell CLL *(6,8)*, chronic T-cell lymphocytosis with neutropenia *(9)*, T-gamma proliferations *(10)*, T8 CLL *(11)*, NK and suppressor T-cell CLL *(12)*, neutropenia with T lymphocytosis *(13)*, T-gamma lymphoproliferative disease *(14)*, T-suppressor-cell CLL *(15)*, granulated T-cell lymphocytosis with neutropenia *(16)*, T-gamma lymphocytosis *(17)*, LGL leukemia *(18)*, T8 hyperlymphocytosis *(19)*, lymphoproliferative disease of granular lymphocytes *(20,21)*, and granular lymphocyte proliferative disorder *(22)*. In 1993, Loughran proposed the terms T-cell LGL leukemia and NK-cell LGL leukemia for the CD3+ and CD3− subsets of the disease, respectively *(2)*.

Classification

In 1989, the French-American-British (FAB) Cooperative Group classified T-cell CLL or LGL leukemia as one of the four subgroups of chronic T-cell lymphoid leukemias *(23)*. The Morphologic, Immunologic and Cytogenetic (MIC) Cooperative Study Group accepted the term LGL leukemia to replace T-CLL in 1990 *(24)*. The Revised European-American Lymphoma (REAL) classification (1994) includes LGL leukemia, T-cell and NK-cell types, under the category of peripheral T-cell and NK-cell neoplasms *(4)*.

T-CELL LGLD

Clinical Features

T-LGLD constitutes approx 80% of cases of LGLD, whereas NK-LGLD represents only 20%. The median age of T-LGLD patients has ranged from 55 to 65 years in different studies *(2,25–28)*. Although affected individuals are typically older adults, approx 10% are below the age of 40 yr, and anecdotal pediatric cases have been reported *(29)*. Males and females have generally been found to be equally affected, although a slight female preponderance has been suggested in some series *(2,26,27)*.

The clinical course of T-LGLD is generally indolent, with some spontaneous regressions *(16,26,30)*. Approximately 25% of patients are asymptomatic, and are diagnosed based on the incidental detection of lymphocytosis of granular lymphocytes on examination of a routine blood smear. The most common presenting features in symptomatic patients are fever and infections in the setting of neutropenia, with or without anemia or thrombocytopenia *(21)*. Patients experience recurrent bacterial infections, including cellulitis, perirectal abscesses, upper respiratory tract infections, and sinusitis. Pneumonia and neutropenic sepsis are observed in severe cases. In contrast, opportunistic infections with viral, fungal, and parasitic pathogens are very rare. Constitutional symptoms are present in 60% of patients; B symptoms including fever, night sweats, and weight loss are present in 15–25%. Although T-LGLD is generally indolent, cases that are rapidly progressive and highly malignant are also observed *(20,21,25,26)*. A CD3+CD56+ variant of T-LGLD has been reported to be more aggressive *(31)*.

Physical findings in T-LGLD include splenomegaly in 20–50% of patients and hepatomegaly in 5–20%. Lymphadenopathy is less common. In the largest study of T-LGLD reported to date, splenomegaly, hepatomegaly, and lympadenopathy were present in 50%, 30% and 12% of patients, respectively *(21)*.

RA is present in 25–30% of T-LGLD patients *(25,32–37)*. Patients with T-LGLD and RA present similarly to patients with Felty's syndrome (FS), which is characterized by RA, neutropenia, and splenomegaly *(38–43)*. The two disorders are also difficult to distinguish because LGL lymphocytosis is present in 30–35% of patients with FS, and analysis of LGL from these FS patients using monoclonal antibodies (MAbs) against TCR Vβ chains demonstrates clonal LGL proliferations *(42)*. The demonstration of a homology of TCR-α and -β chain-junctional hypervariable region motifs in patients with FS has suggested an antigen-driven process in these patients *(43)*. Expansion of CD8+ CD57+ LGL was suggested to be responsible for neutropenia in FS, by suppression of neutrophil precursors *(44)*. Moreover, HLA-DR4 is equally common in patients with FS and with T-LGLD and RA, suggesting that both disorders have a similar immunogenetic basis and are components of a single disease entity *(40,41)*.

Hematologic Features

The cardinal hematologic feature of T-LGLD is the presence of lymphocytosis of LGL in the peripheral blood. LGL are the predominant lymphocyte population in patients with T-LGLD. They have a unique appearance, with eccentric nuclei, abundant cytoplasm, and numerous large azurophilic cytoplasmic granules (Fig. 1). In normal control populations, the LGL count is $0.223 \pm 0.099 \times 10^9$/L *(28)*, and the number of T-LGL cells, identified by multiparameter flow cytometry, is $0.128 \pm 0.118 \times 10^9$/L *(45)*. The average LGL count in patients with T-LGLD is 4×10^9/L, with a range of 0.1 to 50×10^9/L *(25,26)*. The diagnosis of T-LGLD is more difficult to establish in patients with low LGL counts, and more careful examination of the peripheral blood smear is required. Furthermore, the paucity or absence of azurophilic granules in some cases may also make the diagnosis more difficult *(46,47)*. Immunophenotyping studies showing clonal expansion of LGL are necessary to diagnose these patients.

Most patients with T-LGLD have chronic neutropenia, which is the primary cause of morbidity and mortality in the disease *(25)*. Neutropenia is present in 85% of patients, and severe neutropenia, defined by an absolute neutrophil count of less than 0.5×10^9/L, is seen in 50% *(2,28)*. Adult-onset cyclic neutropenia has also been associated with clonal LGL proliferation, indicating that LGL may also play a role in the pathogenesis of this disorder *(48,49)*.

Anemia is present in 20–50% of patients with T-LGLD. Anemia can be normocytic or macrocytic *(14,25,50)*, and may result from a number of mechanisms, including Coombs' positive autoimmune hemolysis *(18,51,52)*, erythroid hypoplasia, and pure red cell aplasia (PRCA) *(25,26,50,53–57)*.

PRCA has been reported in association with T-LGLD with increasing frequency in recent years. There may be geographic variation in the incidence of PRCA: a Japanese study reported PRCA in 12 of 21 patients with T-LGLD (57%) *(26)*, and PRCA was also noted to be a major cause of morbidity in Chinese

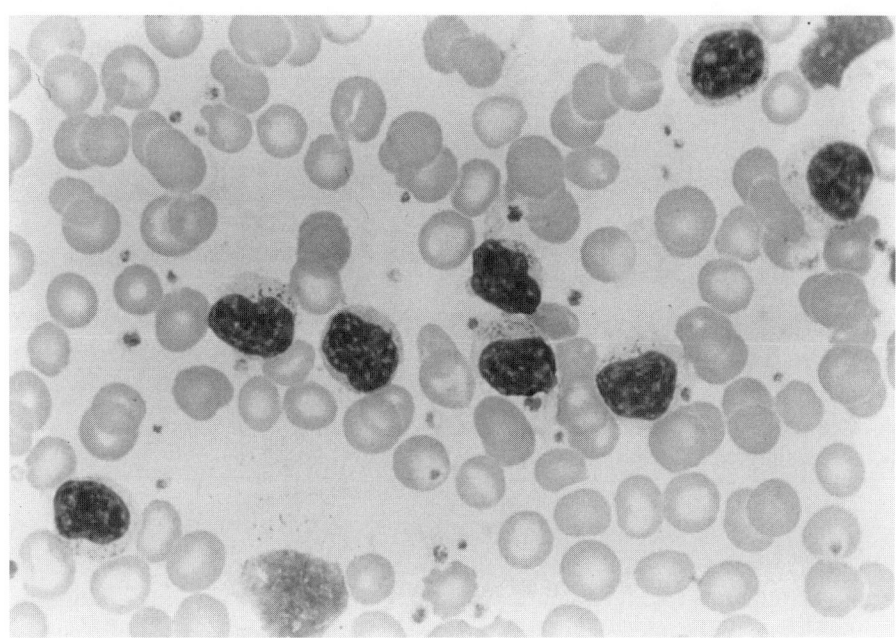

Fig. 1. LGL in the peripheral blood of a patient with T-LGL leukemia (×100 magnification). (Photograph courtesy of Dr. Maurice Barcos, Department of Pathology, Roswell Park Cancer Institute, Buffalo, New York.)

patients with T-LGLD *(56)*. T-LGLD was the most common disorder associated with PRCA in a series from the Mayo Clinic; it was present in 9 of 47 patients (19%), but its true frequency may have been even higher, since only 14 patients were tested for clonal TCR gene rearrangements *(57)*.

Most patients have normal platelet counts; only 20% have thrombocytopenia *(25)*. Idiopathic thrombocytopenic purpura and Evans' syndrome are causes of thrombocytopenia in T-LGLD *(18,51,52)*. Amegakaryocytic thrombocytopenic purpura has also been reported *(53)*.

T-LGLD may also present as pancytopenia in the setting of marrow hypocellularity *(58)*. This presentation is distinguishable from aplastic anemia only by the presence of an increase in CD3+CD8+CD57+ cells in the blood and/or marrow, with TCR gene rearrangements. T-LGLD should be considered in the differential diagnosis of acquired aplastic anemia *(58)*.

T-LGLD has also been reported in association with hematologic malignancies, including hairy cell leukemia (HCL) and multiple myeloma *(59–62)*.

Immunologic Abnormalities

Autoimmune disorders associated with T-LGLD include RA *(25,32–37)*, idiopathic thrombocytopenic purpura *(18,51,52)*, Coombs-positive autoimmune

Table 2
Immunologic Abnormalities in T-LGLD

Immunologic abnormalities in T-LGLD
Polyclonal hypergammaglobulinemia
Hypogammaglobulinemia
Rheumatoid factor with and without RA
Coombs positive hemolytic anemia
Idiopathic thrombocytopenic purpura
PRCA
Antinuclear antibody
Anti-neutrophil antibodies
Circulating immune complexes
Elevated beta-2 microglobulin
B-cell lymphoproliferative disease

hemolytic anemia *(18,51,52)*, and PRCA *(25,26,50,53–57)* (Table 2). Humoral immunologic abnormalities are frequent; they include the presence of rheumatoid factor in patients with and without RA *(63)*, antinuclear antibodies *(63)*, antineutrophil antibodies *(63–65)*, immune complexes *(18,63,64)*, hypoglobulinemia or polyclonal hypergammaglobulinemia *(63,64,66)*, elevated beta-2 microglobulin levels *(64,66)*, and monoclonal gammopathy *(19)*.

Immunologic abnormalities are attributed to altered B-cell function *(65)*. The exact cause of B-cell dysfunction in T-LGLD is unknown. LGL have been shown to inhibit normal B-cell proliferation in B-cell CLL *(67)*. The presence of abnormal LGL may lead to disordered B-cell immunoregulation, since the normal counterparts of LGL are suggested to regulate B-cell activity *(67–69)*.

Pathology and Morphology

Increased numbers of LGL are consistently present in the peripheral blood of patients with T-LGLD *(13,46,70)*. Morphologically, these cells are medium to large in size and have a low nuclear/cytoplasmic ratio. The nucleus is slightly eccentric and is usually round or oval, with moderately condensed chromatin and sparse nucleoli. The cells have abundant, slightly basophilic cytoplasm with numerous azurophilic granules (Fig. 1). They stain in a granular pattern with acid phosphatase, and stain weakly or do not stain at all with alpha-naphthyl acetate esterase (ANAE) and periodic-acid Schiff (PAS) *(13)*.

At the ultrastructural level, the lymphocytes contain abundant membrane-bound, electron-dense granules, corresponding to the granules seen by light microscopy *(13,46)*. These granules form parallel tubular arrays in some cases *(7,14)*. Electron microscopy also demonstrates many well-developed organelles

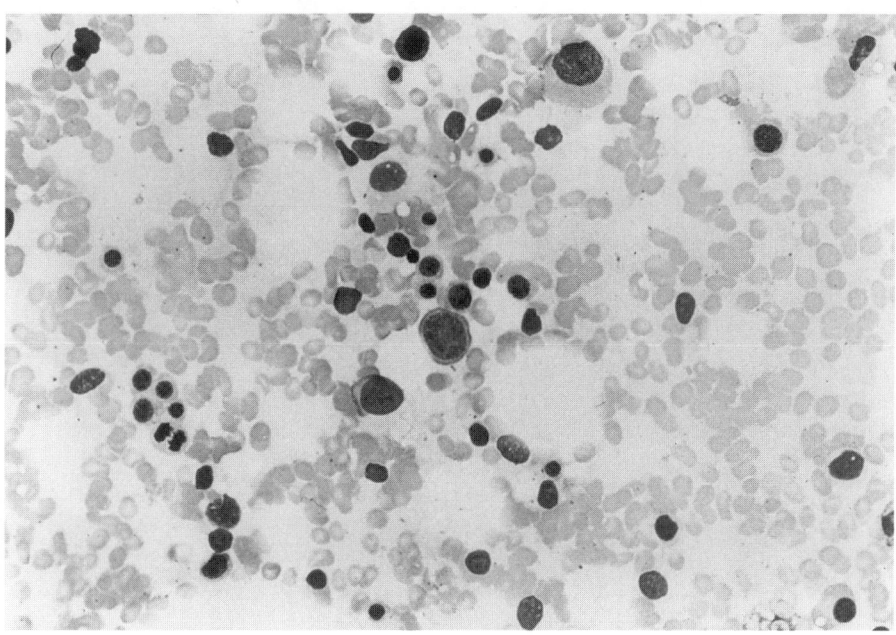

Fig. 2. Bone-marrow aspirate smear from a patient with T-LGL leukemia, showing granulocytic hypoplasia and sparse lymphocytic infiltration (×100 magnification). (Photograph courtesy of Dr. Maurice Barcos, Department of Pathology, Roswell Park Cancer Institute, Buffalo, New York.)

that are centrally placed in the cytoplasm, including a Golgi apparatus, several mitochondria, ribosomes, and rough and smooth endoplasmic reticulum.

Bone marrow infiltration is close to universal, but is usually not extensive, and may be subtle in some cases. The amount of bone marrow infiltration does not correlate with the degree of cytopenias. Lymphocytic infiltration by LGL may be either diffuse interstitial or focal nodular, presenting as lymphoid aggregates (Figs. 2 and 3) *(18,71–73)*. Infiltration is usually sparse, and may be subtle and easily missed unless specifically searched for. Rare patients appear to have normal marrow histology; this is attributable to very small size of lymphoid aggregates, rendering them undetectable by light microscopy. Flow cytometry is usually useful in demonstrating marrow infiltration with LGL, even in cases with subtle or inapparent involvement. Granulocyte maturation is generally normal and orderly *(16,71)*, but maturation arrest at the myelocyte stage has been reported in some cases *(9,13,59)*. Bone marrow fibrosis is occasionally seen *(13)*.

Lymphocytic infiltration of the splenic red pulp cords and hepatic sinusoids is common in cases with involvement of these organs *(71)*. Germinal follicles of the spleen are prominent; they consist of polyclonal reactive B cells. Portal areas

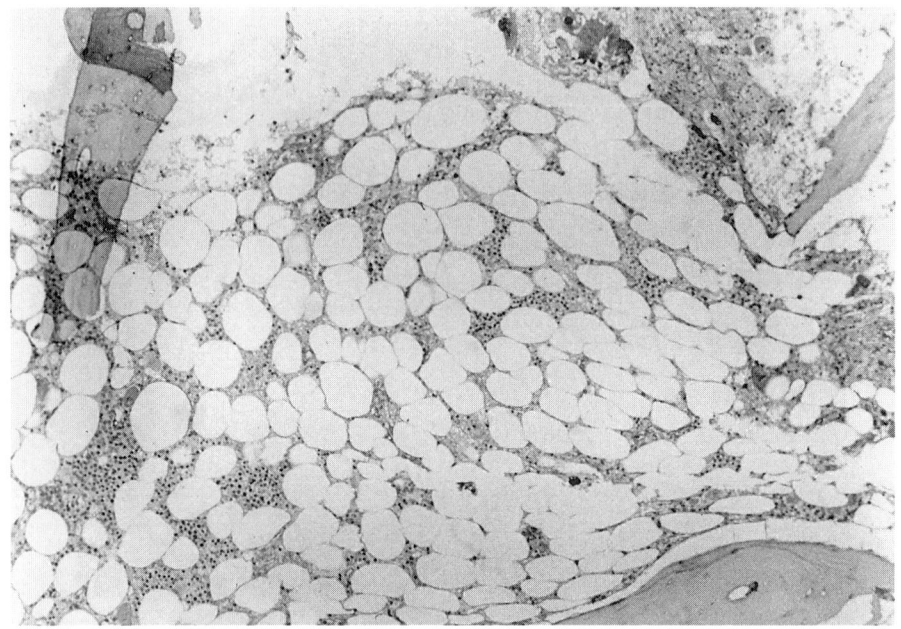

Fig. 3. Bone marrow biopsy from a patient with T-LGL leukemia, showing hypocellularity and focal lymphocytic infiltration (×250 magnification). (Photograph courtesy of Dr. Maurice Barcos, Department of Pathology, Roswell Park Cancer Institute, Buffalo, New York.)

of the liver may be involved in more advanced disease. Cutaneous infiltration and lymph node involvement are very rare.

Immunophenotype

Two major subtypes of LGLD have been defined—T-LGLD and NK-LGLD. In T-LGLD, the cells characteristically express CD3, CD8 and CD57 (Fig. 4); expression of the NK antigen CD16 is variable. CD4, CD5, CD7, CD25, CD56 are usually not expressed (74,75), although CD5 and CD7 were present in one study (76). A high ratio of CD16 to CD56 expression correlated with presence of a clonal CD3 + LGL population with TCR gene rearrangement in 82% of cases in one study (77). Rare cases of T-LGLD with CD4 and CD8 antigen co-expression have also been reported (78). NK-LGL cells lack CD3 expression, but express CD56 (Fig. 5), and may also express CD2, CD7 and CD16 (74,75).

Clonality

Monoclonal proliferation is the *sine qua non* of hematologic malignancies, and is crucial in differentiating reactive vs neoplastic states. The presence of clonal cytogenetic abnormalities serves to demonstrate clonality in hematologic

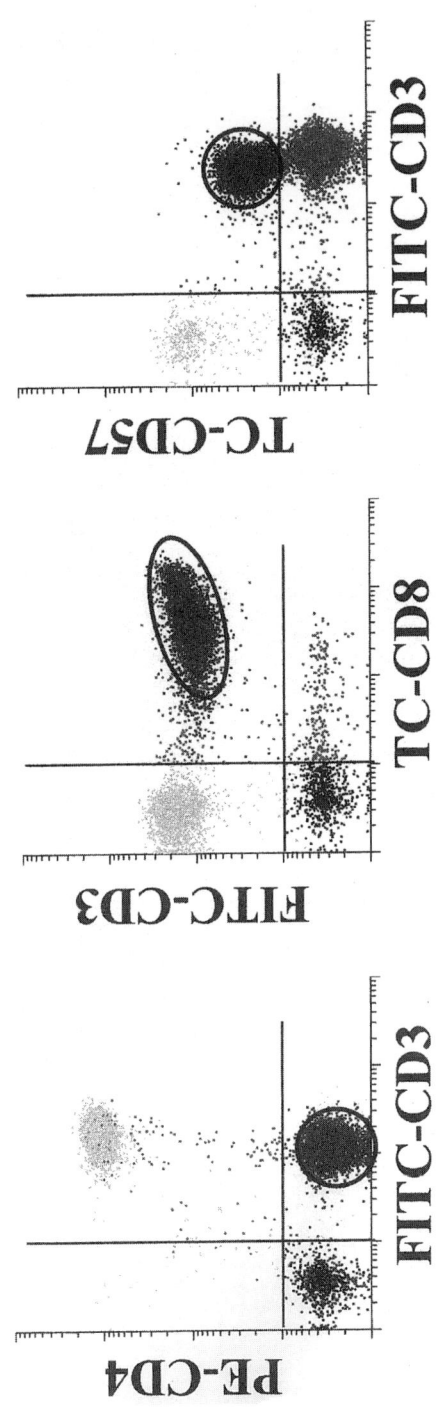

Fig. 4. Immunophenotype of T-LGL leukemia cells, studied by multiparameter flow cytometry. (Courtesy of Dr. Carleton Stewart, Laboratory of Flow Cytometry, Roswell Park Cancer Institute, Buffalo, New York.)

161

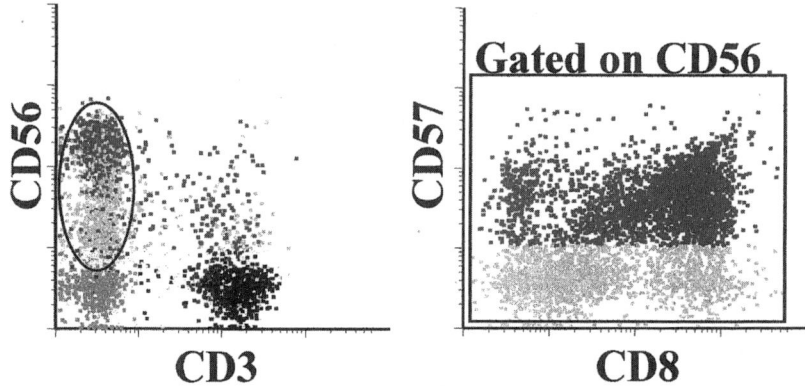

Fig. 5. Immunophenotype of NK-LGL leukemia cells, studied by multiparameter flow cytometry. (Courtesy of Dr. Carleton Stewart, Laboratory of Flow Cytometry, Roswell Park Cancer Institute, Buffalo, New York.)

malignancies with abnormal karyotypes. Molecular analysis of immunoglobulin and TCR gene rearrangements is the method most commonly used to evaluate clonality in lymphoid disorders.

Cytogenetic analysis shows a normal karyotype in 90% of cases of T-cell LGLD *(25,26)*. Chromosomal changes reported in cases with abnormal karyotypes include trisomy 3, del(5q), trisomy 8, inversion 12, and trisomy 14 *(18,25,26)*.

The detection of TCR gene rearrangement through Southern blot or polymerase chain reaction (PCR) techniques has provided evidence for the clonal origin of most cases of CD3+ T-LGLD (Fig. 6) *(79–84)*. In contrast, a germline pattern is observed in NK-LGLD. T-cells usually express TCR αβ heterodimers *(84–86)*. The expression of TCR-α, -β, and -χ gene transcripts has been demonstrated in CD3+ LGL *(84,85)*. Clonality in T-LGLD is further confirmed by TCR Vβ expression determined by the use of anti-TCR Vβ MAbs against variable domains of TCR-β genes *(52,81)*. Lymphocytes in CD3+ T-LGLD utilize diverse TCR Vβ genes *(81,86)*. Since TCR Vβ expression is heterogenous, leukemic CD3+ LGL cells are believed to be clonally transformed in a random fashion with respect to the TCR-β chain.

Etiology and Pathogenesis

ETIOLOGY

The etiology of clonal proliferation of LGL and the mechanisms by which it occurs are unclear. Even the neoplastic nature of this entity has been questioned. Some authors have claimed that most cases of clonal T-LGLD have a chronic reactive rather than a neoplastic etiology *(76,87)*. It was suggested that clonal expansions may occur as manifestations of highly restricted immune responses. Reaction against infectious agents such as human T-lymphotropic virus (HTLV)

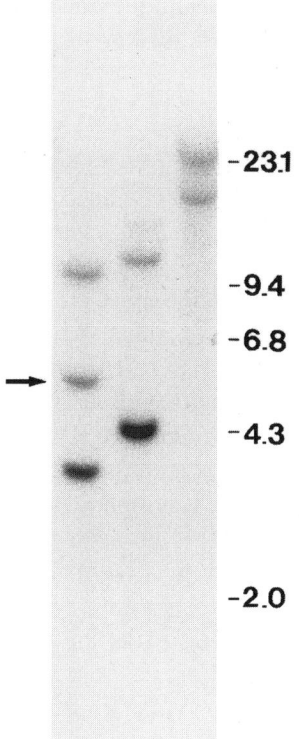

Fig. 6. T-cell-receptor gene rearrangement demonstrated by Southern blot analysis in a patient with T-LGL leukemia. Lanes 1, 2, and 3 show *Hind*III, *Eco*RI and *Bam*HI digests, respectively. The arrow indicates the abnormal band. (Courtesy of the Molecular Diagnostics Laboratory, Roswell Park Cancer Institute, Buffalo, New York.)

I/II, Epstein-Barr virus (EBV) and cytomegalovirus (CMV) has been postulated. Nonspecific expansion of cells in response to an unknown stimulus, or to a B-cell disorder, has also been proposed as a mechanism.

There is a body of evidence suggesting a viral etiology for T-LGLD *(35,88–91)*. Several viruses have been studied, with conflicting results *(92–94)*. The most extensively studied virus is HTLV-I, which is known to be the causative agent in adult T-cell leukemia *(88)*. A number of patients with T-LGLD have seroreactivity to the HTLV-I p24 gag and gp21e envelope proteins *(89,90)*. The immunoreactivity to gp21e is primarily against the BA21 epitope of the protein *(90)*. There is a close association between T-LGLD and BA21 epitope seroreactivity, suggesting a causal relationship, and crossreactivity with an antigen with homology to BA21 was proposed as the pathogenesis of the disease. However, prototypical HTLV infection is rare *(90)*. A recent study also failed to demonstrate a causative role for the unique oncogenic retroviral genus, which includes primate T-cell lymphoma/leukemia viruses (PTLV) and bovine leukemia virus (BLV) *(91)*.

PATHOGENESIS

Like normal CD3+ cytotoxic T-lymphocytes *(95)*, T-LGL cells are antigen-activated cytotoxic T-lymphocytes, as evidenced by their CD3+ CD8+ CD57+ phenotype and rapid triggering of non-MHC-restricted cytotoxicity by anti-CD3 MAb *(96)*.

Cytotoxicity of both normal and leukemic CD3+ LGL can be induced by anti-CD3 MAb and TCR interaction in a manner that mimicks antigen binding and stimulation in vivo *(97–99)*. Anti-CD3 MAb also activates the proliferative response, either alone or in combination with IL-2 or IL-4 *(100)*, suggesting that binding of a foreign stimulatory antigen to TCR in the presence of lymphokines may trigger proliferation of LGL. Expanding LGL in patients with T-LGLD may represent in vivo primed cytotoxic T-lymphocytes responding to an unknown antigen *(97)*. A foreign antigenic stimulus such as a virus may initiate the proliferative response in conjunction with upregulation of IL-2 receptors and IL-2 secretion.

Because T-LGL cells in T-LGLD are in the G0/G1 phase of the cell cycle *(100)*, their increased numbers appear to be a result of prolonged survival rather than increased production. Extended survival of T-LGL in T-LGLD has been attributed to dysregulation of Fas-mediated apoptosis *(101,102)*. Fas ligand (CD95L) is a member of the tumor necrosis factor (TNF) family, which induces apoptosis by binding to its receptor, Fas (CD95) *(103–105)*. CD95/CD95L interactions play a pivotal role in the activation-induced programmed cell death of human T-lymphocytes *(106)*. Like their normal counterparts, T-LGL cells from patients with T-LGLD constitutively express high levels of CD95 *(102)* and CD95L *(101,102)*. However, despite of high levels of CD95 expression, LGL are resistant to CD95-dependent cell death induced by incubation with anti-CD95 MAbs. The mechanism underlying resistance to CD95-induced apoptosis is still obscure. Resistance to Fas-induced apoptosis is not caused by mutation of the CD95 gene *(102)*. Moreover, T-LGL undergo apoptosis after activation by phytohemagglutinin and IL-2, indicating that their resistance to apoptosis is not intrinsic.

LGL cells are capable of undergoing apoptosis after activation with IL-2, and lack of IL-2 in vivo may therefore explain the resistance of T-LGL cells to apoptosis in T-LGLD *(102,104)*. IL-2 is a proliferative signal for T lymphocytes through interaction with a heterodimeric high-affinity receptor consisting of an alpha subunit (*p55*, Tac) and a beta subunit (*p75*) *(107)*, and also predisposes T-cells to CD95- and anti-CD3-mediated cell death *(108)*. IL-2 stimulates proliferation and cytotoxicity of LGL *(109–111)*, which constitutively express high levels of functional intermediate-affinity *p75* IL-2 receptor (R), but not *p55*, at resting state *(109–112)*. IL-2 mediates LGL activation by the *p75* IL-2R, rather than by *p55* peptide *(109–111)*, and induces *p55* IL-2R expression only at the mRNA level, with no generation of antigen *(97)*. Anti-CD3 MAb upregulates *p75* IL-2R on LGL by mimicking antigen activation, without *p55* IL-2R expression *(98)*, and induces *p55* IL-2R expression at both the mRNA and the antigen level *(97)*, but does not induce IL-2 gene transcription or IL-2 secretion, suggesting an IL-2-independent pathway *(98)*. This hypothesis is also supported by the inability of anti-IL-2R MAb to inhibit anti-CD3 MAb-mediated cytotoxicity in CD3+ LGL *(99)*.

TNF-α may be involved as a cofactor in in vitro growth and cytotoxicity of LGL from T-LGLD patients *(113,114)*. TNF receptor (R) *p75*, but not *p55*, is expressed on LGL in the resting state. IL-2 and both anti-CD3 and anti-CD16 antibodies induce expression of *p75* receptor as well as slight upregulation of *p55* receptor *(113)*. Anti-TNF-R and anti-TNF-α MAbs inhibit proliferation of both CD3+ and CD3− LGL induced by these stimuli. Thus TNF-α is directly involved in LGL expansion in vitro, suggesting that endogenous TNF-α may play a role in the pathogenesis of T-LGLD. Recently, Zambello et al. demonstrated that T-LGL from most T-LGLD patients expresses different TNF-R and TNF-ligand (L) antigens, indicating a peculiar cell activation status *(114)*: the CD40, CD40L, CD30, CD70, CD95, and CD95L antigens were expressed on the surface of LGL cells, but CD27 and CD30L were absent. They speculated that the persistent expression of costimulatory molecules of the TNF superfamily on LGL cells may represent different phases of disease in which clonality was established *(114)*. TNF-α upregulates IL-2 receptor in normal lymphocytes, suggesting a relationship between TNF-α and IL-2 in T-LGLD *(115)*.

IL-12 functions as a costimulatory cytokine for in vitro proliferation of LGL stimulated via the TCR *(116,117)*. The combination of anti-CD3 MAb and IL-12 induces a greater proliferative response than either molecule alone. Upregulation of IL-12 receptors on LGL by anti-CD3 MAb and inhibition of proliferation by neutralizing antibody to IL-12 suggests a role for IL-12 in the activation of leukemic T-LGL *(116,117)*. The activity of IL-12 appears to be independent of IL-2, since blockage of the *p55* and *p75* chains of IL-2R does not affect IL-12-mediated LGL proliferation *(117)*.

IL-15 may also facilitate the clonal expansion of LGL *(118)*. Antibodies against the *p75* and *p64* IL-2R chains inhibit IL-15 activity, indicating that IL-15 stimulates proliferation and cytotoxicity of LGL through both chains of the IL-2R.

The multidrug resistance (MDR) phenotype may be responsible for chemoresistance in T-LGLD *(119–121)*. The MDR1 gene on chromosome 7 encodes a 170-KD glycoprotein, P-glycoprotein (Pgp), which functions as an energy-dependent transmembrane drug efflux pump *(122)*. MDR1 mRNA is detected by RT-PCR in LGL *(121)*. Yamamoto et al. demonstrated high levels of Pgp expression on the surface of both T-LGL and NK-LGL, and suggested that Pgpmodulating agents may be beneficial in the reversion of drug resistance in patients with these disorders *(119)*. Pgp function, as demonstrated by the rhodamine 123 dye efflux assay is consistently present in T-LGL *(119–121)*, and is inhibited by the MDR modulator verapamil in most cases *(121)*. Expression of lung resistance protein (LRP), another protein which contributes to the MDR phenotype, was also detected in 75% of the patients with T-LGLD *(121)*.

Perforin or pore-forming protein is a major cytolytic protein mediating T-lymphocyte cytotoxicity. Perforin was shown to be expressed on LGL cells of a patient with CD3+ CD4+ T-LGLD *(123)*. T-cell stimulatory signals such as IL-2 or anti-CD3 MAb induce perforin mRNA in T-cells, and IL-2-induced cytotoxic potential correlates directly with perforin mRNA levels in LGL cells from patients with T-LGLD and NK-LGLD, suggesting that perforin may mediate cytolytic functions of granular lymphocytes in patients with LGLD *(124,125)*. Also supporting this hypothesis is the observation that peripheral blood mononuclear cell cytotoxicity is reduced when perforin is downregulated in long-term cultures in the presence of IL-2 and IL-12 *(126)*.

The platelet-type thrombin receptor designated as PAR-1, the first member of the protease-activated receptors (PARs) family, is expressed on the surface of LGL, and the degree of expression correlates with CD57 expression in T-LGLD *(127)*. PAR-1 may play a role in LGL migration, since thrombin is a chemo-attractant for LGL. However, the functional significance of this association is unclear.

PATHOGENESIS OF CYTOPENIAS ASSOCIATED WITH T-LGLD

The mechanism by which severe neutropenia occurs in T-LGLD remains unknown. Bone marrow infiltration by LGL is usually not extensive, and is insufficient to explain severe neutropenia; moreover, the extent of infiltration does not correlate with the degree of neutropenia *(59)*. Additionally, neutropenia is more common and more severe than anemia and thrombocytopenia. Maturation arrest of the myeloid series at the myelocyte stage is seen in some patients, but is not universal and does not provide a sufficient explanation for severe neutropenia *(16)*.

There is convincing evidence that LGL play a pivotal role in the regulation of hematopoiesis. LGL inhibit granulopoiesis and granulocyte-macrophage colony formation in vitro *(128–131)*. However, granulocytopenia in T-LGLD does not appear to be caused by direct suppression of hematopoietic progenitors in vivo, since suppression of granulocyte-macrophage colony formation has not been observed when LGL from patients with T-LGLD have been co-cultured with bone marrow cells from normal donors *(14,18,66)* or with autologous marrow *(19)*.

Antibody-mediated peripheral immune destruction of granulocytes has also been suggested *(18,66,132)*. Antineutrophil antibodies associated with a short-ened neutrophil life span have been reported *(66)*, and the demonstration of complement fixation by the IgG fraction *(132)* and antibody-dependent cell-mediated cytotoxicity *(14)* supports this hypothesis. However, these findings have not been consistently reproduced in all studies *(9)*. Moreover, the peripheral destruction of neutrophils cannot be the only mechanism responsible for severe neutropenia, because granulocytic hypoplasia in the bone marrow is a common feature and antineutrophil antibodies have been clearly shown to persist after neutrophil counts return to normal following therapy *(133)*.

A lymphokine-associated mechanism may explain the presence of neutropenia and anemia in T-LGLD and the response of these cytopenias to cyclosporine (CSA) therapy, as covered in the Treatment section. LGL from patients with T-LGLD produce a number of immunoreactive lymphokines, including interferon (IFN)-γ, TNF-α and IL-2, which have various effects on hematopoiesis and may mediate the development of cytopenias *(134,135)*. Suppression of T-cell activation by CSA may not only affect the synthesis of IL-2, but also suppress mediators of neutropenia including IFN-γ (135) and TNF-α *(113)*.

Neutropenia in T-LGLD may be caused by the activation of the Fas pathway in the presence of high levels of FasL *(101,102,104,136,137)*. Normal neutrophils express CD95, constitutively express CD95L and undergo spontaneous apoptosis, with death of one-half of the population within 48 h *(138)*. Liu et al. recently demonstrated the presence of high levels of circulating CD95L in serum from 39 of 44 T-LGLD patients *(137)*. A significant association between detectable FasL levels and neutropenia was found, since FasL levels were elevated in 31 of 34 serum samples from patients with T-LGLD associated with neutropenia, but there was no direct correlation between the levels of FasL and the degree of neutropenia. Serum from patients with elevated FasL levels triggered apoptosis of neutrophils from healthy controls, and this effect was inhibited by the addition of a neutralizing antibody to Fas, proving that the Fas pathway is involved in the genesis of neutropenia. Nevertheless, inhibition by Fas antibody was incomplete, indicating the possible role of other mechanisms in addition to Fas-dependent apoptosis. Finally, it was also shown that serum FasL levels decreased with the resolution of neutropenia following therapy for T-LGLD, providing further support for the hypothesis that FasL overproduction is involved in the pathogenesis of neutropenia in T-LGLD *(137)*.

Several mechanisms have been suggested in the pathogenesis of anemia in T-LGLD. These include IL-2-dependent cell-mediated suppression of erythropoiesis and the presence of cytotoxic antibodies against erythroid precursors *(50)*. Moreover, abnormal production of IFN-γ and TNF-α has been implicated in the development of PRCA. LGL can inhibit human erythroid stem cell proliferation in vitro *(139)*, and LGL suppress the in vitro growth of erythroid colony-forming units (CFU) in PRCA associated with B-cell CLL *(140)*. These cells have also been proposed to play a role in the pathogenesis of aplastic anemia *(141)*.

Table 3
Diagnostic Criteria for T-LGLD

Diagnostic criteria for T-LGLD

1. Increased numbers of LGL in peripheral-blood smears
                                            AND
2. Demonstration of a CD3+CD8+CD57+ immunophenotype by multiparameter
   flow cytometry
                                            AND
3. a. ≥2 × 10^9/L CD3+CD57+ mononuclear cells
                                            OR
   b. $0.5 × 10^9/L CD3+CD57+ mononuclear cells with clonal T-cell receptor
   (TCR) beta gene rearrangement

Diagnosis

The diagnosis of T-LGLD should be suspected in every patient who presents with unexplained neutropenia. A detailed history and physical examination constitute the first steps in approaching these patients.

Evaluation of the peripheral blood smear is essential in the initial work-up of patients in whom the diagnosis of T-LGLD is suspected. Lymphocytosis of LGL is the characteristic finding, with or without neutropenia *(13,46,70)*. The bone marrow almost always exhibits diffuse or nodular infiltration by atypical lymphocytes *(71)*. Immunophenotype analysis by multiparameter flow cytometry shows characteristic immunophenotypic findings of expression of the CD3, CD8, and CD57 antigens on LGLs *(74,75)*. Cytogenetic analysis is not very helpful in the diagnosis, as 90% of cases exhibit a normal karyotype *(18,25)*, but demonstration of TCR gene rearrangements by Southern blotting or PCR serves to demonstrate clonality *(79–84)*.

The classical diagnostic criterion for T-LGLD is granular lymphocytosis greater than 2 × 10^9/L, lasting at least 6 mo *(20,21,26,28)*. However, many studies have included patients with granular lymphocyte counts below this cutoff limit *(2,142)*. A new set of criteria was established by Semenzato et al. to incorporate the use of new molecular techniques *(142)* (Table 3). An absolute lymphocytosis greater than 2 × 10^9/L is no longer required to establish the diagnosis of T-LGLD, as long as clonal expansion of an LGL population is proven with the use of molecular techniques. Similarly, 6 mo follow-up is not necessary if clonality is convincingly established. Demonstration of clonal dominance in an expanded granular lymphocyte population was suggested to be a mandatory criterion for establishing the diagnosis of T-LGLD *(142)*, but clonality alone is not a sufficient diagnostic criterion, since minor clonal proliferations of cells without classical cytoplasmic granules can be detected by sensitive techniques such as PCR during autoimmune processes.

Differential Diagnosis

T-LGLD should always be considered in the differential diagnosis of cytopenias. Patients with T-LGLD are usually diagnosed with myelodysplastic syndromes initially, since they typically present with one or more cytopenias in the setting of a cellular marrow with trilineage hematopoiesis. The diagnosis of T-LGLD should be considered in any patient with chronic neutropenia, adult-onset cyclic neutropenia or PRCA. It should also be considered in patients with acquired aplastic anemia, as it may present as pancytopenia and marrow hypocellularity (58).

Other clinical disorders associated with atypical lymphocytosis should be excluded, including solid tumors, lymphomas, idiopathic thrombocytopenic purpura, hemophagocytosis, viral infections, and connective tissue diseases such as systemic lupus erythematosus. Viral infections should be given particular consideration in the differential diagnosis. EBV and CMV infections are known to cause atypical lymphocytosis in the peripheral blood. Immunophenotyping of peripheral blood lymphocytes and demonstration of clonality differentiate T-LGLD from reactive viral lymphocytosis. Furthermore, a 6-mo follow-up period is necessary to rule out transient reactive proliferations if clonality is not demonstrated.

T-LGLD should be differentiated from CD56+ lymphoproliferative diseases, including NK-cell LGLD and chronic NK-cell lymphocytosis. NK-cell non-Hodgkin's lymphoma, NK-like T-cell lymphoma, γδ T-cell lymphoma, and rare cases of CD56+ and/or CD16+ acute lymphocytic leukemia are other disease entities that should be considered in the differential diagnosis.

Treatment

Treatment decisions should be individualized. The clinical course of T-LGLD is typically indolent. Approximately 30% of patients are asymptomatic and do not require treatment (20). Spontaneous regressions have also been reported (26). The major indication for therapy is correction of cytopenias. Specifically, treatment is indicated in patients with severe or life-threatening neutropenia, symptomatic anemia, thrombocytopenia, or clinically aggressive disease (Table 4).

Treatment modalities used for T-LGLD have included corticosteroids, splenectomy, cytotoxic agents such as cyclophosphamide, methotrexate, and nucleoside analogs, hematopoietic growth factors, and CSA (Table 5). The most encouraging results have been reported in recent studies utilizing low-dose oral methotrexate (37,133) and CSA (45). Optimal therapy has not yet been defined.

Corticosteroid therapy is usually ineffective in the treatment of T-LGLD; the response to steroids is generally partial and temporary (21,25,28,50,133,143). Prednisone usually cannot alleviate neutropenia. Moreover, an abnormal lymphocyte population persists in patients in whom neutropenia improves. Additionally, steroid therapy is associated with significant toxicity (25).

Table 4
Indications for Treatment of T-LGLD

Indications for treatment of T-LGLD

Severe neutropenia (ANC $<0.5 \times 10^9$/L)
Neutropenia (ANC $<1 \times 10^9$/L) with recurrent infections
Anemia (Hb <9 g/dL)
Thrombocytopenia (platelets $<50 \times 10^9$/L)

Table 5
Treatment Modalities for T-LGLD

Treatment modalities for T-LGLD

Glucocorticoids
Splenectomy
Hematopoietic growth factors
Cyclophosphamide alone or in combination chemotherapy
Nucleoside analogs
Oral low-dose methotrexate
Cyclosporine
Allogeneic bone marrow transplantation

Splenectomy is another treatment modality for T-LGLD that was discussed in early reports. Since neutropenia was believed to be antibody-mediated and splenectomy was known to be effective in other autoimmune cytopenias, it was theorized that splenectomy should be effective in T-LGLD. No benefit was seen in most patients reported in the literature *(21,27,52)*. Splenectomy has been effective in the resolution of symptomatic anemia or neutropenia associated with T-LGLD only in isolated cases *(25,144)*; it resulted in transient improvement in cytopenias in these patients, but had no effect on the underlying lymphopro–liferative disorder *(145,146)*. In fact, the number of circulating LGL frequently increased in the postoperative period *(21,27,146,147)*. In a report of four patients who underwent splenectomy for T-LGLD, two patients experienced sustained resolution of neutropenia, but one of the two later died of progressive disease *(146)*.

The benefit of hematopoietic growth factors in T-LGLD is controversial, with conflicting reports in the literature. Successful treatment of neutropenia has been described in isolated cases *(148–155)*, and no clear benefit has been seen in others *(156,157)*. In one report, three of four patients showed favorable responses to GM-CSF *(155)*. Notably, leukemic clones persist after treatment with either G-CSF or GM-CSF, even in responsive patients in whom neutrophil counts normalize. There is no clear difference between the response of neutropenia in T-LGLD to G-CSF or GM-CSF, although a direct comparative trial has not been performed. A transient response to GM-CSF was reported in a patient who failed G-CSF therapy, suggesting variable patterns of growth-factor response in different patients *(158)*.

Cyclophosphamide, used alone or in combination with prednisone, has been reported to be effective in T-LGLD in some cases *(25,26)* but not in others *(159)*. Cyclophosphamide used alone was less toxic and was associated with more durable remissions *(25)*. Single-agent oral cyclophosphamide was especially effective in patients with PRCA associated with T-LGLD *(26,54,57,61)*. Combination chemotherapy regimens that include cyclophosphamide, such as cyclophosphamide, vincristine, and prednisone (CVP) or cyclophosphamide, doxorubicin, vincristine, and prednisone (CHOP), have been employed in aggressive disease, but have generally been unsuccessful. Single-agent chlorambucil therapy has also produced occasional sustained responses *(143)*. Other immunosuppressive agents, including anti-lymphocyte globulin, anti-thymocyte globulin, and azathioprine, have been used with some success *(53,56,160)*.

Nucleoside analogs including fludarabine *(159)*, 2-chlorodeoxyadenosine *(161,162)* and 2'-deoxycoformycin *(163,164)* have been used in the treatment of T-LGLD with variable success. Reports have generally included only a few cases, and it is very difficult to draw conclusions based on this limited experience.

Low-dose oral methotrexate therapy has been reported to induce durable complete clinical remissions in patients with T-LGLD *(37,133)*. In a series of 10 patients, five achieved complete clinical remission, with normalization of both neutrophil and CD3+CD57+ LGL counts, and one had a partial response, with normalization of neutrophil counts but persistence of the abnormal LGL clone *(133)*. Three of the five complete responders achieved molecular remission, with disappearance of TCR gene rearrangement *(133)*. In a second series, three of four patients with T-LGLD and associated RA had clinical responses defined by resolution of joint pain and swelling and disappearance of recurrent infections, and two of the three achieved complete hematologic and molecular remission, with normalization of the LGL count and disappearance of TCR gene rearrangement *(37)*. Response to methotrexate is rather slow, with a 2-wk to 4-mo interval from initiation of therapy to attainment of a clinical response *(133,160)*, and maintenance therapy is required after the response is attained. Notably, not all patients treated with methotrexate respond *(133,144,159)*. Methotrexate may be especially effective in the setting of RA *(37)*. The exact mechanism of action of methotrexate in T-LGLD is unknown. Liu et al. demonstrated reduction in circulating FasL levels associated with clinical response to methotrexate *(137)*. Furthermore, FasL levels increased in a patient at disease relapse.

CSA is an immunosuppressive agent that suppresses both cellular and humoral immunity by inhibiting activation of CD4+ lymphocytes. CSA also inhibits expression of genes coding for IL-2, the IL-2 receptor, and other cytokines *(165)*. CSA has been reported to successfully treat neutropenia and anemia in patients with T-LGLD both in case reports *(52,55,166–168)* and in recent series *(45,50,56)*. In most patients, cytopenias respond to CSA despite persistence of the leukemic clone *(45,50,56)*, but there is one case report of disappearance of TCR rearrangement in a patient treated with a combination of CSA and G-CSF *(157)*. PRCA associated with T-LGLD also responds to CSA *(50,55–57)*. In the largest series reported to date, five T-LGLD patients with severe neutropenia were treated with CSA, which was initiated at doses of 1 to 1.5 mg/kg orally every 12 h *(45)*. Four of the five responded to CSA alone, and the fifth responded following the addition of low-dose GM-CSF. Ongoing CSA therapy was required to sustain responses. Three patients were alive with normal neutrophil counts on continuous low-dose CSA therapy, with follow-ups of two, eight, and eight-and-a-half yr, and the other two died of unrelated causes despite maintaining normal neutrophil counts. In another report, two patients with T-LGLD and one with NK-LGLD with treatment-refractory anemia displayed rapid and sustained responses to CSA *(50)*. In all reports, maintenance therapy has been necessary once the desired response is obtained, although doses can be reduced in the maintenance phase *(45,50,55)*.

The mechanism by which neutropenia associated with T-LGLD responds to CSA is unclear. CSA is known to inhibit the expression of genes coding for IL-2 and the IL-2 receptor *(165)*; thus, cytokine-mediated pathogenetic events in the neutropenia and anemia associated with T-LGLD may be altered by CSA *(45,50,60)*. An alternative hypothesis is suggested by the recent demonstration of Pgp overexpression in T-LGL leukemia cells in T-LGLD, with Pgp-mediated drug efflux *(119,121)*. The Pgp modulator verapamil is beneficial in the reversion of Pgp-mediated resistance in patients with T-LGLD *(119,121)*. CSA is another MDR modulator that reverses Pgp-mediated drug efflux *(169)*, and the effects of CSA on T-LGL cells may occur through Pgp modulation. Pgp is also involved in the transmembrane transport of cytokines, including IL-2 and IFN-γ, in normal T-lymphocytes *(170,171)*, and inhibition of Pgp-mediated transport of these cytokines may considerably reduce IL-2 production by activated lymphocytes.

Allogeneic bone-marrow transplantation (Allo-BMT) represents a potentially curative therapeutic modality in patients with T-LGLD who are of appropriate age and have an HLA-compatible donor. There is a single case report of successful treatment of T-LGLD with Allo-BMT in a 23-yr-old patient with significant visceral involvement and recurrent life-threatening infections, who had not responded to corticosteroids, splenectomy, or growth factors *(172)*.

Prognosis

T-LGLD is a heterogenous disorder that usually runs an indolent course. Our knowledge about the clinical course of the disease is limited by the limited number of reports of its natural history published to date. Patients' clinical characteristics and prognoses appear to be highly variable. The main cause of mortality is the infections that occur in the setting of neutropenia *(2,28)*. Rapid progression of the lymphoproliferative disorder has also been recognized as the cause of death in a small number of patients.

The largest series investigating the natural history of T-LGLD published to date was a multicenter study that included 151 cases *(21)*. The 4-yr mortality was 17%; lymph node and liver involvement, fever at the time of initial diagnosis, skin infiltration, and low or high white blood cell (WBC) counts were the adverse prognostic factors. Dhodapkar et al. reported a 10% mortality in 68 patients seen at the Mayo Clinic, with a median follow-up of 44 mo. The 10-yr actuarial survival was greater than 80%, with an actuarial median survival of 161 mo for the entire cohort *(25)*. Anemia was the most common indication for treatment, followed by B-symptoms and neutropenia. There was no prognostic factor predictive of short survival, but the presence of neutropenia, infections, or B-symptoms correlated with a low probability of achieving complete remission. Oshimi et al. reported a variable survival, ranging from 3 mo to more than 14 yr, in a follow-up study of 33 patients, including two with spontaneous regressions *(26)*. In another report, 38 patients with a median follow-up of 17 mo had an 18% mortality; most deaths were from neutropenic sepsis *(28)*.

A CD3+ CD56+ subset of T-LGLD has been described, with an aggressive clinical course and a poor prognosis. Combination chemotherapy is generally employed in these patients, but the outcome is usually poor, and the majority of patients died within 1 yr of diagnosis *(31)*.

NK-CELL LGLD

Approximately 20% of cases of LGLD are NK-cell type *(2,5,173)*. Most patients have been reported from the Far East, especially Japan. The clinical picture is totally different from that of T-LGLD. Patients are younger: most patients are diagnosed in their third or early fourth decade; the median age is 39 yr *(2)*. NK-cell LGLD usually pursues a more aggressive course than T-LGLD, with frequent visceral organ involvement *(174,175)*. Patients commonly present with hepatosplenomegaly and systemic B-symptoms, including fever, night sweats, and weight loss. Involvement of the gastrointestinal system has been reported, with bowel ulcers, jaundice, and ascites *(174–177)*. Anemia and thrombocytopenia are more severe than in T-LGLD, but neutropenia is less severe. Immunologic abnormalities are not observed.

The peripheral blood smear in NK-LGLD is similar to that in T-LGLD, with increased numbers of lymphocytes showing the characteristic features of LGL by light microscopy. At the ultrastructural level, however, these cells are deficient in the parallel tubular arrays that are usually present in T-LGL cells *(178)*. The bone marrow is almost universally involved in NK-LGLD.

NK-LGLD is characterized by a CD3-negative phenotype *(2–4)*, with expression of CD56, as well as CD2, CD7, and CD16 (74, 75). NK-LGL display a germline TCR gene pattern. Because TCR gene rearrangements are absent, the clonal nature of NK-LGLD is not readily demonstrated. Cytogenetic abnormalities may be useful in demonstrating clonality, but no characteristic chromosomal abnormalities exist *(174,175,179)*. Aberrations involving the long arm of chromosome 6 are the changes most frequently found in these patients, either alone or in association with other chromosome changes *(180)*. Most cases with chromosomal abnormalities have complex karyotypes. X-linked polymorphism gene analysis has been suggested as a technique for demonstrating clonality in female patients with NK-LGLD *(181)*.

A viral etiology has been strongly implicated in the clonal expansion of NK-cells; EBV has been of particular interest *(177,182–185)*. Most patients with EBV-associated NK-LGLD have been reported from Japan, but there are rare reports from the United States *(185)*. EBV viral DNA integration in leukemia cells was demonstrated in some patients, indicating the clonal origin of NK-LGLD and a possible direct involvement of EBV in LGL transformation *(177,183–186)*. An etiological relationship similar to that in EBV-associated B-cell lymphomas was suggested *(184)*, but the presence of EBV DNA could not be confirmed in large-scale studies in patients from the United States and Europe *(182,187,188)*. A specific subgroup of NK cells that evolve as a direct response to EBV infection was suggested in another study, although EBV sequences were detected in peripheral blood mononuclear cells of only six of 19 patients with NK-LGLD *(92)*.

Treatment is usually not effective in NK-LGLD. Combination chemotherapy, which has generally consisted of cyclophosphamide-containing regimens, yields poor results; survival is short, with rare long-term survival. Patients usually die within a few months of diagnosis because of disseminated aggressive disease and associated coagulopathy. There are case reports of successful treatment of patients with EBV-associated NK-LGLD with BMT *(177,186)*.

MDR mediated by Pgp has been implicated in the drug-resistance associated with the aggressive clinical course of NK-LGLD *(119,189)*. MDR modulators including CSA and its analog PSC833 are less effective in inhibiting Pgp function in aggressive than in indolent NK-LGLD *(189)*. This lack of efficacy might be caused by the presence of other mechanisms of drug resistance *(189)*.

CONCLUSION

LGL proliferative diseases include T-cell and NK-cell LGLD, two diseases that differ markedly in their presentation, therapy, and prognosis. The diagnosis of T-LGLD should be considered in any patient with cytopenias. In particular, T-LGLD is a highly treatable cause of life-threatening severe neutropenia. Patients with T-LGLD respond to two recently reported therapies, low-dose oral methotrexate and cyclosporine. Mechanisms of treatment response must be elucidated, and optimal therapy must be defined.

REFERENCES

1. Timonen T, Ortaldo JR, Herberman RB. Characteristics of human large granular lymphocytes and relationship to natural killer and K cells. *J Exp Med* 1981; 153:569–582.
2. Loughran TP. Clonal diseases of large granular lymphocytes. *Blood* 1993; 82:1–14.
3. Chan WC, Link S, Mawle A, et al. Heterogeneity of large granular lymphocyte populations: delineation of two major subtypes. *Blood* 1986; 68:1142–1153.
4. Harris NL, Jaffe ES, Stein H, et al. A revised European-American classification of lymphoid neoplasms: a proposal from the International Lymphoma Study Group. *Blood* 1994; 84: 1361–1392.
5. Scott CS, Richards SJ, Sivakumaran M, et al. Transient and persistent expansions of large granular lymphocytes (LGL) and NK-associated (NKa) cells: the Yorkshire Leukaemia Group Study. *Br J Haematol* 1993; 83:505–515.
6. Brouet J-C, Flandrin G, Sasportes M, et al. Chronic lymphocytic leukemia of T-cell origin: immunological and clinical evaluation in eleven patients. *Lancet* 1975; 2:890–893.
7. McKenna RW, Parkin J, Kersey JH, et al. Chronic lymphoproliferative disorder with unusual clinical, morphological, ultrastructural and membrane surface marker characteristics. *Am J Med* 1977; 62:588–596.
8. Matutes E, Brito-Babapulle V, Worner I, et al. T-cell chronic lymphocytic leukemia: the spectrum of mature T-cell disorders. *Nouv Rev Fr Hematol* 1988; 30:347–351.
9. Aisenberg AC, Wilkes BM, Harris NL, et al. Chronic T-cell lymphocytosis with neutropenia. Report of a case studied with monoclonal antibody. *Blood* 1981; 58:818–822.
10. Rumke HC, Miedema F, Ten Berge IJM, et al. Functional properties of T cells in patients with chronic T lymphocytosis and chronic T cell neoplasia. *J Immunol* 1982; 129:419–426.
11. Brisbane JU, Berman LD, Osband ME, Neiman RS. T8 chronic lymphocytic leukemia. A distinctive disorder related to T8 lymphocytosis. *Am J Clin Pathol* 1983; 80:391–396.
12. Palutke M, Eisenberg L, Kaplan J, et al. Natural killer and suppressor T-cell chronic lymphocytic leukemia. *Blood* 1983; 62:627–634.
13. Chan WC, Check I, Schick C, et al. A morphologic and immunologic study of the large granular lymphocyte in neutropenia with T lymphocytosis. *Blood* 1984; 63:1133–1140.
14. Reynolds CW, Foon KA. T-gamma lymphoproliferative disease and related disorders in humans and experimental animals: a review of the clinical, cellular and functional characteristics. *Blood* 1984; 64:1146–1158.
15. Bakri K, Ezdinli EZ, Wasser LP, et al. T suppressor cell chronic lymphocytic leukemia. Phenotypic characterization by monoclonal antibodies. *Cancer* 1984; 54:284–292.
16. McKenna RW, Arthur DC, Gajl-Peczalska KJ. Granulated T-cell lymphocytosis with neutropenia: malignant or benign chronic lymphoproliferative disorder? *Blood* 1985; 66:259–266.
17. Miedema F, Terpstra FG, Smith JW, et al. T-γ lymphocytosis is clinically non-progressive but immunologically heterogenous. *Clin Exp Immunol* 1985; 61:440–449.
18. Loughran TP, Kadin ME, Starkebaum G, et al. Leukemia of large granular lymphocytes: association with clonal chromosomal abnormalities and autoimmune neutropenia, thrombocytopenia and hemolytic anemia. *Ann Intern Med* 1985; 102:169–175.
19. Grillot-Courvalin C, Vinci G, Tsapis A, et al. The syndrome of T8 hyperlymphocytosis: variation in phenotype and cytotoxic activities of granular cells and evaluation of their role in associated neutropenia. *Blood* 1986; 69: 1204–1210.
20. Semenzato G, Pandolfi F, Chisesi T, et al. The lymphoproliferative disease of granular lymphocytes: a heterogenous disorder ranging from indolent to aggressive conditions. *Cancer* 1987; 60:2971–2978.
21. Pandolfi F, Loughran TP, Starkebaum G, et al. Clinical course and prognosis of the lymphoproliferative disease of granular lymphocytes: a multicenter study. *Cancer* 1990; 65:341–348.

22. Oshimi K. Granular lymphocyte proliferative disorders: report of 12 cases and review of the literature. *Leukemia* 1988; 2:617–627.

23. Bennett JM, Catovski D, Daniel MT, et al. Proposals for the classification of chronic (mature) B and T lymphoid leukaemias: French-American-British (FAB) Cooperative Group. *J Clin Pathol* 1989; 42:567–584.

24. Bennett JM, Juliusson G, Mecucci C. Morphologic, immunologic, and cytogenetic classification of the chronic (mature) B and T lymphoid leukemias: Fourth meeting of the MIC Cooperative Study Group. *Cancer Res* 1990; 50:2212.

25. Dhodapkar MV, Li C-Y, Lust JA, et al. Clinical spectrum of clonal proliferations of T-large granular lymphocytes: a T-cell clonopathy or undetermined significance? *Blood* 1994; 84:1620–1627.

26. Oshimi K, Yamada O, Kaneko T, et al. Laboratory findings and clinical courses of 33 patients with granular lymphocyte-proliferative disorders. *Leukemia* 1993;7:782-788.

27. Newland AC, Catovski D, Linch D, et al. Chronic T-cell lymphocytosis: a review of 21 cases. *Br J Haematol* 1984; 58:433–446.

28. Loughran TP, Starkebaum G. Large granular lymphocyte leukemia: report of 38 cases and review of the literature. *Medicine* 1987; 66:397–405.

29. De Rossi G, Pasqualetti D, De Sancti G, et al. Childhood abnormal expansion of large granular lymphocytes. *Acta Haematol* 1985; 73:206–209.

30. Sun T, Brody J, Koduru P, et al. Study of the major phenotype of large granular T-cell lymphoproliferative disorder. *Am J Clin Pathol* 1992; 98:516–521.

31. Gentile TC, Uner AH, Hutchison RE, et al. CD3+, CD56+ aggressive variant of large granular lymphocyte leukemia. *Blood* 1994; 84:2315–2321.

32. Barton JC, Prasthofer EF, Egan ML, et al. Rheumatoid arthritis associated with expanded populations of granular lymphocytes. *Ann Intern Med* 1986; 104: 314–323.

33. Samanta A, Grant I, Nichol FE, et al. Large granular lymphocytosis associated with rheumatoid arthritis. *Ann Rheum Dis* 1988; 47:873–875.

34. Loughran TP, Starkebaum G, Kidd P, Neiman P. Clonal proliferation of large granular lymphocytes in rheumatoid arthritis. *Arthritis Rheum* 1988; 31:31–36.

35. Horiuchi T, Hirokawa M, Satoh K, et al. Clonal expansion of gammadelta-T lymphocytes in an HTLV-I carrier, associated with chronic neutropenia and rheumatoid arthritis. *Ann Hematol* 1999; 78:101–104.

36. Starkebaum G. Leukemia of large granular lymphocytes and rheumatoid arthritis. *Am J Med* 2000; 108:744–745.

37. Hamidou MA, Sadr FB, Lamy T, et al. Low-dose methotrexate for the treatment of patients with large granular lymphocyte leukemia associated with rheumatoid arthritis. *Am J Med* 2000; 108:730–732.

38. Wallis WJ, Loughran TP Jr, Kadin M, et al. Polyarthritis and neutropenia associated with circulating large granular lymphocytes. *Ann Intern Med* 1985; 103:357–362.

39. Bowman SJ, Corrigall V, Panayi GS, Lanchbury JS. Hematologic and cytofluorographic analysis of patients with Felty's syndrome: a hypothesis that a discrete event leads to large granular lymphocyte expansions in this condition. *Arthritis Rheum* 1995; 38:1252–1259.

40. Bowman SJ, Sivakumaran M, Snowden N, et al. The large granular lymphocyte syndrome with rheumatoid arthritis. Immunogenetic evidence for a broader definition of Felty's syndrome. *Arthritis Rheum* 1994; 37:1326–1330.

41. Starkebaum G, Loughran TP, Gaur LK, et al. Immunogenetic similarities between patients with Felty's syndrome and those with clonal expansions of large granular lymphocytes in rheumatoid arthritis. *Arthritis Rheum* 1997; 40:624–626.

42. Bowman SJ, Bhavnani M, Geddes GC, et al. Large granular lymphocyte expansions in patients with Felty's syndrome: analysis using anti-T cell receptor V beta-specific monoclonal antibodies. *Clin Exp Immunol* 1995; 101:18–24.

43. Bowman SJ, Hall MA, Panayi GS, Lanchbury JS. T cell receptor alpha-chain and beta-chain junctional region homology in clonal CD3+, CD8+ T lymphocyte expansions in Felty's syndrome. *Arthritis Rheum* 1997; 40:615–623.

44. Coakley G, Iqbal M, Brooks D, et al. CD8+, CD57+ T cells from healthy elderly subjects suppress neutrophil development in vitro: implications for the neutropenia of Felty's and large granular lymphocyte syndromes. *Arthritis Rheum* 2000; 43:834–843.

45. Sood R, Stewart CC, Aplan PD, et al. Neutropenia associated with T-cell large granular lymphocyte leukemia: long-term response to cyclosporine therapy despite persistence of abnormal cells. *Blood* 1998; 91:3372–3378.

46. McDaniel HL, MacPherson BR, Tindle BH, Lunde JH. Lymphoproliferative disorder of granular lymphocytosis: a heterogenous disease. *Arch Pathol Lab Med* 1992; 116:242–248.

47. Bassan R, Introna M, Rambaldi A, et al. Large granular lymphocyte/natural killer cell proliferative disease: clinical and laboratory heterogeneity. *Scand J Hematol* 1986; 37:91–93.

48. Loughran TP, Hammond WP. Adult onset cyclic neutropenia is a benign neoplasm associated with clonal proliferation of large granular lymphocytes. *J Exp Med* 1986; 164:2089–2094.

49. Loughran TP, Clark EA, Price TH, Hammond WP. Adult-onset cyclic neutropenia is associated with increased large granular lymphocytes. *Blood* 1986; 68:1082–1087.

50. Bible KC, Tefferi A. Cyclosporine A alleviates severe anemia associated with refractory large granular lymphocytic leukemia and chronic natural killer cell lymphocytosis. *Br J Haematol* 1996; 93:406–408.

51. Akashi K, Shibuya T, Taniguchi S, et al. Multiple hematopoietic disorders and insidious clonal proliferation of large granular lymphocytes. *Br J Haematol* 1999; 107:670–673.

52. Brinkman K, van Doggen JJ, van Lom K, et al. Induction of remission in T-large granular lymphocyte leukemia with cyclosporin A, monitored by use of immunophenotyping with V beta antibodies. *Leukemia* 1998; 12:150–154.

53. Kouides PA, Rowe JM. Large granular lymphocyte leukemia presenting with both amegakaryocytic thrombocytopenic purpura and pure red cell aplasia: clinical course and response to immunosuppressive therapy. *Am J Hematol* 1995; 49:232–236.

54. Masuda M, Arai Y, Nishina H, et al. Large granular lymphocyte leukemia with pure red cell aplasia in a renal transplant recipient. *Am J Hematol* 1998; 57:72–76.

55. Coutinho J, Lima M, dos Anjos Teixeira M, et al. Pure red cell aplasia associated to clonal CD8+ T-cell large granular lymphocytosis: dependence on cyclosporin therapy. *Acta Haematol* 1998; 100:207–210.

56. Kwong YL, Wong KF. Association of pure red cell aplasia with T large granular lymphocyte leukemia. *J Clin Pathol* 1998; 51:672–675.

57. Lacy MQ, Kurtin PJ, Tefferi A. Pure red cell aplasia: association with large granular lymphocyte leukemia and the prognostic value of cytogenetic abnormalities. *Blood* 1996; 87:3000–3006.

58. Go RS, Tefferi A, Li C-Y, Lust JA, Phyliky RL. Lymphoproliferative disease of granular T lymphocytes presenting as aplastic anemia. *Blood* 2000; 96:3644–3646.

59. Amparo E, Kaplan L, Rosenbloom B, Lee S. T-gamma-lymphoproliferative disorder arising in a background of autoimmune disease and terminating in plasma cell dyscrasia with primary amyloidosis. *Arch Pathol Lab Med* 1991; 115:74–77.

60. Marolleau JP, Henni T, Gaulard P, et al. Hairy cell leukemia associated with large granular lymphocyte leukemia: immunologic and genomic study, effect of interferon treatment. *Blood* 1988; 72:655–660.

61. Bassan R, Rambaldi A, Allavena P, et al. Association of large granular lymphocyte/natural killer cell proliferative disease and second hematologic malignancy. *Am J Hematol* 1988; 29:85–93.

62. Hanada T, Ishida T, Kojima H, Tsuchiya T. Granular lymphocyte leukaemia in association with multiple myeloma. *Br J Haematol* 1992; 80:127–129.

63. Sivakumaran M, Richards S. Immunological abnormalities of chronic large granular lymphocytosis. *Clin Lab Haematol* 1997; 19:57–60.

64. Gentile TC, Wener MH, Starkebaum G, Loughran TP. Humoral immune abnormalities in T-cell large granular lymphocyte leukemia. *Leuk Lymphoma* 1996; 23:365–70.

65. Starkebaum G, Martin PJ, Singer JW, et al. Chronic lymphocytosis with neutropenia: evidence for a novel, abnormal T-cell population associated with antibody-mediated neutrophil destruction. *Clin Immunol Immunopathol* 1983; 27:110–123.

66. Bassan R, Pronesti M, Buzzetti M, et al. Autoimmunity and B-cell dysfunction in chronic proliferative disorders of large granular lymphocytes/natural killer cells. *Cancer* 1989; 63:90–95.

67. Perri RT, Kay NE. Large granular lymphocytes from B-chronic lymphocytic leukemia patients inhibit normal B cell proliferation. *Am J Hematol* 1989; 31:166–172.

68. Dhodapkar MV, Lust JA, Phyliky RL. T-cell large granular lymphocytic leukemia and pure red cell aplasia in a patient with type I autoimmune polyendocrinopathy: Response to immunosuppressive therapy. *Mayo Clin Proc* 1994; 69:1085–1088.

69. Brieva JA, Targan S, Stevens RH. NK and T cell subsets regulate antibody production by human in vitro antigen-induced lymphoblastoid B cells. *J Immunol* 1984; 132:611–615.

70. McKenna RW. Lymphoproliferative disorder of granular lymphocytosis: more questions than answers. *Arch Pathol Lab Med* 1992; 116:235–237.

71. Agnarsson BA, Loughran TP, Starkebaum G, Kadin M. The pathology of large granular lymphocyte leukemia. *Hum Pathol* 1989; 20:643–651.

72. Iizuka Y, Nishinarita S, Ohshima T, Sawada S. Hematopoiesis in patients with acute natural killer cell leukemia and large granular lymphocytosis: relationship between clinical features and hematopoietic inhibitor activity of peripheral mononuclear cells. *Eur J Haematol* 1989; 43:257–258.

73. Merlio JP, De Mascarel A, Goussot JF. Bone marrow involvement in large granular lymphocyte leukemia. *Hum Pathol* 1990; 21:458–459.

74. Jennings CD, Foon KA. Recent advances in flow cytometry: application to the diagnosis of hematologic malignancy. *Blood* 1997; 90:2863–2892.

75. Borowitz MJ, Bray R, Gascoyne R, et al. US-Canadian consensus recommendations on the immunophenotypic analysis of hematologic neoplasia by flow cytometry: Data analysis and interpretation. *Cytometry* 1997; 30:236–244.

76. Richards SJ, Short M, Scott CS. Clonal CD3+CD8+ large granular lymphocyte (LGL)/NK-associated expansions: primary malignancies or secondary reactive phenomena? *Leuk Lymphoma* 1995; 17:303–311.

77. Sivakumaran M, Richards SJ, Hunt KM, et al. Patterns of CD16 and CD56 expression in persistent expansions of CD3+Nka+ lymphocytes are predictive for clonal T-cell receptor gene rearrangements. *Br J Haematol* 1991; 78:368–377.

78. Richards SJ, Sivakumaran M, Parapia LA, et al. A distinct large granular lymphocyte (LGL)/NK-associated (Nka) abnormality characterised by membrane CD4 and CD8 coexpression. The Yorkshire Leukaemia Group. *Br J Haematol* 1992; 82:494–501.

79. Loiseau P, Divine M, Le Paslier D, et al. Phenotypic and genotypic heterogeneity of large granular lymphocyte expansion. *Leukemia* 1987; 1:205–209.

80. Rambaldi A, Pelicci PG, Allavena P, et al. T cell receptor B chain gene rearrangements in lymphoproliferative disorders of large granular lymphocytes/natural killer cells. *J Exp Med* 1995; 162:2156–2162.

81. Zambello R, Trentin L, Facco M, et al. Analysis of the T cell receptor in the lymphoproliferative disease of granular lymphocytes: superantigen activation of clonal CD3+ granular lymphocytes. *Cancer Res* 1995; 55:6140–6145.

82. Chan WC, Winton EF, Waldmann TA. Lymphocytosis of large granular lymphocytes. *Arch Intern Med* 1986; 146:1201–1203.

83. Ryan DK, Alexander HD, Morris TC. Routine diagnosis of large granular lymphocytic leukemia by Southern blot and polymerase chain reaction analysis of clonal T cell receptor gene rearrangement. *Mol Pathol* 1997; 50: 77–81.

84. Loughran TP, Starkebaum G, Aprile JA, et al. Rearrangement and expression of T-cell receptor genes in large granular lymphocyte leukemia. *Blood* 1988; 71:822–824.
85. Pelicci PG, Allavena P, Subar M, et al. T cell receptor (alpha, beta, gamma) gene rearrangements and expression in normal and leukemic large granular lymphocytes/natural killer cells. *Blood* 1987; 70:1500–1508.
86. Davey MP, Starkebaum G, Loughran TP. CD3+ leukemic large granular lymphocytes utilize diverse T-cell receptor V beta genes. *Blood* 1995; 85:146–150.
87. Semenzato G, Pizzolo G, Ranucci A, et al. Abnormal expansions of polyclonal large to small size granular lymphocytes: reactive or neoplastic process? *Blood* 1984; 63:1271–1277.
88. Starkebaum G, Loughran TP, Kalyanaraman VS, et al. Serum reactivity to human T-cell leukemia/lymphoma virus type I proteins in patients with large granular lymphocyte leukemia. *Lancet* 1987; 1:596–598.
89. Loughran TP, Sherman MP, Ruscetti FW, et al. Prototypical HTLV-I/II infection is rare in LGL leukemia. *Leuk Res* 1994; 18:423–429.
90. Loughran TP, Hadlock KG, Perzova R, et al. Epitope mapping of HTLV envelope seroreactivity in LGL leukemia. *Br J Haematol* 1998; 101:318–324.
91. Perzova R, Loughran TP, Dube S, et al. Lack of BLV and PTLV DNA sequences in the majority of patients with large granular lymphocyte leukemia. *Br J Haematol* 2000; 109:64–70.
92. Pellenz M, Zambello R, Semenzato G, Loughran TP. Detection of Epstein-Barr virus by PCR analyses in lymphoproliferative disease of granular lymphocytes. *Leuk Lymphoma* 1996; 23:371–374.
93. Pawson R, Schulz TF, Matutes E, Catovski D. The human T-cell lymphotropic viruses types I/II are not involved in T prolymphocytic leukemia and large granular lymphocytic leukemia. *Leukemia* 1997; 11:1305–1311.
94. Fouchard N, Flageul B, Bagot M, et al. Lack of evidence of HTLV-I/II infection in T CD8 malignant or reactive lymphoproliferative disorders in France: a serological and/or molecular study of 169. *Leukemia* 1995; 9:2087–2092.
95. Phillips JH, Lanier LL. Lectin-dependent and anti-CD3-induced cytotoxicity are preferentially mediated by peripheral blood cytotoxic T lymphocytes expressing Leu-7 antigen. *J Immunol* 1986; 136:1579–1585.
96. Spits H, Yssel H, Leeuwenberg J, DeVries JE. Antigen-specific cytotoxic T cell and antigen-specific proliferating T cell clones can be induced to cytolytic activity by monoclonal antibodies against T3. *Eur J Immunol* 1985; 15:88–91.
97. Zambello R, Cassatella MA, Trentin L, et al. Different mechanisms of activation of proliferating CD3+ cells in patients with lymphoproliferative disease of granular lymphocytes. *Leukemia* 1991; 5:942–950.
98. Loughran TP, Aprile JA, Ruscetti FW. Anti-CD3 monoclonal antibody mediated cytotoxicity occurs through an interleukin-2 independent pathway in CD3+ large granular lymphocytes. *Blood* 1990; 75:935–940.
99. Yoon HJ, Aprile JA, Loughran TP. Interleukin-2 receptor monoclonal antibodies have no effect on anti-CD3 monoclonal antibody-mediated cytotoxicity in CD3+ leukemic large granular lymphocytes. *Cell Immunol* 1990; 131:404–408.
100. Aprile JA, Russo M, Pepe MS, Loughran TP. Activation signals leading to proliferation of normal and leukemic CD3+ large granular lymphocytes. *Blood* 1991; 78:1282–1285.
101. Perzova R, Loughran TP. Constitutive expression of Fas ligand in large granular lymphocyte leukemia. *Br J Haematol* 1997; 97:123–126.
102. Lamy T, Liu JH, Landowski TH, et al. Dysregulation of CD95/CD95 ligand-apoptotic pathway in CD3+ large granular lymphocyte leukemia. *Blood* 1998; 92:4771–4777.
103. Nagata S, Golstein P. The Fas death factor. *Science* 1995;267:1449–1456.
104. Tanaka M, Suda T, Haze K, et al. Fas ligand in human serum. *Nat Med* 1996; 2:317–322.

105. Ashkenazi A, Dixit WM. Death receptors: signaling and modulation. *Science* 1998; 281: 1305–1308.
106. Alderson MR, Tough TW, Davis-Smith T, et al. Fas ligand mediates activation-induced cell death in human T lymphocytes. *J Exp Med* 1995; 181:71–77.
107. Robb RJ, Munck A, Smith KA. T cell growth factor receptors. Quantitation, specificity and biological relevance. *J Exp Med* 1981; 154:1455–1474.
108. Owen-Schaub LB, Yonehara S, Crimp WL, Grimm EA. DNA fragmentation and cell death is selectively triggered in activated human lymphocytes by Fas antigen engagement. *Cell Immunol* 1992; 140:197–205.
109. Tsudo M, Goldman CK, Bongiovanni KF, et al. The p75 peptide is the receptor for interleukin 2 expressed on large granular lymphocytes and is responsible for the IL-2 activation of these cells. *Proc Natl Acad Sci USA* 1987; 84:5394–5398.
110. Zambello R, Trentin L, Pizzolo G, et al. Cell membrane expression and functional role of the p75 subunit of the interleukin-2 receptor in lymphoproliferative disease of granular lymphocytes. *Blood* 1990; 76:2080–2085.
111. Colamonici OR, Quinones R, Rosolen A, et al. The beta subunit of interleukin-2 receptor mediated interleukin-2 induction of anti-CD3 redirected cytotoxic capability in large granular lymphocytes. *Blood* 1988; 71:825–828.
112. Yoon HJ, Sugamura K, Loughran TP. Activation of leukemic large granular lymphocytes by interleukin-2 via the p75 interleukin-2 receptor. *Leukemia* 1990; 4:848–850.
113. Zambello R, Trentin L, Bulian P, et al. Role of tumor necrosis factor alpha and its specific 55-kd and 75-kd receptors in patients with lymphoproliferative disease of granular lymphocytes. *Blood* 1992; 80:2030–2037.
114. Zambello R, Trentin L, Facco M, et al. Analysis of TNF-receptor and ligand superfamily molecules in patients with lymphoproliferative disease of granular lymphocytes. *Blood* 2000; 96:647–654.
115. Owen-Schaub L, Crump W, Morin GI, Grimm EA. Regulation of lymphocyte tumor necrosis factor receptors by IL-2. *J Immunol* 1989; 143:2236–2241.
116. Gentile TC, Loughran TP. Interleukin-12 is a costimulatory cytokine for leukemic CD3+ large granular lymphocytes. *Cell Immunol* 1995; 166:158–161.
117. Zambello R, Trentin L, Cassatella MA, et al. IL-12 is involved in the activation of CD3+ granular lymphocytes in patients with lymphoproliferative disease of granular lymphocytes. *Br J Haematol* 1996; 92:308–314.
118. Zambello R, Facco M, Trentin L, et al. Interleukin-15 triggers the proliferation and cytotoxicity of granular lymphocytes in patients with lymphoproliferative disease of granular lymphocytes. *Blood* 1997; 89:201–211.
119. Yamamoto T, Iwasaki T, Watanabe N, et al. Expression of multidrug resistance P-glycoprotein on peripheral blood mononuclear cells of patients with granular lymphocyte-proliferative disorders. *Blood* 1993; 81:1342–1346.
120. Drenou B, Amiot L, Lamy T, et al. Multidrug resistance in aggressive lymphoproliferative disorders of T and natural killer origin. *Leuk Lymphoma* 1998; 30:381–387.
121. Lamy T, Drenou B, Fardel O, et al. Multidrug resistance analysis in lymphoproliferative disease of large granular lymphocytes. *Br J Haematol* 1998; 100:509–515.
122. Endicot JA, Ling V. The biochemistry of P-glycoprotein mediated multidrug resistance. *Annu Rev Biochem* 1989; 58:137–171.
123. Yasukawa M, Utsunomiya Y, Inoue Y, et al. Monoclonal proliferation of CD4+ large granular lymphocytes with cytolytic activity. *Br J Haematol* 1995; 91:419–420.
124. Oshimi K, Shinkai Y, Okumura K, et al. Perforin gene expression in granular lymphocyte proliferative disorders. *Blood* 1990; 75:704–708.
125. Smyth MJ, Ortaldo JR, Shinkai Y, et al. Interleukin-2 induction of pore-forming protein gene expression in human peripheral blood CD8+ T cells. *J Exp Med* 1990; 171:1269–1281.

126. Facchetti P, Tacchetti C, Prigione I, et al. Ultrastructural and functional studies of the inter-action between IL-12 and IL-2 for the generation of lymphokine-activated killer cells. *Exp Cell Res* 1999; 253:440–453.

127. Macey MG, Hou L, Milne T, et al. A CD4+ proliferation of large granular lymphocytes expresses the protease activated receptor-1. *Br J Haematol* 1998; 101:78–81.

128. Barr RD, Stevens CA. The role of autologous helper and suppressor T cells in the regulation of human granulopoiesis. *Am J Hematol* 1982; 12:323–326.

129. Morris TCM, Vincent PC, Sutherland R, Hersey P. Inhibition of normal human granulopoie-sis in vitro by non-B and non-T lymphocytes. *Br J Haematol* 1980; 45:541–550.

130. Spitzer G, Verma DS. Cells with Fc gamma receptors from normal blood donors suppress granulocytic macrophage colony formation. *Blood* 1982; 60:758–766.

131. Hansson M, Beran M, Andersson B, Kiessling R. Inhibition of in vitro granulopoiesis by autologous allogeneic human NK cells. *J Immunol* 1982; 129:126–132.

132. Rustagi PK, Han T, Ziolkowski L, et al. Granulocyte antibodies in leukemic chronic lymphoproliferative disorders. *Br J Haematol* 1987; 66:461–465.

133. Loughran TP, Kidd PG, Starkebaum G. Treatment of large granular lymphocyte leukemia with oral low-dose methotrexate. *Blood* 1994; 84:2164–2170.

134. Kasahara T, Djeu JY, Dougherty SF, Oppenheim JJ. Capacity of human large granular lymphocytes to produce multiple lymphokines: interleukin-2, interferon, and colony stimu-lating factors. *J Immunol* 1983; 131:2379–2385.

135. Hooks JJ, Haynes BF, Detrick-Hooks B, et al. Gamma interferon production by lymphocytes from a patient with TG cell proliferative disease. *Blood* 1982; 59:198–201.

136. Cifone MG, De Maria R, Roncaioli P, et al. Apoptotic signaling through CD95 (Fas/Apo-1) activates an acidic sphingomyelinase. *J Exp Med* 1994; 180:1547–1552.

137. Liu JH, Wei S, Lamy T, et al. Chronic neutropenia mediated by Fas ligand. *Blood* 2000; 95:3219–3222.

138. Liles WC, Kiener PA, Ledbetter JA, et al. Differential expression of Fas (CD95) and Fas ligand on normal human phagocytes: implications for the regulation of apoptosis in neutro-phils. *J Exp Med* 1996; 184:429–440.

139. Mangan KF, Hartnett ME, Matis SA, et al. Natural killer cells suppress human erythroid stem cell proliferation in vitro. *Blood* 1984; 63:260–269.

140. Mangan KF, Chikkappa G, Farley PC. T gamma cells suppress growth of erythroid colony forming units in vitro in the pure red cell aplasia of the B-cell chronic lymphocytic leukemia. *J Clin Invest* 1982; 70:1148–1156.

141. Bacigalupo A, Podesta M, Mingaria MC, et al. Immune suppression of hematopoiesis in aplastic anemia: activity of T-γ lymphocytes. *J Immunol* 1980; 125:1449–1453.

142. Semenzato G, Zambello R, Starkebaum G, et al. The lymphoproliferative disease of granular lymphocytes: updated criteria for diagnosis. *Blood* 1997; 89:256–260.

143. Kwong YL, Wong KF, Chan LC, et al. Large granular lymphocyte leukemia: a study of nine cases in a Chinese population. *Am J Clin Pathol* 1995; 103:76–81.

144. Gentile TC, Loughran TP. Resolution of autoimmune hemolytic anemia following splenec-tomy in CD3+ large granular lymphocyte leukemia. *Leukemia Lymphoma* 1996; 23:405–408.

145. Imamura N, Kuramoto A. Effect of splenectomy in aggressive large granular lymphocyte leukaemia. *Br J Haematol* 1988; 69:577–578.

146. Loughran TP, Starkebaum G, Clark E, et al. Evaluation of splenectomy in large granular lymphocyte leukemia. *Br J Haematol* 1987; 67:135–140.

147. Kelemen E, Gergely P, Lehoczky D, et al. Permanent large granular lymphocytosis in the blood of splenectomized individuals without concomitant increase of in vitro natural killer cell cytotoxicity. *Clin Exp Immunol* 1986; 63:696–702.

148. Kaneko T, Ogawa Y, Hirata Y, et al. Agranulocytosis associated with granular lymphocyte leukemia: improvement of peripheral blood granulocyte count with human recombinant granulocyte colony stimulating factor (G-CSF). *Br J Haematol* 1990; 74:121–122.

149. Weide R, Heymanns J, Koppler H, et al. Successful treatment of neutropenia in T-LGL leukemia (T(-lymphocytosis) with granulocyte colony-stimulating factor. *Ann Hematol* 1994; 69:117–119.
150. Vickers M, Stross P, Millard P, Barton C. Response of T-beta CD8+ lymphocytosis-associated neutropenia to G-CSF. *Br J Haematol* 1994; 87:431–433.
151. Walls J, Dessypris EN, Krantz SB. Granulocyte colony-stimulating factor overcomes severe neutropenia of large granular lymphocytosis. *Am J Med Sci* 1992; 304:363–365.
152. Cooper DL, Henderson-Bakas M, Berliner N. Lymphoproliferative disorder of granular lymphocytes associated with severe neutropenia: response to granulocyte colony-stimulating factor. *Cancer* 1993; 72:1607–1611.
153. Genvresse I, Spath-Schwalbe E, Lukowsky A, Possinger K. Delayed response to granulocyte colony-stimulating factor (G-CSF) in a case of severe neutropenia associated with large granular lymphocyte (LGL) leukemia. *Eur J Haematol* 1998; 60:133–134.
154. Folk SM, Tefferi A. Granulocyte-macrophage colony-stimulating factor for the treatment of neutropenia associated with large granular lymphocyte leukemia. *Am J Hematol* 1992; 39:316.
155. Mulder AB, de Wolf JTM, Smit JW, et al. Correction of neutropenia by GM-CSF in patients with large granular lymphocyte proliferation. *Ann Hematol* 1992; 65:91–95.
156. Thomssen C, Nissen C, Gratwohl A, et al. Agranulocytosis associated with T-gamma lymphocytosis: no improvement of peripheral blood granulocyte count with human recombinant granulocyte-macrophage colony-stimulating factor (GM-CSF). *Br J Haematol* 1989; 71:157–158.
157. Jakubowski A, Winton EF, Gencarelli A, Gabrilove J. Treatment of chronic neutropenia associated with large granular lymphocytosis with cyclosporine A and filgastrim. *Am J Hematol* 1995; 50:288–291.
158. Lamy T, LePrise P-Y, Amiot L, et al. Response to granulocyte-macrophage colony-stimulating factor (GM-CSF) but not to G-CSF in a case of agranulocytosis associated with large granular lymphocyte leukemia. *Blood* 1995; 85:3352–3353.
159. Witzig TE, Weitz JJ, Lundberg JH, Tefferi A. Treatment of refractory T-cell chronic lymphocytic leukemia with purine nucleoside analogs. *Leuk Lymphoma* 1994; 14:137–139.
160. Bargetzi MJ, Wortelboer M, Pabst T, et al. Severe neutropenia in T-large granular lymphocyte leukemia corrected by intensive immunosuppression. *Ann Hematol* 1996; 73:149–151.
161. Edelman MJ, O'Donnell RT, Meadows I. Treatment of refractory large granular lymphocytic leukemia with 2-chlorodeoxyadenosine. *Am J Hematol* 1997;54:329–331.
162. O'Brien S, Kurzrock R, Duvic M, et al. 2-chlorodeoxyadenosine therapy in patients with T-cell lymphoproliferative disorders. *Blood* 1994; 84:733–738.
163. Mercieca J, Matutes E, Dearden C, et al. The role of pentostatin in the treatment of T-cell malignancies: analysis of response rate in 145 patients according to disease subtype. *J Clin Oncol* 1994; 12:2588–2593.
164. Dearden C, Matutes E, Catovsky D. Deoxycoformycin in the treatment of mature T-cell leukemias. *Br J Cancer* 1991; 64:903–906.
165. Kahan BD. Cyclosporine. *N Engl J Med* 1989; 321:1725–1738.
166. Gabor PE, Mishalani S, Lee S. Rapid response to cyclosporine therapy and sustained remission in large granular cell leukemia. *Blood* 1995; 87:1199–1200.
167. Pastor E, Sayas MJ. Severe neutropenia associated with large granular lymphocyte lymphocytosis: successful control with cyclosporin A. *Blut* 1989; 59:501–502.
168. Garipidou V, Tsatalas C, Sinacos Z. Severe neutropenia in a patient with large granular lymphocytosis: prolonged successful control with cyclosporin A. *Haematologica* 1991; 76:424–425.
169. Foxwell BM, Mackie A, Ling V, Ryffel B. Identification of the multidrug resistance-related P-glycoprotein as a cyclosporine binding protein. *Mol Pharmacol* 1989; 36:543–546.

170. Drach J, Gsur A, Hamilton G, et al. Involvement of P-glycoprotein in the transmembrane transport of interleukin-2 (IL-2), IL-4 and interferon-gamma in normal human T lymphocytes. *Blood* 1996; 88:1747–1754.

171. Raghu G, Park SW, Roninson IB, Metcheter EB. Monoclonal antibodies against P-glycoprotein and MDR1 gene product inhibit interleukin-2 release from PHA-activated lymphocytes. *Exp Hematol* 1996; 24:1258–1264.

172. Seebach J, Speich R, Gmur J. Allogeneic bone marrow transplantation for CD3+/TCRγδ+ large granular lymphocyte proliferation. *Blood* 1995; 85:853.

173. Scott CS, Richards SJ. Classification of large granular lymphocyte (LGL) and NK-associated (NKa) disorders. *Blood Rev* 1992; 6:220–233.

174. Macon WR, Williams ME, Greer JP, et al. Natural killer-like T-cell lymphomas: aggressive lymphomas of T-large granular lymphocytes. *Blood* 1996; 87:1474–1483.

175. Taniwaki M, Tagawa S, Nishigaki H, et al. Chromosomal abnormalities define clonal proliferation in CD3- large granular lymphocyte leukemia. *Am J Hematol* 1990; 33:32–38.

176. Ohno T, Kanoh T, Arita Y, et al. Fulminant clonal expansion of large granular lymphocytes. Characterization of their morphology, phenotype, genotype, and function. *Cancer* 1988; 62:1918–1927.

177. Takami A, Nakao S, Yachie A, et al. Successful treatment of Epstein-Barr virus-associated natural killer cell large granular lymphocytic leukaemia using allogeneic peripheral blood stem cell transplantation. *Bone Marrow Transplant* 1998; 21:1279–1282.

178. Prasthofer EF, Barton JC, Zarcone D, Grossi CE. Ultrastructural morphology of granular lymphocytes (GL) from patients with immunophenotypically homogeneous expansions of GL populations (GLE). *J Submicrosc Cytol* 1987; 19:345–354.

179. Shimodaira S, Ishida F, Kobayashi H, et al. The detection of clonal proliferation in granular lymphocyte-proliferative disorders of natural killer cell lineage. *Br J Haematol* 1995; 90:578–584.

180. Wong KF, Zhang YM, Chan JKC. Cytogenetic abnormalities in natural killer cell lymphoma/leukaemia—is there a consistent pattern? *Leuk Lymphoma* 1999; 34:241–250.

181. Kelly A, Richards SJ, Sivakumaran M, et al. Clonality of CD3 negative large granular lymphocyte proliferations determined by PCR based X-inactivation studies. *J Clin Pathol* 1994; 47:399–404.

182. Zambello R, Loughran TP Jr, Trentin L, et al. Serologic and molecular evidence for a possible pathogenetic role of viral infection in CD3-negative natural killer-type lymphoproliferative disease of granular lymphocytes. *Leukemia* 1995; 9:1207–1211.

183. Kawa-Ha K, Ishihara S, Ninomiya t, et al. CD3-negative lymphoproliferative disease of granular lymphocytes containing Epstein-Barr viral DNA. *J Clin Invest* 1989; 84:51–55.

184. Hart DNJ, Baker BW, Inglis MJ, et al. Epstein-Barr viral DNA in acute large granular lymphocyte (natural killer) leukemic cells. *Blood* 1992; 79:2116–2123.

185. Gelb AB, van de Rijn M, Regula DP, et al. Epstein-Barr virus-associated natural killer-large granular lymphocyte leukemia. *Hum Pathol* 1994; 25:953–960.

186. Teshima T, Miyaji R, Fukuda M, Ohshima K. Bone marrow transplantation for Epstein-Barr virus-associated natural killer cell-large granular lymphocyte leukaemia. *Lancet* 1996; 347:1124.

187. Loughran TP, Zambello R, Ashley R, et al. Failure to detect Epstein-Barr viral DNA in peripheral blood mononuclear cells of most patients with large granular lymphocyte leukemia. *Blood* 1993;81:2723–2727.

188. Chan WC, Gu LB, Masih A, et al. Large granular lymphocyte proliferation with the natural killer-cell phenotype. *Am J Clin Pathol* 1992;97:353–358.

189. Egashira M, Kawamata N, Sugimoto K, et al. P-glycoprotein expression on normal and abnormally expanded natural killer cells and inhibition of P-glycoprotein function by cyclosporin A and its analogue, PSC833. *Blood* 1999;93:599–606.

8 Myeloproliferative Syndromes

Nelida N. Sjak-Shie, MD, PhD
and Gary J. Schiller, MD

Contents

INTRODUCTION

The chronic myeloid disorders are pathologically and clinically divided into two major categories: the myelodysplastic syndromes and the chronic myeloproliferative disorders. The myelodysplastic syndromes (MDS) are characterized by trilineage myeloid bone-marrow dysplasia with variable degrees of associated peripheral cytopenias. In contrast, the chronic myeloproliferative disorders (CMPDs) are characterized by the presence of varying degrees of peripheral leukocytosis, thrombocytosis, or erythrocytosis and splenomegaly. The classic myeloproliferative disorders first described by Dameshek *(1)* in 1951 included: polycythemia rubra vera (PCV), essential thrombocythemia (ET), agnogenic myeloid metaplasia with myelofibrosis (AMMM), and chronic myelogenous leukemia (CML). Several other clinical entities may be considered myeloproliferative as well (Table 1). It may not be possible to definitively classify a chronic myeloid disorder as either MDS or CMPDs because of overlapping clinical and pathologic features.

All chronic myeloproliferative disorders possess an inherent potential to evolve into more aggressive disease states. However, the rate of transformation to leukemia or fibrosis varies significantly among the different myeloprolifera-

From: *Current Clinical Oncology: Chronic Leukemias and Lymphomas:*
Biology, Pathophysiology, and Clinical Management
Edited by: G. J. Schiller © Humana Press Inc., Totowa, NJ

Table 1
Classification of Myeloproliferative Disorders and Myelodysplastic Syndromes

Myeloproliferative disorders	Overlap disorders	Myelodysplastic syndromes
Chronic myeloid leukemia	Chronic myelomonocytic leukemia	Refractory anemia
Essential thrombocythemia		Refractory anemia with ringed sideroblasts
Agnogenic myeloid metaplasia with myelofibrosis		Refractory anemia with excess blasts
Polycythemia rubra vera		Refractory anemia with excess blasts in transformation
Primary familial polycythemia		
Chronic neutrophilic leukemia		
Chronic monocytic leukemia		
Chronic basophilic leukemia		
Systemic mastocytosis		
Hypereosinophilic syndrome		

tive subtypes. It is generally accepted that the CMPDs are clonal stem-cell disorders, but the exact molecular pathogenesis of these diseases is not well-characterized. CML is the focus of discussion in Chapter 5, which summarizes the vast amount of information generated regarding its pathogenesis as well as novel available therapies. This chapter reviews our current knowledge of the clinical features and available therapeutic options for PCV, ET, AMMM, and chronic myelomonocytic leukemia (CMML).

POLYCYTHEMIA RUBRA VERA

Polycythemia rubra vera (PCV) was first described by Vaquez in 1892, and subsequently outlined in greater detail in 1903 by Osler *(2,3)*. PCV is an acquired clonal stem-cell disorder typically characterized by trilineage bone-marrow hyperplasia, pronounced peripheral erythrocytosis, as well as variable degrees of leukocytosis and thrombocytosis. PCV presents with a wide spectrum of clinical and hematological findings, and no single disease-specific diagnostic marker is available.

Pathogenesis

Although the exact molecular etiology of PCV remains unknown, recent progress has been made in characterizing the erythroid progenitor cells. In PCV these cells are hypersensitive to a number of growth factors, including interleukin-3, (IL-3) granulocyte-macrophage colony-stimulating factor (GM-SCF), stem-cell factor, and thrombopoietin *(4–6)*. With regard to erythropoietin,

Table 2
The Polycythemia Vera Study Group Diagnostic Criteria
for Polycythemia Rubra Vera[a]

A1 Raised red-cell mass (male >36mL/kg; female >32mL/kg)	B1 Thrombocytosis (platelet count >400 × 10^9/L)
A2 Normal arterial oxygen (saturation >92%)	B2 Leukocytosis >12 × 10^9/L (no fever or infection)
A3 Splenomegaly	B3 Raised neutrophil alkaline phosphatase score >100 or raised B_{12} (>900 ng/L) or raised B_{12} binding capacity (>2200 ng/L)

[a] The diagnosis of PCV requires the following combinations: A1 1 A2 1 A3 or A1 1 A2 1 any two from category B (ref. 70).

scientists debated whether PCV cells were hypersensitive or independent of this growth factor. Using a serum-free medium devoid of any burst-promoting activity, Correa et al. (6) convincingly demonstrated that PCV erythroid precursors are independent of erythropoietin, but very hypersensitive to insulin-like growth factor-(IGF)-I. Interestingly, PCV patients also have significantly elevated levels of IGF-binding-protein-1, which is involved in the promotion of erythroid burst formation in vitro (7). These observations suggest that signal-transduction pathways may be altered in patients with PCV.

Recent studies by Silva et al. (8) demonstrate that in PCV, erythroid precursors express higher levels of the anti-apoptotic protein Bcl-x_L compared to normal precursors. They also found Bcl-x_L in an abnormally high proportion of relatively mature erythroid precursors in PCV patients. These observations suggest the presence of defects in programmed cell death, which may explain the proliferation and accumulation of PCV cells without the need for growth factors.

Using subtractive hybridization techniques, Temerinac (9) and colleagues have recently isolated a novel gene, PRV-1, which is overexpressed in PCV, but not detectable in normal subjects or patients with other myeloproliferative disorders. PVR-1 is a member of the uPAR receptor superfamily, and appears to be a novel hematopoietic receptor selectively found in PCV. The consistency with which this gene is overexpressed in PCV suggests that it may play a role in the pathogenesis of this disease.

Diagnostic Criteria and Differential Diagnosis

The Polycythemia Vera Study Group (PVSG) established the first set of diagnostic criteria for distinguishing PCV from other myeloproliferative disorders in 1975 (10) (Table 2). These stringent criteria—the false-positive rate is less than 0.5% (11)—may exclude patients with mild clinical manifestations or

Table 3
Modified Diagnostic Criteria for Polycythemia Rubra Vera
as Proposed by Messinezy[b]

A1 Raised red-cell mass (.25% above mean normal predicted value)	B1 Thrombocytosis (platelet count $>400 \times 10^9$/L)
A2 Absence of secondary polycythemia	B2 Neutrophil leukocytosis (neutrophil count $>10 \times 10^9$/L)
A3 Palpable splenomegaly	B3 Splenomegaly on ultrasound/isotope scanning
A4 Clonality marker (i.e., abnormal marrow karyotype)	B4 Characteristic BFU-E growth or reduced serum erythropoietin

[b]The diagnosis of PCV requires the following combinations: A1 + A2 + A3 or A4 as well as A1 + A2 + any two from category B (ref. *14*).

early stage disease. The most important conventional criterion for PCV is the presence of an elevated red blood cell (RBC) mass *(12,13)*, which helps to distinguish between true and spurious erythrocytosis. Once the presence of true erythrocytosis is confirmed, the diagnosis of PCV is established by the presence of an increased RBC mass, splenomegaly, and a lack of tissue hypoxia (criterias A1 + A2 + A3), or by the presence of an increased RBC mass, the lack of tissue hypoxia, and evidence of either thrombocytosis, leukocytosis, elevated leukocyte alkaline phosphatase score, vitamin B_{12} level, or serum unbound B_{12}-binding capacity (criterias A1 + A2 + any two criteria from category B) *(10,11)*.

Although the original PVSG criteria for PCV have been reasonably reliable, minor modifications to incorporate new and more specific techniques may permit even greater diagnostic accuracy *(14,15)*. The proposed modifications are summarized in Table 3 and include: 1) the use of mean normal predicted red-cell mass values for each patient; 2) a more rigorous exclusion of all potential causes of secondary erythrocytosis (Table 4); 3) the evaluation for the presence of splenomegaly by physical examination or using other objective means; 4) a demonstration of clonal proliferation; 5) a demonstration of spontaneous endogenous erythroid colony growth; 6) evidence of granulocytosis instead of leukocytosis; and 7) evidence of reduced or low-normal levels of erythropoietin. Documentation of increased splenic size, reduced levels of erythropoietin, and the characteristic BFU-E growth are more specific for PCV than raised serum B12 levels or neutrophil alkaline phosphatase scores *(14,15)*.

Clinical Features

PCV usually occurs in the sixth and seventh decades of life *(16–19)*, although rare instances of childhood PCV *(20)* have been described and approximately 5–7% of adults are diagnosed before the age of 40 *(21,22)*. The yearly incidence of PCV varies considerably in different parts of the world, with incidence rates

Table 4
Causes of Erythrocytosis

Primary	Secondary	Spurious
Polycythemia rubra vera	Decreased tissue oxygenation:	Reduced plasma volume
Familial polycythemia	1. High altitude	
Sporadic polycythemia	2. Chronic lung disease	
	3. Alveolar hypoventilation	
	4. Cardiovascular right-to-left shunt	
	5. High-oxygen-affinity hemo-globinopathy	
	6. Carboxyhemoglobinemia	
	7. Congenitally decreased erythrocyte 2,3-DPG	
	Normal tissue oxygenation:	
	1. Tumors producing erythropoietin or other erythropoietic substances	
	2. Renal diseases	
	3. Adrenal cortical hypersecretion	
	4. Exogenous androgens	

ranging from 0.2/million in Japan up to 16/million in Rochester, Minnesota *(18,19)*. There appears to be a slight male preponderance and ethnic variation among PCV patients by a ratio of 1.1-2:1 *(16–19,22)*, and 17–26% of PCV patients are diagnosed incidentally *(21,23)*. Common signs and symptoms at presentation include headaches, generalized weakness, epigastric discomfort, dizziness, sweating, pruritus, visual disturbances, plethora, splenomegaly, hepatomegaly, and hypertension *(10,23)*. In addition, patients frequently present with signs and symptoms associated with thrombosis, and less frequently with hemorrhage. The median survival of untreated PCV patients is approx 18 mo *(23)*, but with current management the median survival exceeds 10 yr.

In patients with PCV, both hemorrhagic and thrombotic complications often occur. Thrombotic complications are present in 20% of patients at diagnosis, and develop in 30% more patients during the course of PCV despite therapy *(24)*. In 14% of PCV patients thrombotic complications were identified before the overt development of PCV *(22)*. Most of these thrombotic events (46%) occurred during the 2 yr preceding the diagnosis of PCV, suggesting a causal relationship between the progressive expansion of this clonal disorder and the increased risk of thrombosis. A wide spectrum of thrombotic complications are seen in PCV, ranging from major arterial thromboses such as myocardial infarction and cere-brovascular occlusion to peripheral arterial and venous thrombosis, such as peripheral gangrene and deep venous thrombosis.

Three manifestations—erythromelalgia, Budd-Chiari syndrome, and neurological complications—merit special attention. Erythromelalgia consists of recurrent bouts of burning pain in the feet or hands associated with warmth and erythema of the affected area. Eighteen percent of all patients with erythromelalgia have underlying PCV *(25–27)*. Moreover, erythromelalgia may precede the diagnosis of PCV by as many as 12 yr *(25–27)*. This symptom usually occurs in the setting of thrombocytosis and responds to treatment with low-dose aspirin *(26–28)*. Another unusual complication seen in PCV, Budd-Chiari syndrome, has been documented in 6% of PCV patients at autopsy *(29)*. Furthermore, 10–13% of patients with this syndrome have underlying PCV *(30,31)*. Cerebrovascular complications ranging from transient ischemic attacks *(22,32)* (2–20%) to ischemic strokes *(22,32)* (9–9.5%) frequently occur in PCV, and are often overlooked as early clues of this disease *(27)*.

Hemorrhagic complications occur less frequently, and primarily involve the gastrointestinal system. Vascular distension from the increased blood volume, functional platelet abnormalities, and severe thrombocytosis all appear to play a role in the risk of bleeding associated with PCV *(24)*. In a single, small clinical trial, the use of high-dose aspirin was associated with an excessive risk of gastrointestinal bleeding *(33)*. Although lower doses of aspirin are well-tolerated in patients with vascular disease *(34)*, their long-term efficacy and safety in preventing thromboses in PCV have not been rigorously evaluated.

Several factors appear to increase the risk of thrombosis in PCV. Advancing age is associated with an increased risk of thrombosis *(35,36)*, from a rate of 1.8 events/100 patients per yr in patients younger than 40 yr to a rate of 5.1 events/ 100 patients per yr in patients older than 70 yr *(22)*. In addition, a previous history of thrombosis *(35,36)* or frequent phlebotomy *(35,37)* increases the risk. However, it has been suggested that the patients with higher phlebotomy requirements differ in disease severity from those patients in whom relatively infrequent phlebotomy is sufficient to maintain stable blood levels. Surprisingly, the degree of thrombocytosis or erythrocytosis has not been consistently correlated with the risk of thrombosis of PCV *(24,38)*. Furthermore, no correlation has been established between the numerous, well-documented abnormalities in platelet function and coagulation factors in PCV and the risk of thrombosis or bleeding *(23)*.

Natural Course of the Disease

Our knowledge regarding the natural history of PCV remains limited because of the rarity of the disease itself and the influence of commonly used methods of treatment on the course of the disease, especially in terms of the rate of conversion to leukemia. Regardless of the leukemogenic effects of therapy, PCV itself clearly is a progressive disease. Four stages of disease can be recognized in PCV, although it should be emphasized that individual patients do not proceed through these stages in sequential fashion. Incidentally diagnosed patients may remain in an "asymptomatic phase" for many years. Patients become increasingly symptomatic as they enter a "proliferative phase" characterized by the increased incidence of thrombohemorrhagic complications. After an interval of 15 yr, approx 10–15% of PCV patients develop post-polycythemia myeloid metaplasia, also known as the "spent phase" because of the waning of bone-marrow proliferative activity *(24,39,40)*. Myelosuppressive therapy does not appear to influence the risk of transformation to the spent phase *(11,39)*. The risk of progression to post-polycythemia myeloid metaplasia continues to rise with time regardless of therapy, and reaches 50% after 20 yr *(41)*. The spent phase is characterized by progressive bone-marrow fibrosis, increasing extramedullary hematopoiesis, a leukoerythroblastic peripheral blood picture, and normalization of the RBC mass independent of therapy *(24,40,41)*. Unfortunately, there is no effective therapy for this phase of the disease. Patients with life-threatening thrombocytopenia, marked symptomatic splenomegaly, or severe hemolytic anemia may be considered candidates for palliative splenectomy or splenic irradiation if their overall medical condition permits. Post-polycythemia myeloid metaplasia is associated with a shorter survival compared to patients with agnogenic myeloid metaplasia. Most patients die within 3 yr of recognition of this phase, and the transformation to acute leukemia is a frequent cause of death.

Finally, approx 1–2 % of PCV patients treated with phlebotomy alone will develop acute leukemia, suggesting that the transformation to leukemia is part of the natural history of this disease *(42)*. Myelosuppressive therapy appears to increase the risk of transformation to leukemia in patients with PCV to a variable degree, depending on the therapeutic agent in question *(42–45)*. Typically, PCV transforms into a myeloid leukemia, although a few cases of acute lymphoblastic leukemia have been described *(46)*. Treatment of leukemia in the setting of PCV has generally been disappointing, although rare cases of complete remission and prolonged disease-free-survival have been reported *(42,47)*.

Therapeutic Options

Despite several carefully conducted clinical trials, including a few randomized trials, no unequivocal best treatment guidelines are agreed upon, particularly for younger patients. Clearly, current management of PCV has profoundly improved the natural history of this disease, because the current median survival is estimated to exceed 10 yr compared to the median survival of 18 mo in untreated patients *(23)*. Consensus has been reached regarding the need to phlebotomize PCV patients as rapidly as clinically feasible to an optimal hematocrit level of 45% or less for men, or 42% or less for women *(48)*. In patients considered at low risk for thrombotic complications, defined as younger patients without a known history of prior thrombotic events, no additional therapy may be required. In high-risk patients (older patients with a prior history of thrombotic complications and those requiring frequent phlebotomy to maintain stable blood counts) additional myelosuppressive therapy may be indicated. Myelo-suppressive therapy has been shown to reduce the risk of thrombosis, reduce the size of the spleen, and reduce peripheral blood thrombocytosis and erythrocytosis *(11,49)*. Furthermore, the PVSG-01 study clearly demonstrated a greater incidence of thrombosis during the first 3–5 yr of therapy with phlebotomy only compared to patients treated with phlebotomy and either P^{32} or chlorambucil *(11,38)*. A greater incidence of leukemia and other malignancies in patients receiving therapy with these myelosuppressive agents was also documented *(11,38)*. Therefore, P^{32}, chlorambucil, or similar alkylating agents are largely reserved for use in older patients for whom considerations of convenience sometimes outweigh concerns of an increased risk of transformation to leukemia. Several studies using hydroxyurea also suggest that this agent is leukemogenic in patients with PCV *(43,50)*, although its leukemogenicity appears to be less pronounced.

A recent review of experience with interferon-(IFN) α in 279 patients with PCV confirmed its therapeutic efficacy and safety in this disease *(51)*. IFN at doses ranging from 3–35 million IU/wk resulted in a complete remission (defined by a stable hematocrit of 45% without the need for concomitant phlebotomies) in 50% of patients evaluated. Furthermore, a reduction in splenomegaly was observed in 77%, and control of pruritus was achieved in 81% of patients. It remains to be seen whether IFN-α impacts favorably on the clinical course of PCV, particularly its late sequelae. IFN-α has no known mutagenic or teratogenic properties, which is of particular importance to younger patients with PCV. Unfortunately, IFN-α is unlikely to become first-line treatment for most PCV patients, mainly because of the high degree of intolerance to the drug itself. In 21% of patients, IFN-α therapy was discontinued because of excessive side effects *(51)*. IFN's mode of administration and high cost further limit its generalized use in PCV.

Anagrelide is a novel nonmyelosuppressive, nonleukemogenic, generally well-tolerated, and selective platelet-lowering agent *(52)*. Although the risk of thrombosis in PCV does not correlate with the degree of thrombocytosis, as discussed here, the risk of bleeding and the development of erythromelalgia are greater with significant thrombocytosis. Anagrelide may be useful in PCV in these settings, and it may also help ameliorate the transient increased risk of thrombosis associated with treatment with phlebotomy alone. We therefore encourage continued evaluation of the role of anagrelide in PCV in clinical trials.

ESSENTIAL THROMBOCYTHEMIA

Essential thrombocythemia (ET) is a myeloproliferative disorder characterized by persistent thrombocytosis in the periphery and excessive proliferation of megakaryocytes in the bone marrow. Epstein et al. first described ET as a hemorrhagic thrombocytosis in 1934 *(53)*. There is no cytogenetic or molecular abnormality that definitively establishes the diagnosis of ET. Although it is

Table 5
Causes of Thrombocytosis

Primary	Secondary
Essential thrombocytosis	Post-splenectomy state
	Chronic iron deficiency
	Neoplastic disease (especially with metastasis)
	Chronic inflammation
	Chronic infection
	Associated with other myeloproliferative disorder
	Postsurgical rebound
	Acute blood loss

formally considered a monoclonal stem-cell disorder, recent evidence suggests that many patients with ET (57%) have polyclonal hematopoiesis *(54)*. This observation illustrates the heterogeneity of patients diagnosed with ET using current clinical diagnostic criteria. Notably, the incidence of thrombotic, rather than hemorrhagic complications appeared to be less in patients with polyclonal hematopoiesis. Therefore, future clinical studies will need to explore these differences in greater detail to allow improved individualized therapy for patients with ET.

Pathogenesis

The molecular pathogenesis of ET remains unknown. Thrombopoietin and its receptor stimulate the growth of megakaryocyte progenitors as well as more primitive hematopoietic progenitors both in vivo and in vitro *(55)*. In ET, serum levels of thrombopoietin are normal or elevated *(56,57)*. In addition, mRNA expression and c-Mpl, the thrombopoietin receptor, are significantly reduced in ET *(58)*, although this reduction is also seen in PCV and AMMM *(59)*. The discovery that familial thrombocythemia is associated with a mutation in the thrombopoietin gene *(60)* has stimulated a search for similar alterations in ET. However, the search for mutations in the thrombopoietin gene, or c-Mpl, has been unsuccessful to date.

Diagnostic Criteria and Differential Diagnosis

Because of the lack of a specific diagnostic marker, the diagnostic criteria established by the PVSG are directed primarily at the exclusion of reactive thrombocytosis (Table 5) and of other myeloproliferative disorders *(61)* (Table 6). Approximately 5% of patients who present with ET will evolve to a diagnosis of PCV *(62)*, but the reverse is very rare *(63)*.

Table 6

The PCV Study Group Diagnostic Criteria for Essential Thrombocythemia[c]

1.	Platelet count >600,000/μL
2.	Normal RBC mass (males <36mL/kg; females <32 mg/kg)
3.	No evidence of iron deficiency
4.	No Philadelphia chromosome or bcr-abl gene rearrangement
5.	Lack of extensive bone-marrow fibrosis
6.	No cytogenetic or morphologic evidence of MDS
7.	No cause for secondary thrombocytosis

[c]*See* ref. *61.*

Clinical Features

ET usually occurs in the sixth and seventh decades of life *(64–68)*. With the advent of automated Coulter counters, ET has been diagnosed with increasing frequency in asymptomatic patients, including young adults and children *(69–71)*. More recent studies suggest that up to 25% of patients diagnosed with ET are less than 40 yr of age *(72,73)*. There is a slight female preponderance noted in most studies *(64–68)*, with a ratio of 1.18 to 1.76:1. ET is one of the most common myeloproliferative disorders, with an annual incidence ranging from 7 to 25/million *(69,74)*. Approximately one-third of ET patients are asymptomatic at diagnosis. The remaining patients commonly present with vasomotor disturbances (paresthesias, erythromelalgia, acrocyanosis), headaches, dizziness, visual disturbances, atypical transient ischemic attacks, and splenomegaly, as well as signs and symptoms associated with thrombosis and hemorrhage *(69,75,76)*. Since life-threatening complications are relatively rare in this disease, most patients with ET enjoy a near-normal life expectancy *(77)*.

Like PCV, ET is characterized by an increased risk of thrombotic complications compared to a control population matched for age, sex, and cardiovascular risk factors (1% vs 7% patient/yr) *(78)*. The risk of thrombosis is highest for patients older than 60 yr (15%) and for those with a prior history of thrombosis (31%) *(78)*. Major thrombotic episodes rarely occur unexpectedly in previously diagnosed, asymptomatic patients. Generally, serious thromboses are either present at diagnosis or are preceded by minor thrombotic signs and symptoms in patients with ET *(24,62)*. The thrombogenic effects of advanced age *(79)* and prior history of thrombosis *(80)* have been confirmed by other large studies. Additional risk factors for thrombosis may include the presence of cardiovascular risk factors *(81)*, especially smoking *(82)*. Similar to PCV, the degree of thrombocytosis or abnormalities in platelet function do not correlate with the risk of thrombosis *(83)*. Although both venous and arterial thromboses occur, the incidence of venous thrombosis is less frequent in ET than in PCV *(62)*.

Special mention should be made of the potential complications in pregnant patients with ET. This situation is likely to arise more frequently as more patients are diagnosed at younger ages. Pregnancy in ET is often complicated by recurrent spontaneous abortions, premature deliveries, and fetal growth retardation, possibly because of multiple placental infarctions that lead to placental insufficiency *(50,84,85)*. The risk of miscarriage is greatest during the first trimester (up to 36%), after which complications are much less frequent *(83)*. Unfortunately, the at-risk population for complications during pregnancy cannot be predicted, and published information regarding the management of ET during pregnancy is extremely limited. Cytotoxic therapy carries the risk of congenital malformation, especially when used in the first trimester of pregnancy. Considering these caveats, a few pregnancies have been managed successfully with the use of low-dose aspirin when platelet counts were only modestly elevated *(86)*. IFN has also been used successfully in a limited number of pregnant ET patients *(50,87)*. IFN has an advantage because it has never been shown to be teratogenic and does not cross the placenta *(50,87)*. It should be emphasized that because of the paucity of information, no definitive treatment recommendations can be made.

Major bleeding complications, in the absence of platelet anti-aggregating therapy, are very rare in ET (<1%), and when present are usually not clinically significant *(78,80,83,88,89)*. Easy bruising and bleeding from mucous membranes such as the gastrointestinal tract are generally noted in association with severe thrombocytosis and an acquired deficiency of von Willebrand's factor *(90,91)*.

Natural Course of the Disease

Although ET is a chronic progressive disease, it has a low incidence (range <2% to 5%) of transformation into acute leukemia *(78,80,88,89)*. Leukemia transformation in ET is primarily observed in patients who have received treatment with P^{32} or alkylating agents, which themselves are leukemogenic *(61,92)*. Similarly, ET also has a low rate of progression to myelofibrosis, estimated at 2–3% *(65)*.

Therapeutic Options

Although there are no substantial differences in life expectancy when comparing ET patients to normal controls, there is a high rate of morbidity associated with this disease. The risk of long-term treatment for management of symptoms must be weighed carefully against the risk of leukemia for each individual patient. The morbidity associated with microvascular occlusive complications typically resolves dramatically with the use of platelet anti-aggregating agents and/or reduction in platelet counts *(76,93,94)*. These ischemic symptoms are attributed to in vivo platelet activation in the arterioles, with or without thrombosis, which may explain the lack of efficacy of coumadin therapy. Although platelet anti-aggregating agents relieve the symptoms associated with microvascular occlusive complications, their efficacy in the prevention of major thrombosis in ET has never been definitively demonstrated. These agents certainly have the potential to increase the inherent risk of bleeding associated with ET, although recent studies with low-dose aspirin have not noted an increase in frequency or severity of hemorrhagic complications *(75,88)*.

In patients considered at low risk for major thrombotic complications, defined as patients less than 60 yr of age without a prior history of major thrombosis, careful monitoring without active treatment may be appropriate, especially considering that in ET catastrophic thromboses are usually preceded by less severe thrombotic complications. In high-risk patients, the use of hydroxyurea in comparison with no treatment has been shown to significantly reduce the risk of thrombosis (3.6% vs 24% during a median follow-up of 27 mo) *(82,95)*. Although other myelosuppressive drugs can also effectively reduce the risk of thrombosis, their use is limited by their leukemogenic properties *(92)*. Hydroxyurea may also increase the risk of transformation to leukemia in ET *(43,61)*, although the available data are equivocal *(39)*. At this time, the long-term safety of hydroxyurea in ET is still uncertain, and prospective controlled studies are required before reaching definitive conclusions regarding the potential hazards associated with hydroxyurea.

IFN is a potentially nonmutagenic and nonleukemogenic alternative to conventional therapy with cytotoxic drugs. Although IFN has demonstrated therapeutic activity in ET *(96,97)*, no prospective trials comparing IFN to standard treatments have been performed. The therapeutic effects of IFN include platelet reduction *(97–102)* (80–100% response rates), resolution of splenomegaly *(97,99,102)*, and control of disease-related symptoms *(98–100,102,103)*. Long-term studies have confirmed the ability of IFN to maintain disease control for over 5 yr, and lower doses may be sufficient to maintain control *(87)*. Several studies also reported sustained remissions following discontinuation of long-term IFN therapy *(98,102,103)*. The problems associated with IFN are similar to those discussed for its use in PCV: prohibitive side effects, cost, and inconvenient mode of administration.

Anagrelide, an oral quinazolin derivative, produces a durable, dose-dependent reduction in circulating platelets in over 90% of patients with ET, regardless of the presence or absence of prior therapy *(72)*. Although originally developed as an inhibitor of platelet function, platelet aggregation remains unaffected at the doses used to treat thrombocytosis. Anagrelide has no appreciable effect on other hematologic variables *(104,105)*. Most of the side effects of anagrelide are cardiovascular and stem from the direct peripheral vasodilatory effect and the positive inotropic activity of the drug. Up to 16% of patients treated with anagrelide have discontinued its use because of side effects *(105)*.

Table 7
Causes of Bone-Marrow Fibrosis

Myeloid disorders	Lymphoid disorders	Non-hematologic disorders
Chronic myeloproliferative disorders	Lymphomas	Metastatic carcinoma
Myelodysplastic syndromes	Hairy cell leukemia	Connective tissue disease
Acute myelofibrosis	Multiple myeloma	Infections
Acute myeloid leukemia		Vitamin D-deficiency
Mast-cell disease		Renal osteodystrophy
Malignant histiocytosis		Gray platelet syndrome
		Gaucher's disease
		Osteopetrosis
		Hypo/hyperthyroidism

AGNOGENIC MYELOID METAPLASIA WITH MYELOFIBROSIS

Agnogenic myeloid metaplasia with myelofibrosis (AMMM), also known as primary myelofibrosis or idiopathic myelofibrosis, is a myeloproliferative disorder characterized by progressive bone-marrow fibrosis, clonal myelopro-liferation, extramedullary hematopoiesis in multiple organs, and a leukoerythroblastic peripheral-blood picture *(106)*. AMMM is a rare disorder that was first described by Heuck in 1879 *(107)*. The differential diagnosis of AMMM encompasses the many causes of secondary bone-marrow fibrosis (Table 7), the inclusion of which may account for the many conflicting reports on the natural history, prognosis, and karyotypic patterns characteristic of AMMM.

Pathogenesis

Bone-marrow fibrosis results from the abnormal deposition of excess collagen derived from fibroblasts. In AMMM, bone-marrow fibrosis develops in response to growth factors secreted by the monoclonal megakaryocytes and monocytes that are part of the neoplastic process. The collagen-producing fibroblasts in ET are functionally and morphologically normal, and are polyclonal *(108)*. Alterations in the expression of several cytokines with fibrogenic, angiogenic, and osteogenic properties have been reported *(109–111)*. However, it remains unclear whether the observed alterations in cytokine production are pathogenic or merely reactive in nature.

Of interest are the recent reports of an AMMM-like syndrome in mice exposed to high concentrations of thrombopoietin, the primary growth factor for megakaryocytes *(112)*. A similar AMMM-like syndrome is also observed in thrombopoietin-transfected mice *(113)*. The bone-marrow fibrosis appears to be

Table 8
The Cologne criteria for AMMM[d]

A. No evidence of other CMPDs or MDS
B. Splenomegaly (palpable or >11cm on ultrasound)
C. Thrombocythemia (platelet count >500 × 10^9/L)
D. Anemia (hemoglobin <12g/dL)
E. Peripheral-blood leukoerythroblastosis
F. Histopathology: granulocytic and megakaryocytic myeloproliferation with large, multilobulated nuclei containing megakaryocytes with evidence of abnormal clustering, maturation defects, and
   1) no reticulin fibrosis
   2) slight reticulin fibrosis
   3) marked increased density of reticulin fibers, collagen fibrosis, and
   4) osteosclerosis (endophytic bone formation).
The diagnosis of AMMM is established with the following combinations:
   Stage 1   A+B+C+F1: hypercellular, prefibrotic stage clinically similar to ET
   Stage 2   A+B+C+D+F$_2$: early AMMM
   Stage 3   A+B+D+F$_3$: classic AMMM
   Stage 4   A+B+D+E+F$_{3+4}$: advanced AMMM

[d]See ref. 116.

mediated by increased levels of TNF-β activity because of the increased megakaryocyte mass induced by thrombopoietin (114). The pathogenic interactions of TNF-β and thrombopoietin in patients with ET remain unknown.

Diagnostic Criteria and Differential Diagnosis

As with all CMPDs, there is no single biologic, clinical, or pathologic characteristic that is specific for AMMM. Again, the PVSG was the first to develop a set of diagnostic criteria for AMMM (115) requiring: myelofibrosis involving over one-third of the bone marrow, a leukoerythroblastic peripheral-blood picture, splenomegaly, the absence of diagnostic criteria for other CMPDs, and no evidence of a systemic disorder. Since then two different proposals delineating diagnostic criteria for AMMM have been suggested. The Cologne criteria proposed by Thiele et al. (116) combined accepted clinical characteristics of AMMM with histopathologic bone-marrow characteristics to define the disease itself and its different stages. The authors postulate that AMMM evolves progressively from an early stage in which minimal or no bone-marrow fibrosis is present to the later stages, with increasing myelofibrosis, anemia, peripheral-blood erythroblastosis, and osteosclerosis (Table 8).

The Italian Cooperative Group on Myeloproliferative Disorders, a group of 12 Italian experts, arrived at a consensus on the diagnostic definition of AMMM

Table 9
The Italian Consensus Criteria for AMMM[e]

Necessary criteria	Optional criteria
1. Diffuse bone-marrow fibrosis	1. Splenomegaly
2. Absence of Philadelphia chromosome or bcr-abl rearrangement in peripheral blood cells	2. Anisopoikilocytosis with teardrop erythrocytes
	3. Presence of circulating immature myeloid cells
	4. Presence of circulating erythroblasts
	5. Presence of clusters of megakaryoblasts and anomalous megakaryocytes in bone-marrow sections
	6. Myeloid metaplasia

The diagnosis of AMMM is established with the following combinations:
  The two necessary criteria with any two optional criteria if splenomegaly is present.
  The two necessary criteria with any four optional criteria if splenomegaly is absent.

[e]*See* ref. *149.*

based on a review of the available information in the literature. The panel identified six optional and two mandatory criteria to establish the diagnosis of AMMM (Table 9). The mandatory criteria consisted of: diffuse bone-marrow fibrosis and absence of Philadelphia chromosome or breakpoint-cluster region/Abelson leukemia virus (bcr-abl) rearrangement in peripheral blood. The six optional criteria included: splenomegaly, anisopoikilocytosis with teardrop erythrocytes, the presence of circulating immature myeloid cells, circulating erythroblasts, clusters of megakaryoblasts and anomalous megakaryocytes in bone-marrow sections, and myeloid metaplasia. It should be noted that unlike the Cologne criteria, the Italian consensus criteria purposefully include both patients with idiopathic disease as well as those that transform from other chronic myeloproliferative disorders. Since the latter condition appears to carry a worse prognosis than AMMM, inclusion of these patients may influence our understanding of the natural history of those patients with true idiopathic myelofibrosis if such a distinct disease entity indeed exists.

Clinical Features

AMMM is a rare disease with an estimated incidence of 0.5 to 1.5/100,000. *(117,118)*. No consistent differences in distribution according to sex have been identified *(119–121)*. Although the disease affects mostly older individuals with a median age at diagnosis of 65 yr *(119–121)*, a childhood form of AMMM exists that may have a more favorable prognosis compared to its adult equivalent

(122,123). Approximately one-third of patients are virtually asymptomatic at diagnosis, but with time all patients become symptomatic and commonly suffer variable degrees of cachexia, severe fatigue, night sweats, and low-grade fevers, dyspnea, bone pain, pruritus, and abdominal discomfort *(119,124)*. Most of these symptoms can be attributed to one of the following mechanisms: progressive bone-marrow failure, hypermetabolism, hepato/splenomegaly, thromboembolic complications, and autoimmune diseases *(119,124,125)*.

Autoimmune phenomena are uniquely associated with AMMM among the myeloproliferative disorders, and include Coombs-positive autoimmune hemolytic anemia, nephrotic syndrome, cutaneous vasculitis, Sweet's syndrome, and pyoderma gangrenosum *(126–129)*. Patients have also demonstrated the presence of antinuclear antibodies, rheumatoid factor, lupus-anticoagulant antibody, and hypocomplementemia *(130,131)*. Unusual symptoms directly related to extramedullary hematopoiesis include lymphadenopathy, acute cardiac tamponade, hematuria, pleural effusion, ascites, papular skin lesions, and spinalcord compression *(125,132–136)*. Thrombohemorrhagic complications, portal hypertension, and infections also contribute significantly to morbidity and mortality in AMMM *(125)*. AMMM, like ET and PCV, has an inherent risk of transformation to acute leukemia. Approximately 20% of patients with AMMM will transform during the first 10 yr after diagnosis *(137)*.

Natural Course of the Disease

The clinical spectrum of AMMM is very broad, ranging from nearly asymptomatic patients with chronic stable disease to patients with severe constitutional symptoms at presentation and a rapidly fatal course. This variation may be a result of the heterogeneity of patients included under the diagnosis of myelofibrosis. The most recent studies report median survival times ranging from 3.5–5.5 yr *(119,120,138–141)*, but for a given individual, survival may range from 1 yr to over 30 yr. These observations have stimulated evaluation of potential prognostic factors in AMMM to identify subgroups of patients with different clinical outcomes. Several clinical and biologic factors have been evaluated, with varying and often conflicting results. The hemoglobin concentration at diagnosis has emerged as an important prognostic indicator in most studies. However, other parameters, including constitutional symptoms, platelet count, the presence of osteomyelosclerosis, reticulocyte count, spleen size, the presence of normal megakaryocytes, circulating blasts, bone-marrow angiogenesis and the percentage of granulocyte precursors, have been used in varying combinations as prognostic scoring systems *(125,139,141–143)*.

A recent system proposed by Dupriez et al. *(119)* was able to identify three distinct prognostic groups using a hemoglobin level <10 g/dL and white-bloodcell (WBC) counts <4 or >30 × 10^9/L as adverse prognostic factors (Table 10). Patients with no adverse prognostic factors had a median survival of 93 mo (low

Table 10
The Lille Scoring System for AMMM[f]

Number of adverse prognostic factors*	Risk group	Median survival (months)
0	Low	93
1	Intermediate	26
2	High	13

*Adverse prognostic factors include: hemoglobin <10g/dL, WBC count <4 or >30 × 10^9/L.
[f]See ref. 119.

risk), compared to a median survival of 26 mo for patients with one adverse prognostic factor (intermediate risk) and 13 mo for patients with two adverse prognostic factors (high risk). Two additional factors have emerged as important prognostic indicators in AMMM: age at diagnosis (120,144) and abnormal cytogenetics (119,138). By combining age, hemoglobin concentration, and karyotype, Reilly et al. (138) identified risk groups with median survival times varying from 16 mo (poor risk) to 180 mo (good risk).

Accurate prognostic information would certainly facilitate therapeutic decisions, especially when considering aggressive treatment options that are associated with considerable up-front morbidity and mortality. At present, it is unclear which prognostic scoring model more accurately predicts clinical outcome in AMMM. It may be reasonable to suggest that patients who lack any of the identified poor prognostic indicators may expect a median survival greater than 10 yr, and the median survival for those with any adverse factors may not even reach 3 yr.

Therapeutic Options

No medical therapy has yet been demonstrated to improve overall survival in patients with AMMM. Therefore, therapeutic interventions are mainly directed at the alleviation of symptoms. Many different agents, including androgens (145), erythropoietin (146), and danazol (145) have been used to ameliorate the symptoms associated with anemia in AMMM, typically with limited success. Notably, there have been occasional reports of aggravation of splenomegaly because of stimulation of extramedullary hematopoiesis in addition to bone-marrow erythrocytosis. Immunosuppression with cyclosporine (CSA) (147) or corticosteroids (148) has also been reported to alleviate symptoms associated with anemia in some patients (149).

For patients whose symptoms are mainly caused by myeloproliferation such as thrombocytosis, leukocytosis, or organomegaly, cytotoxic agents may be considered. The use of cytotoxic agents may be associated with a higher risk of transformation to acute leukemia, although no long-term studies are available to address this theoretical concern. IFN has also been evaluated as an alternative to cytotoxic agents in AMMM. IFN was considered ideally suited for treatment of AMMM based on its ability to preferentially inhibit megakaryocyte lineages *(150)*. IFN did result in clinical improvement in about 50% of the patients reported in small studies *(149)*. The problems associated with IFN remain similar to those discussed for its use in PCV: prohibitive side effects, cost, and inconvenient mode of administration. Progressive enlargement of the spleen—with concurrent thrombocytopenia, anemia, portal hypertension, and splenic pain—warrants consideration of splenectomy or splenic irradiation to alleviate symptoms. Splenectomy in AMMM is associated with significant surgical morbidity (31–39%) and mortality (8.4–9%), as well as an increased postoperative risk of venous or portal thrombosis. In addition, some patients develop massive hepatomegaly and severe thrombocytosis post-splenectomy *(151,152)*. The most troubling post-splenectomy complication, however, is the increased incidence of leukemia transformation *(151)*. A recent multicenter historical cohort study of 549 patients with AMMM confirmed that the risk of transformation to leukemia is significantly higher in patients who underwent splenectomy, with a cumulative incidence of 55% in splenectomized patients compared to 27% in nonsplenectomized patients. Furthermore, the risk of transformation to leukemia appears to be independent of factors related to spleen removal assignment *(153)*. However, splenectomy did alleviate constitutional symptoms, portal hypertension, splenic pain, and anemia in some patients with AMMM *(151,152)*. We conclude that splenectomy in AMMM is associated with substantial risks that should be carefully weighed against its palliative potential for each patient.

An alternative to splenectomy is splenic irradiation, which has resulted in reversal of splenomegaly and associated splenic pain in 59–94% of patients with a median duration of response ranging from 6–10 mo *(154,155)*. Of concern is the prolonged and severe myelosuppression observed in 26% of patients after a single dose of splenic irradiation, which resulted in fatal bleeding and infectious complications in 13% *(155)*. In addition, splenectomy after splenic irradiation was associated with an increased risk of postoperative bleeding *(155)*. Therefore, splenic irradiation should only be considered in patients for whom splenectomy is not a suitable option.

None of the therapeutic interventions discussed here have been shown to prolong the survival of patients with AMMM. These palliative approaches are unsatisfactory for younger, intermediate- to high-risk patients whose predicted median survival is less than 3 yr. The role of allogeneic transplantation in AMMM has been studied, with increasing reports of encouraging results. A recent retrospective multicenter study of 55 patients with myelofibrosis (AMMM and ET transformed into myelofibrosis with myeloid metaplasia) reported a 91% rate of engraftment with pretransplant splenectomy, absence of grade-three myelofibrosis, and a high number of nucleated cells infused, associated with a significantly shorter time to engraftment *(156)*. Complete hematologic remission reported in 70% of patients was associated with significant reversal of myelofibrosis in 40%. The overall estimated 5-yr survival for those patients who received a histocompatible matched related graft was 54%. Overall, 44% patients died from infections, chronic and acute graft vs host disease, disease progression, solid organ failure, and graft failure, as well as lymphoproliferative disorders. Considering that the predicted 5-yr survival for AMMM patients treated with supportive measures is 40%, allogeneic transplant appears to offer a survival advantage to a select group of young patients. A hemoglobin level less than 100 g/L before transplant and the absence of grade-three myelofibrosis were significantly associated with a better outcome. Nine patients were alive more than 5 yr after transplantation in this study, and the same authors have previously reported two patients who are alive and disease free 10 yr and 15 yr after allogeneic bone-marrow transplantation (Allo-BMT) *(157)*. These observations suggest that Allo-BMT offers a chance for long-term survival and possibly cure in young patients with AMMM. However, for low-risk AMMM patients for whom predicted median survival exceeds 10 yr, it may not be reasonable to propose Allo-BMT in light of the substantial morbidity and mortality associated with this procedure.

CHRONIC MYELOMONOCYTIC LEUKEMIA

Chronic myelomonocytic leukemia (CMML) is considered a variant of MDS, although it is frequently biologically and clinically distinct from MDS because of its pronounced proliferative rather than dysplastic features and frequent extramedullary involvement *(158–161)*, characteristics it shares with the CMPDs discussed in this chapter. Therefore, we propose to classify CMML as a variant of the chronic myeloproliferative disorders.

Diagnostic Criteria and Differential Diagnosis

CMML appears to be a heterogeneous disease characterized by isolated monocytosis with a mild degree of dysplasia in some patients, severe cytopenias in others, and most frequently with proliferative symptoms dominating the clinical picture *(159)*. The latter group thus shares the principal clinical feature common to the chronic myeloproliferative disorders, and perhaps this clinical entity should be classified as such. The classification of CMML is further complicated by the possibility of evolution from one subgroup into another, and by the finding that it can arise secondary to other recognized myeloproliferative or myelodysplastic syndromes *(159)*. Because no specific biologic or molecular markers of the disease have been identified, diagnosis is based on clinical characteristics. Zittoun et al. first described CMML in 1972 *(162)* and the French-American-British Cooperative Group (FAB) subsequently classified the disease as a subdivision of MDS *(163)*. The FAB defined CMML as a myelodysplastic disorder with peripheral monocytosis of greater than $1 \times 10^9/L$; the appearance of monocytic cells in the bone marrow; dysplasia of either the erythroid, megakaryocytic, or granulocytic precursors; and less than 5% circulating blasts with less than 30% marrow blasts *(163,164)*.

Clinical Features and Natural Course of the Disease

CMML is a disease of the elderly, with a median age at presentation ranging from 64–72 yr and a significant male predominance of 2-3.3:1 *(165–167)*. At presentation, most patients are asymptomatic, but others have symptoms associated with anemia and variable degrees of cachexia. Signs of proliferation including leukocytosis, splenomegaly, hepatomegaly, lymphadenopathy, gingival hyperplasia, and cutaneous infiltration are frequently observed in patients with CMML *(166–168)*. Hypergammaglobulinemia has been reported in more than 50% of patients with CMML *(161,166,169)*. It is usually polyclonal, although monoclonal gammopathies have been reported in less than 10% of patients as well. Median survival in CMML ranges from 8 mo to 3 yr *(161,168)*. It has been suggested that patients with abnormal cytogenetics at diagnosis appear to present earlier in life and may have a shorter survival compared to CMML patients with normal cytogenetics. In particular, in CMML monosomy 7 is associated with a more aggressive disease and a poor survival *(167)*. The percentage of bone-marrow blast cells also strongly influences survival in patients with CMML, with significantly better survival in patients with less than 5% marrow blasts *(165,166)*. Many CMML patients die from complications associated with progressive cytopenias (infection or bleeding) before the transformation to acute leukemia occurs. The risk of leukemia transformation is high (24–53%), and the outcome of treatment after transformation is disappointing *(166,167)*.

Therapeutic Options

Currently, no effective therapy exists for either CMML or the acute leukemia that may develop following CMML. Supportive measures are widely considered to be the standard of care. Results with hematopoietic growth factors, low-dose chemotherapy with cytarabine, and combination anti-leukemia chemotherapy in MDS have been unsatisfactory *(170–176)*. Few studies have specifically addressed the efficacy of chemotherapy in patients with CMML, and the number of CMML patients included in studies of MDS has been small. The most promising results are those reported by Kantarjian and colleagues *(177,178)*, who noted conversion to a diploid karyotype in MDS/CMML patients who achieved a complete remission with a well-tolerated regimen of topotecan and cytarabine. However, it remains unclear how this cytogenetic remission may impact on the natural history or overall survival of CMML, since this was a single-treatment-arm study. Considering the efficacy of topotecan, oral topoisomerase I inhibitors such as camptothecin *(179)* may also offer therapeutic benefit in patients with CMML.

CONCLUSION

More than 100 yr have passed since the description of the first myeloproliferative disorder by Vaquez in 1892 *(2)*. Several studies have been performed; many under the auspices of the PVSG, and our diagnostic and therapeutic strategies—particularly for ET and PCV—rely heavily on the results of these studies. Given the low incidence of the CMPDs, cooperative study groups such as the PVSG are essential to the advancement of our understanding of these diseases. A greater understanding of the unique pathogenetic mechanisms underlying the CMPDs will not only facilitate more accurate classification of the individual disease entities, but may also allow for the design of targeted therapeutic interventions. Our descriptions of PCV, ET, AMMM, and CMML are a summary of our current understanding of these myeloproliferative disorders.

REFERENCES

1. Dameshek W. Some speculations on the myeloproliferative syndromes. *Blood* 1951; 6:372.
2. Vaquez H. Sur une forme speciale de cyanose s' accompagnant d' hyperglobulie excessive et persistente. *Compt Rend Soc Biol* 1892; 44:384–388.
3. Osler W. Chronic cyanosis, with polycythemia and enlarged spleen: a new disease entity. *Am J Med Sci* 1903; 126:187–201.
4. Dai CH, Krantz SB, Means RT, Jr., Horn ST, Gilbert HS. Polycythemia vera blood burst-forming units-erythroid are hypersensitive to interleukin-3. *J Clin Invest* 1991; 87:391–396.
5. Dai CH, Krantz S. Vanadate mimics the effect of stem cell factor on highly purified human erythroid burst-forming units in vitro, but not the effect of erythropoietin. *Exp Hematol* 1992; 20:1055–1060.
6. Martin JM, Ghandi K, Jackson WR, Dessypris EN. Hypersensitivity of polycythemia vera megakaryocytic progenitors to thrombopoietin. *Blood* 1996; 88:94. (absract 363)
7. Mirza AM, Ezzat S, Axelrad AA. Insulin-like growth factor binding protein-1 is elevated in patients with polycythemia vera and stimulates erythroid burst formation in vitro. *Blood* 1997; 89:1862–1869.
8. Silva M, Richard C, Benito A, Sanz C, Olalla I, Fernandez-Luna JL. Expression of Bcl-x in erythroid precursors from patients with polycythemia vera. *N Engl J Med* 1998; 338:564–571.
9. Temerinac S, Klippel S, Strunck E, et al. Cloning of PRV-1, a novel member of the uPAR receptor superfamily, which is overexpressed in polycythemia rubra vera. *Blood* 2000; 95:2569–2576.
10. Berlin NI. Diagnosis and classification of the polycythemias. *Semin Hematol* 1975; 12:339–351.
11. Berk PD, Goldberg JD, Donovan PB, Fruchtman SM, Berlin NI, Wasserman LR. Therapeutic recommendations in polycythemia vera based on Polycythemia Vera Study Group protocols. *Semin Hematol* 1986; 23:132–143.
12. Pearson TC, Glass UH, Wetherley-Mein G. Interpretation of measured red cell mass in the diagnosis of polycythaemia. *Scand J Haematol* 1978; 21:153–162.
13. Pearson TC, Botterill CA, Glass UH, Wetherley-Mein G. Interpretation of measured red cell mass and plasma volume in males with elevated venous PCV values. *Scand J Haematol* 1984; 33:68–74.
14. Messinezy M, Pearson TC. The classification and diagnostic criteria of the erythrocytoses (polycythaemias). *Clin Lab Haematol* 1999; 21:309–316.

15. Pearson TC, Messinezy M. The diagnostic criteria of polycythaemia rubra vera. *Leuk Lymphoma* 1996; 22 Suppl 1:87–93.
16. Modan B, Kallner H, Zemer D, Yoran C. A note on the increased risk of polycythemia vera in Jews. *Blood* 1971; 37:172–176.
17. Prochazka AV, Markowe HL. The epidemiology of polycythaemia rubra vera in England and Wales 1968-1982. *Br J Cancer* 1986; 53:59–64.
18. Silverstein MN, Lanier AP. Polycythemia vera, 1935-1969: an epidemiologic survey in Rochester, Minnesota. *Mayo Clin Proc* 1971; 46:751–753.
19. Kurita S. [Epidemiological studies of polycythemia vera in Japan (author's transl)]. *Nippon Ketsueki Gakkai Zasshi* 1974; 37:793–795.
20. Danish EH, Rasch CA, Harris JW. Polycythemia vera in childhood: case report and review of the literature. *Am J Hematol* 1980; 9:421–428.
21. Najean Y, Mugnier P, Dresch C, Rain JD. Polycythaemia vera in young people: an analysis of 58 cases diagnosed before 40 years. *Br J Haematol* 1987; 67:285–291.
22. Polycythemia vera: the natural history of 1213 patients followed for 20 years. Gruppo Italiano Studio Policitemia. *Ann Intern Med* 1995; 123:656–664.
23. Bilgrami S, Greenberg BR. Polycythemia rubra vera. *Semin Oncol* 1995; 22:307–326.
24. Murphy S. Therapeutic dilemmas: balancing the risks of bleeding, thrombosis, and leukemic transformation in myeloproliferative disorders (MPD). *Thromb Haemost* 1997; 78:622–626.
25. Babb RR, Alarcon-Segovia D, Fairbairn JR. Erythermalgia. Review of 51 cases. *Circulation* 1964; 29:136–141.
26. van Genderen PJ, Michiels JJ. Erythromelalgia: a pathognomonic microvascular thrombotic complication in essential thrombocythemia and polycythemia vera. *Semin Thromb Hemost* 1997; 23:357–363.
27. Michiels JJ. Erythromelalgia and vascular complications in polycythemia vera. *Semin Thromb Hemost* 1997; 23:441–454.
28. Michiels JJ, Abels J, Steketee J, van Vliet HH, Vuzevski VD. Erythromelalgia caused by platelet-mediated arteriolar inflammation and thrombosis in thrombocythemia. *Ann Intern Med* 1985; 102:466–471.
29. Wanless IR, Peterson P, Das A, Boitnott JK, Moore GW, Bernier V. Hepatic vascular disease and portal hypertension in polycythemia vera and agnogenic myeloid metaplasia: a clinico-pathological study of 145 patients examined at autopsy. *Hepatology* 1990; 12:1166–1174.
30. Tavill AS, Wood EJ, Kreel L, Jones EA, Gregory M, Sherlock S. The Budd-Chiari syndrome: correlation between hepatic scintigraphy and the clinical, radiological, and pathological findings in nineteen cases of hepatic venous outflow obstruction. *Gastroenterology* 1975; 68:509–518.
31. Valla D, Casadevall N, Lacombe C, et al. Primary myeloproliferative disorder and hepatic vein thrombosis. A prospective study of erythroid colony formation in vitro in 20 patients with Budd-Chiari syndrome. *Ann Intern Med* 1985; 103:329–334.
32. Silverstein A, Gilbert H, Wasserman LR. Neurologic complications of polycythemia. *Ann Intern Med* 1962; 57:909–916.
33. Tartaglia AP, Goldberg JD, Berk PD, Wasserman LR. Adverse effects of antiaggregating platelet therapy in the treatment of polycythemia vera. *Semin Hematol* 1986; 23:172–176.
34. Patrono C. Aspirin as an antiplatelet drug. *N Engl J Med* 1994; 330:1287–1294.
35. Barbui T, Finazzi G. Risk factors and prevention of vascular complications in polycythemia vera. *Semin Thromb Hemost* 1997; 23:455–461.
36. Landolfi R, Rocca B, Patrono C. Bleeding and thrombosis in myeloproliferative disorders: mechanisms and treatment. *Crit Rev Oncol Hematol* 1995; 20:203–222.
37. Najean Y, Rain JD. The very long-term evolution of polycythemia vera: an analysis of 318 patients initially treated by phlebotomy or 32P between 1969 and 1981. *Semin Hematol* 1997; 34:6–16.

38. Berk PD, Wasserman LR, Fruchtman SM. Treatment of polycythemia vera: a summary of clinical trials conducted by the polycythemia vera study group. In: Wasserman LR, Berk PD, Berlin NI, eds. *Polycythemia Vera and the Myeloproliferative Disorders*. WB Saunders, Philadelphia, PA, 1995; 166–194.

39. Fruchtman SM, Mack K, Kaplan ME, Peterson P, Berk PD, Wasserman LR. From efficacy to safety: a Polycythemia Vera Study group report on hydroxyurea in patients with polycythemia vera. *Semin Hematol* 1997; 34:17–23.

40. Silverstein MN. The evolution into and the treatment of late stage polycythemia vera. *Semin Hematol* 1976; 13:79–84.

41. Najean Y, Dresch C, Rain JD. The very-long-term course of polycythaemia: a complement to the previously published data of the Polycythaemia Vera Study Group. *Br J Haematol* 1994; 86:233–235.

42. Landaw SA. Acute leukemia in polycythemia vera. *Semin Hematol* 1986; 23:156–165.

43. Weinfeld A, Swolin B, Westin J. Acute leukaemia after hydroxyurea therapy in polycythaemia vera and allied disorders: prospective study of efficacy and leukaemogenicity with therapeutic implications. *Eur J Haematol* 1994; 52:134–139.

44. Wehmeier A, Sudhoff T, Meierkord F. Relation of platelet abnormalities to thrombosis and hemorrhage in chronic myeloproliferative disorders. *Semin Thromb Hemost* 1997; 23:391–402.

45. Nand S, Messmore H, Fisher SG, Bird ML, Schulz W, Fisher RI. Leukemic transformation in polycythemia vera: analysis of risk factors. *Am J Hematol* 1990; 34:32–36.

46. Braich TA, Grogan TM, Hicks MJ, Greenberg BR. Terminal lymphoblastic transformation in polycythemia vera. *Am J Med* 1986; 80:304–306.

47. Hazani A, Tatarsky I, Barzilai D. Prolonged remission of leukemia associated with polycythemia vera. *Cancer* 1977; 40:1297–1299.

48. Tefferi A. The Philadelphia chromosome negative chronic myeloproliferative disorders: a practical overview. *Mayo Clin Proc* 1998; 73:1177–1184.

49. Kaplan SD. Update of a mortality study of workers in petroleum refineries. *J Occup Med* 1986; 28:514–516.

50. Ravandi-Kashani F, Schafer AI. Microvascular disturbances, thrombosis, and bleeding in thrombocythemia: current concepts and perspectives. *Semin Thromb Hemost* 1997; 23:479–488.

51. Lengfelder E, Berger U, Hehlmann R. Interferon alpha in the treatment of polycythemia vera. *Ann Hematol* 2000; 79:103–109.

52. Petitt RM, Silverstein MN, Petrone ME. Anagrelide for control of thrombocythemia in polycythemia and other myeloproliferative disorders. *Semin Hematol* 1997; 34:51–54.

53. Epstein E, Goedel A. Hammorrhagische thrombozythamie bei vaskularer schrumpfmilz. *Virkows Arch Pathol Anat* 1934; 292:233–248.

54. Harrison CN, Gale RE, Machin SJ, Linch DC. A large proportion of patients with a diagnosis of essential thrombocythemia do not have a clonal disorder and may be at lower risk of thrombotic complications. *Blood* 1999; 93:417–424.

55. Murray LJ, Luens KM, Estrada MF, et al. Thrombopoietin mobilizes CD34+ cell subsets into peripheral blood and expands multilineage progenitors in bone marrow of cancer patients with normal hematopoiesis. *Exp Hematol* 1998; 26:207–216.

56. Cerutti A, Custodi P, Duranti M, Noris P, Balduini CL. Thrombopoietin levels in patients with primary and reactive thrombocytosis. *Br J Haematol* 1997; 99:281–284.

57. Tahara T, Usuki K, Sato H, et al. A sensitive sandwich ELISA for measuring thrombopoietin in human serum: serum thrombopoietin levels in healthy volunteers and in patients with haemopoietic disorders. *Br J Haematol* 1996; 93:783–788.

58. Horikawa Y, Matsumura I, Hashimoto K, et al. Markedly reduced expression of platelet c-mpl receptor in essential thrombocythemia. *Blood* 1997; 90:4031–4038.

59. Moliterno AR, Hankins WD, Spivak JL. Impaired expression of the thrombopoietin receptor by platelets from patients with polycythemia vera. *N Engl J Med* 1998; 338:572–580.

60. Kondo T, Okabe M, Sanada M, et al. Familial essential thrombocythemia associated with one-base deletion in the 5'-untranslated region of the thrombopoietin gene. *Blood* 1998; 92:1091–1096.

61. Murphy S, Peterson P, Iland H, Laszlo J. Experience of the Polycythemia Vera Study Group with essential thrombocythemia: a final report on diagnostic criteria, survival, and leukemic transition by treatment. *Semin Hematol* 1997; 34:29-39.

62. Murphy S. Diagnostic criteria and prognosis in polycythemia vera and essential thrombocythemia. *Semin Hematol* 1999; 36:9-13.

63. Randi ML, Barbone E, Zerbinati P, Soini B, Rossi C, Girolami A. Essential thrombocythemia following polycythemia vera: an unusual sequence. *J Med* 1996; 27:363-8.

64. Van de Pette JE, Prochazka AV, Pearson TC, Singh AK, Dickson ER, Wetherley-Mein G. Primary thrombocythaemia treated with busulphan. *Br J Haematol* 1986; 62:229-237.

65. Bellucci S, Janvier M, Tobelem G, et al. Essential thrombocythemias. Clinical evolutionary and biological data. *Cancer* 1986; 58:2440-2447.

66. Grossi A, Rosseti S, Vannucchi AM, Rafanelli D, Ferrini PR. Occurrence of haemorrhagic and thrombotic events in myeloproliferative disorders: a retrospective study of 108 patients. *Clin Lab Haematol* 1988; 10:167-175.

67. Wehmeier A, Daum I, Jamin H, Schneider W. Incidence and clinical risk factors for bleeding and thrombotic complications in myeloproliferative disorders. A retrospective analysis of 260 patients. *Ann Hematol* 1991; 63:101-106.

68. Randi ML, Stocco F, Rossi C, Tison T, Girolami A. Thrombosis and hemorrhage in thrombocytosis: evaluation of a large cohort of patients (357 cases). *J Med* 1991; 22:213-223.

69. McIntyre KJ, Hoagland HC, Silverstein MN, Petitt RM. Essential thrombocythemia in young adults. *Mayo Clin Proc* 1991; 66:149–154.

70. Millard FE, Hunter CS, Anderson M, et al. Clinical manifestations of essential thrombocythemia in young adults. *Am J Hematol* 1990; 33:27–31.

71. Randi ML, Fabris F, Girolami A. Thrombocytosis in young people: evaluation of 57 cases diagnosed before the age of 40. *Blut* 1990; 60:233–237.

72. Tefferi A, Silverstein MN, Petitt RM, Mesa RA, Solberg LA, Jr. Anagrelide as a new platelet-lowering agent in essential thrombocythemia: mechanism of actin, efficacy, toxicity, current indications. *Semin Thromb Hemost* 1997; 23:379–383.

73. Chistolini A, Mazzucconi MG, Ferrari A, et al. Essential thrombocythemia: a retrospective study on the clinical course of 100 patients. *Haematologica* 1990; 75:537–540.

74. Mesa RA, Tefferi A, Jacobsen SJ. The incidence and epidemiology of essential thrombocythemia and agnogenic myeloid metaplasia: an Olmstead County study. *Blood* 1997; 90:347a. (abst)

75. Hehlmann R, Jahn M, Baumann B, Kopcke W. Essential thrombocythemia. Clinical characteristics and course of 61 cases. *Cancer* 1988; 61:2487–2496.

76. Michiels JJ, Koudstaal PJ, Mulder AH, van Vliet HH. Transient neurologic and ocular manifestations in primary thrombocythemia. *Neurology* 1993; 43:1107–1110.

77. Rozman C, Giralt M, Feliu E, Rubio D, Cortes MT. Life expectancy of patients with chronic nonleukemic myeloproliferative disorders. *Cancer* 1991; 67:2658–2663.

78. Cortelazzo S, Viero P, Finazzi G, D'Emilio A, Rodeghiero F, Barbui T. Incidence and risk factors for thrombotic complications in a historical cohort of 100 patients with essential thrombocythemia. *J Clin Oncol* 1990; 8:556–562.

79. Randi ML, Fabris F, Rossi C, Tison T, Barbone E, Girolami A. Sex and age as prognostic factors in essential thrombocythemia. *Haematologica* 1992; 77:402–404.

80. Colombi M, Radaelli F, Zocchi L, Maiolo AT. Thrombotic and hemorrhagic complications in essential thrombocythemia. A retrospective study of 103 patients. *Cancer* 1991; 67:2926–2930.

81. Watson KV, Key N. Vascular complications of essential thrombocythaemia: a link to cardiovascular risk factors. *Br J Haematol* 1993; 83:198–203.

82. Cortelazzo S, Finazzi G, Ruggeri M, et al. Hydroxyurea for patients with essential thrombocythemia and a high risk of thrombosis. *N Engl J Med* 1995; 332:1132–1136.

83. Tefferi A, Silverstein MN, Hoagland HC. Primary thrombocythemia. *Semin Oncol* 1995; 22:334–340.

84. Beard J, Hillmen P, Anderson CC, Lewis SM, Pearson TC. Primary thrombocythaemia in pregnancy. *Br J Haematol* 1991; 77:371–374.

85. Greisshammer M, Bangerter M, VanVliet H, et al. Aspirin in essential thrombocythemia: status quo and quo vadis. *Semin Thromb Hemost* 1997; 23:371–378.

86. Pearson TC. Primary thrombocythaemia: diagnosis and management. *Br J Haematol* 1991; 78:145–148.

87. Elliott MA, Tefferi A. Interferon-alpha therapy in polycythemia vera and essential thrombocythemia. *Semin Thromb Hemost* 1997; 23:463–472.

88. Fenaux P, Simon M, Caulier MT, Lai JL, Goudemand J, Bauters F. Clinical course of essential thrombocythemia in 147 cases. *Cancer* 1990; 66:549–556.

89. Brandt L, Anderson H. Survival and risk of leukaemia in polycythaemia vera and essential thrombocythaemia treated with oral radiophosphorus: are safer drugs available? *Eur J Haematol* 1995; 54:21–26.

90. Budde U, Schaefer G, Mueller N, et al. Acquired von Willebrand's disease in the myeloproliferative syndrome. *Blood* 1984; 64:981–985.

91. Budde U, Dent JA, Berkowitz SD, Ruggeri ZM, Zimmerman TS. Subunit composition of plasma von Willebrand factor in patients with the myeloproliferative syndrome. *Blood* 1986; 68:1213–1217.

92. Sterkers Y, Preudhomme C, Lai JL, et al. Acute myeloid leukemia and myelodysplastic syndromes following essential thrombocythemia treated with hydroxyurea: high proportion of cases with 17p deletion. *Blood* 1998; 91:616–622.

93. Singh AK, Wetherley-Mein G. Microvascular occlusive lesions in primary thrombocythaemia. *Br J Haematol* 1977; 36:553–564.

94. Michiels JJ, van Joost T. Erythromelalgia and thrombocythemia: a causal relation. *J Am Acad Dermatol* 1990; 22:107–111.

95. Barbui T, Finazzi G, Dupuy E, Kiladjian JJ, Briere J. Treatment strategies in essential thrombocythemia. A critical appraisal of various experiences in different centers. *Leuk Lymphoma* 1996; 22(Suppl 1):149–160.

96. Tefferi A, Elliott MA, Solberg LA, Jr., Silverstein MN. New drugs in essential thrombocythemia and polycythemia vera. *Blood Rev* 1997; 11:1–7.

97. Sacchi S, Tabilio A, Leoni P, et al. Interferon alpha-2b in the long-term treatment of essential thrombocythemia. *Ann Hematol* 1991; 63:206–209.

98. Pogliani EM, Rossini F, Miccolis I, et al. Alpha interferon as initial treatment of essential thrombocythemia. Analysis after two years of follow-up. *Tumori* 1995; 81:245–248.

99. Rametta V, Ferrara F, Marottoli V, Matera C, Mettivier V, Cimino R. Recombinant interferon alpha-2b as treatment of essential thrombocythaemia. *Acta Haematol* 1994; 91:126–129.

100. Middelhoff G, Boll I. A long-term clinical trial of interferon alpha-therapy in essential thrombocythemia. *Ann Hematol* 1992; 64:207–209.

101. Sacchi S, Tabilio A, Leoni P, et al. Sustained complete hematological remission in essential thrombocythemia after discontinuation of long-term alpha-IFN treatment. *Ann Hematol* 1993; 66:245–246.

102. Giles FJ. Maintenance therapy in the myeloproliferative disorders: the current options. *Br J Haematol* 1991; 79(Suppl 1):92–95.

103. Gisslinger H, Chott A, Scheithauer W, Gilly B, Linkesch W, Ludwig H. Interferon in essential thrombocythaemia. *Br J Haematol* 1991; 79(Suppl 1):42–47.

104. Balduini CL, Bertolino G, Noris P, Ascari E. Effect of anagrelide on platelet count and function in patients with thrombocytosis and myeloproliferative disorders. *Haematologica* 1992; 77:40–43.
105. Anagrelide, a therapy for thrombocythemic states: experience in 577 patients. Anagrelide Study Group. *Am J Med* 1992; 92:69–76.
106. Ward HP, Block MH. The natural history of agnogenic myeloid metaplasia (AMM) and a critical evaluation of its relationship with the myeloproliferative syndrome. *Medicine* (Baltimore) 1971; 50:357–420.
107. Heuck G. Zwei falle von leukamie mit eigenthumlichem blut-resp. Knochenmarksbefund. *Virchows Archiv* 1879; 79:475–496.
108. Jacobson RJ, Salo A, Fialkow PJ. Agnogenic myeloid metaplasia: a clonal proliferation of hematopoietic stem cells with secondary myelofibrosis. *Blood* 1978; 51:189–194.
109. Martyre MC, Le Bousse-Kerdiles MC, Romquin N, et al. Elevated levels of basic fibroblast growth factor in megakaryocytes and platelets from patients with idiopathic myelofibrosis. *Br J Haematol* 1997; 97:441–448.
110. Katoh O, Kimura A, Itoh T, Kuramoto A. Platelet derived growth factor messenger RNA is increased in bone marrow megakaryocytes in patients with myeloproliferative disorders. *Am J Hematol* 1990; 35:145–150.
111. Long MW, Robinson JA, Ashcraft EA, Mann KG. Regulation of human bone marrow-derived osteoprogenitor cells by osteogenic growth factors [published erratum appears in *J Clin Invest* 1995 Nov;96(5):2541]. *J Clin Invest* 1995; 95:881–887.
112. Ulich TR, del Castillo J, Senaldi G, et al. Systemic hematologic effects of PEG-rHuMGDF-induced megakaryocyte hyperplasia in mice. *Blood* 1996; 87:5006–5015.
113. Yan XQ, Lacey D, Hill D, et al. A model of myelofibrosis and osteosclerosis in mice induced by overexpressing thrombopoietin (mpl ligand): reversal of disease by bone marrow transplantation. *Blood* 1996; 88:402–409.
114. Yanagida M, Ide Y, Imai A, et al. The role of transforming growth factor-beta in PEG-rHuMGDF-induced reversible myelofibrosis in rats. *Br J Haematol* 1997; 99:739–745.
115. Laszlo J. Myeloproliferative disorders (MPD): myelofibrosis, myelosclerosis, extramedullary hematopoiesis, undifferentiated MPD, and hemorrhagic thrombocythemia. *Semin Hematol* 1975; 12:409–432.
116. Thiele J, Kvasnicka HM, Diehl V, Fischer R, Michiels J. Clinicopathological diagnosis and differential criteria of thrombocythemias in various myeloproliferative disorders by histopathology, histochemistry and immunostaining from bone marrow biopsies. *Leuk Lymphoma* 1999; 33:207–218.
117. McNally RJ, Rowland D, Roman E, Cartwright RA. Age and sex distributions of hematological malignancies in the U.K. *Hematol Oncol* 1997; 15:173–189.
118. Mesa RA, Silverstein MN, Jacobsen SJ, Wollan PC, Tefferi A. Population-based incidence and survival figures in essential thrombocythemia and agnogenic myeloid metaplasia: an Olmsted County Study, 1976-1995. *Am J Hematol* 1999; 61:10–15.
119. Dupriez B, Morel P, Demory JL, et al. Prognostic factors in agnogenic myeloid metaplasia: a report on 195 cases with a new scoring system. *Blood* 1996; 88:1013–1018.
120. Kvasnicka HM, Thiele J, Werden C, Zankovich R, Diehl V, Fischer R. Prognostic factors in idiopathic (primary) osteomyelofibrosis. *Cancer* 1997; 80:708–719.
121. Cervantes F, Pereira A, Esteve J, et al. Identification of "short-lived" and "long-lived" patients at presentation of idiopathic myelofibrosis. *Br J Haematol* 1997; 97:635–640.
122. Sekhar M, Prentice HG, Popat U, et al. Idiopathic myelofibrosis in children. *Br J Haematol* 1996; 93:394–397.
123. Altura RA, Head DR, Wong WC. Prolonged survival of children with idiopathic myelofibrosis (IMF). *Blood* 1999; 94:114a. (abstract 501)

124. Cervantes F, Pereira A, Esteve J, Cobo F, Rozman C, Montserrat E. [Idiopathic myelofibro-sis: initial features, evolutive patterns and survival in a series of 106 patients]. *Med Clin* (Barc) 1997; 109:651–655.

125. Hasselbalch H. Idiopathic myelofibrosis: a clinical study of 80 patients. *Am J Hematol* 1990; 34:291–300.

126. Khumbananda M, Horowitz HI, Eyster ME. Coombs' positive hemolytic anemia in myelofi-brosis with myeloid metaplasia. *Am J Med Sci* 1969; 258:89–93.

127. Akikusa B, Komatsu T, Kondo Y, Yokota T, Uchino F, Yonemitsu H. Amyloidosis compli-cating idiopathic myelofibrosis. *Arch Pathol Lab Med* 1987; 111:525–529.

128. Soppi E, Nousiainen T, Seppa A, Lahtinen R. Acute febrile neutrophilic dermatosis (Sweet's syndrome) in association with myelodysplastic syndromes: a report of three cases and a review of the literature. *Br J Haematol* 1989; 73:43–47.

129. Caughman W, Stern R, Haynes H. Neutrophilic dermatosis of myeloproliferative disorders. Atypical forms of pyoderma gangrenosum and Sweet's syndrome associated with myelopro-liferative disorders. *J Am Acad Dermatol* 1983; 9:751–758.

130. Bernhardt B, Valletta M. Lupus anticoagulant in myelofibrosis. *Am J Med Sci* 1976; 272: 229–231.

131. Gordon BR, Coleman M, Kohen P, Day NK. Immunologic abnormalities in myelofibrosis with activation of the complement system. *Blood* 1981; 58:904–910.

132. Imam TH, Doll DC. Acute cardiac tamponade associated with pericardial extramedullary hematopoiesis in agnogenic myeloid metaplasia. *Acta Haematol* 1997; 98:42–43.

133. Xiao JC, Walz-Mattmuller R, Ruck P, Horny HP, Kaiserling E. Renal involvement in myeloproliferative and lymphoproliferative disorders. A study of autopsy cases. *Gen Diagn Pathol* 1997; 142:147-53.

134. Patel BM, Su WP, Perniciaro C, Gertz MA. Cutaneous extramedullary hematopoiesis. *J Am Acad Dermatol* 1995; 32:805–807.

135. Bartlett RP, Greipp PR, Tefferi A, Cupps RE, Mullan BP, Trastek VF. Extramedullary hemato-poiesis manifesting as a symptomatic pleural effusion. *Mayo Clin Proc* 1995; 70:1161–1164.

136. Cook G, Sharp RA. Spinal cord compression due to extramedullary haemopoiesis in myelofibrosis. *J Clin Pathol* 1994; 47:464–465.

137. Cervantes F, Barosi G, Demory JL, et al. Myelofibrosis with myeloid metaplasia in young individuals: disease characteristics, prognostic factors and identification of risk groups. *Br J Haematol* 1998; 102:684–690.

138. Reilly JT, Snowden JA, Spearing RL, et al. Cytogenetic abnormalities and their prognostic significance in idiopathic myelofibrosis: a study of 106 cases. *Br J Haematol* 1997; 98:96–102.

139. Visani G, Finelli C, Castelli U, et al. Myelofibrosis with myeloid metaplasia: clinical and haematological parameters predicting survival in a series of 133 patients. *Br J Haematol* 1990; 75:4–9.

140. Cervantes F, Pereira A, Esteve J, Cobo F, Rozman C, Montserrat E. The changing profile of idiopathic myelofibrosis: a comparison of the presenting features of patients diagnosed in two different decades. *Eur J Haematol* 1998; 60:101–105.

141. Rupoli S, Da Lio L, Sisti S, et al. Primary myelofibrosis: a detailed statistical analysis of the clinicopathological variables influencing survival. *Ann Hematol* 1994; 68:205–212.

142. Varki A, Lottenberg R, Griffith R, Reinhard E. The syndrome of idiopathic myelofibrosis. A clinicopathologic review with emphasis on the prognostic variables predicting survival. *Medicine* (Baltimore) 1983; 62:353–371.

143. Njoku OS, Lewis SM, Catovsky D, Gordon-Smith EC. Anaemia in myelofibrosis: its value in prognosis. *Br J Haematol* 1983; 54:79–89.

144. Barosi G, Berzuini C, Liberato LN, Costa A, Polino G, Ascari E. A prognostic classification of myelofibrosis with myeloid metaplasia. *Br J Haematol* 1988; 70:397-401.

145. Cervantes F, Hernandez-Boluda JC, Alvarez A, Nadal E, Montserrat E. Danazol treatment of idiopathic myelofibrosis with severe anemia. *Haematologica* 2000; 85:595–599.

146. Rodriguez JN, Martino ML, Dieguez JC, Prados D. rHuEpo for the treatment of anemia in myelofibrosis with myeloid metaplasia. Experience in 6 patients and meta-analytical approach. *Haematologica* 1998; 83:616–621.

147. Pietrasanta D, Clavio M, Vallebella E, Beltrami G, Cavaliere M, Gobbi M. Long-lasting effect of cyclosporin-A on anemia associated with idiopathic myelofibrosis. *Haematologica* 1997; 82:458–459.

148. Paquette RL, Meshkinpour A, Rosen PJ. Autoimmune myelofibrosis. A steroid-responsive cause of bone marrow fibrosis associated with systemic lupus erythematosus. *Medicine* (Baltimore) 1994; 73:145–152.

149. Barosi G. Myelofibrosis with myeloid metaplasia: diagnostic definition and prognostic classification for clinical studies and treatment guidelines. *J Clin Oncol* 1999; 17:2954–2970.

150. Carlo-Stella C, Cazzola M, Gasner A, et al. Effects of recombinant alpha and gamma interferons on the in vitro growth of circulating hematopoietic progenitor cells (CFU-GEMM, CFU-Mk, BFU-E, and CFU-GM) from patients with myelofibrosis with myeloid metaplasia. *Blood* 1987; 70:1014–1019.

151. Barosi G, Ambrosetti A, Buratti A, et al. Splenectomy for patients with myelofibrosis with myeloid metaplasia: pretreatment variables and outcome prediction. *Leukemia* 1993; 7:200–206.

152. Tefferi A, Mesa RA, Nagorney DM, Schroeder G, Silverstein MN. Splenectomy in myelofibrosis with myeloid metaplasia: a single- institution experience with 223 patients. *Blood* 2000; 95:2226–2233.

153. Barosi G, Ambrosetti A, Centra A, et al. Splenectomy and risk of blast transformation in myelofibrosis with myeloid metaplasia. Italian Cooperative Study Group on Myeloid with Myeloid Metaplasia. *Blood* 1998; 91:3630–3636.

154. Bouabdallah R, Coso D, Gonzague-Casabianca L, Alzieu C, Resbeut M, Gastaut J. Safety and efficacy of splenic irradiation in the treatment of patients with idiopathic myelofibrosis: a report on 15 patients. *Leuk Res* 2000; 24:491–495.

155. Elliott MA, Chen MG, Silverstein MN, Tefferi A. Splenic irradiation for symptomatic splenomegaly associated with myelofibrosis with myeloid metaplasia. *Br J Haematol* 1998; 103:505–511.

156. Guardiola P, Anderson JE, Bandini G, et al. Allogeneic stem cell transplantation for agnogenic myeloid metaplasia: a European Group for Blood and Marrow Transplantation, Societe Francaise de Greffe de Moelle, Gruppo Italiano per il Trapianto del Midollo Osseo, and Fred Hutchinson Cancer Research Center Collaborative Study. *Blood* 1999; 93:2831–2838.

157. Guardiola P, Esperou H, Cazals-Hatem D, et al. Allogeneic bone marrow transplantation for agnogenic myeloid metaplasia. French Society of Bone Marrow Transplantation. *Br J Haematol* 1997; 98:1004–1009.

158. Bennett JM, Catovsky D, Daniel MT, et al. The chronic myeloid leukaemias: guidelines for distinguishing chronic granulocytic, atypical chronic myeloid, and chronic myelomonocytic leukaemia. Proposals by the French-American-British Cooperative Leukaemia Group. *Br J Haematol* 1994; 87:746–754.

159. Michaux JL, Martiat P. Chronic myelomonocytic leukaemia (CMML)—a myelodysplastic or myeloproliferative syndrome? *Leuk Lymphoma* 1993; 9:35–41.

160. Cambier N, Baruchel A, Schlageter MH, et al. Chronic myelomonocytic leukemia: from biology to therapy. *Hematol Cell Ther* 1997; 39:41–48.

161. Fenaux P, Beuscart R, Lai JL, Jouet JP, Bauters F. Prognostic factors in adult chronic myelomonocytic leukemia: an analysis of 107 cases. *J Clin Oncol* 1988; 6:1417–1424.

162. Zittoun R, Bernadou A, Bilski-Pasquier G, Bousser J. [Subacute myelo-monocytic leukemia. Study of 27 cases and review of the literature]. *Sem Hop* 1972; 48:1943–1956.

163. Bennett JM, Catovsky D, Daniel MT, et al. Proposals for the classification of the myelodysplastic syndromes. *Br J Haematol* 1982; 51:189–199.
164. Goasguen JE, Bennett JM. Classification and morphologic features of the myelodysplastic syndromes. *Semin Oncol* 1992; 19:4–13.
165. Storniolo AM, Moloney WC, Rosenthal DS, Cox C, Bennett JM. Chronic myelomonocytic leukemia. *Leukemia* 1990; 4:766–770.
166. Tefferi A, Hoagland HC, Therneau TM, Pierre RV. Chronic myelomonocytic leukemia: natural history and prognostic determinants. *Mayo Clin Proc* 1989; 64:1246–1254.
167. Cytogenetics of chronic myelomonocytic leukemia. *Cancer Genet Cytogenet* 1986; 21:11–30.
168. Kantarjian HM, Kurzrock R, Talpaz M. Philadelphia chromosome-negative chronic myelogenous leukemia and chronic myelomonocytic leukemia. *Hematol Oncol Clin N Am* 1990; 4:389–404.
169. Solal-Celigny P, Desaint B, Herrera A, et al. Chronic myelomonocytic leukemia according to FAB classification: analysis of 35 cases. *Blood* 1984; 63:634–638.
170. Greenberg P, Taylor K, Larson R, al. e. Phase III randomized trial of G-CSF vs observation for myelodysplastic syndrome (MDS). *Blood* 1993; 82:196. (abstract 768)
171. Hellstrom-Lindberg E. Efficacy of erythropoietin in the myelodysplastic syndromes: a meta-analysis of 205 patients from 17 studies. *Br J Haematol* 1995; 89:67–71.
172. Miller KB, Kim K, Morrison FS, et al. The evaluation of low-dose cytarabine in the treatment of myelodysplastic syndromes: a phase-III intergroup study [published erratum appears in *Ann Hematol* 1993 Mar;66(3):164]. *Ann Hematol* 1992; 65:162–168.
173. Estey E, Pierce S, Kantarjian H, et al. Treatment of myelodysplastic syndromes with AML-type chemotherapy. *Leuk Lymphoma* 1993; 11:59–63.
174. Ruutu T, Hanninen A, Jarventie G, et al. Intensive chemotherapy of poor prognosis myelodysplastic syndromes (MDS) and acute myeloid leukemia following MDS with idarubicin and cytarabine. *Leuk Res* 1997; 21:133–138.
175. Parker JE, Pagliuca A, Mijovic A, et al. Fludarabine, cytarabine, G-CSF and idarubicin (FLAG-IDA) for the treatment of poor-risk myelodysplastic syndromes and acute myeloid leukaemia. *Br J Haematol* 1997; 99:939–944.
176. Wattel E, De Botton S, Luc Lai J, et al. Long-term follow-up of de novo myelodysplastic syndromes treated with intensive chemotherapy: incidence of long-term survivors and outcome of partial responders. *Br J Haematol* 1997; 98:983–991.
177. Beran M, Estey E, O'Brien S, et al. Topotecan and cytarabine is an active combination regimen in myelodysplastic syndromes and chronic myelomonocytic leukemia. *J Clin Oncol* 1999; 17:2819–2830.
178. Beran M, Kantarjian H. Results of topotecan-based combination therapy in patients with myelodysplastic syndromes and chronic myelomonocytic leukemia. *Semin Hematol* 1999; 36:3–10.
179. Pantazis P. The water-insoluble camptothecin analogues: promising drugs for the effective treatment of haematological malignancies. *Leuk Res* 1995; 19:775–788.

9 Advances in the Biology and Treatment of Multiple Myeloma

James R. Berenson, MD and Robert A. Vescio, MD

INTRODUCTION

Multiple myeloma is the second most common hematologic malignancy, with approximately 15,000 new cases each year in the United States. Our understanding of the pathophysiology underlying myeloma continues to expand, but the etiology of this plasma-cell dyscrasia remains unclear. Although controversy remains regarding a possible viral etiology of myeloma, evidence suggesting a role for the human herpesvirus-8 (HHV-8) is mounting. The roles of cytogenetic abnormalities, as well as aberrant angiogenesis and cytokine expression in the etiology of myeloma continue to be explored, and may lead to future therapeutic strategies. Transplantation in myeloma is rarely curative, but offers clinical benefit for young and possibly older myeloma patients as well. Newer bisphosphonates may offer greater ease of administration, improved efficacy, and possibly even enhanced anti-tumor effect. Finally, thalidomide and other new agents offer new therapeutic alternatives to myeloma patients who were previously refractory to multiple agents.

Multiple myeloma accounts for approximately one-tenth of all hematologic malignancies, and its incidence is rising as our society ages. Multiple myeloma is a malignant plasma-cell dyscrasia (mature B-cell lymphoid neoplasm), character-

From: *Current Clinical Oncology: Chronic Leukemias and Lymphomas:*
Biology, Pathophysiology, and Clinical Management
Edited by: G. J. Schiller © Humana Press Inc., Totowa, NJ

ized by the accumulation of malignant plasma cells in the bone-marrow compart-ment. These terminally differentiated B-lymphocytes produce a single immuno-globulin (Ig) known as a monoclonal protein. Monoclonal proteins are the laboratory hallmark of multiple myeloma, and are also seen in other disorders such as monoclonal gammopathy of undetermined significance and Walden-strom's macroglobulinemia. Although we continue to add to our understanding of the pathophysiology underlying myeloma, the etiology of this plasma-cell dyscrasia remains unclear. Controversy surrounds the possible viral etiology of myeloma, yet evidence suggesting a role for HHV-8 is mounting. There is also increasing understanding of the role of genetic abnormalities, angiogenesis, and cell-signaling pathways in this B-cell malignancy. These developments have resulted in exciting new therapeutic options for patients with this disease. These novel therapeutic approaches are clearly needed, because the median survival of myeloma has not improved during the past several decades. High-dose therapy followed by hematopoietic support for patients with myeloma is rarely curative, but offers some clinical benefit, and now can be safely performed even for patients in their seventies. Bisphosphonates have become part of the standard of care for bone disease and hypercalcemia in myeloma, but newer analogs may offer greater ease of administration, improved efficacy, and possibly even an enhanced anti-tumor effect. In addition, our fundamental understanding of the pathophysiology of bone disease in these patients has changed dramatically, and is leading to new therapeutic approaches. Thalidomide offers significant clinical benefit to myeloma patients who were previously refractory to multiple agents, and its role in early stages of the disease is under investigation. A multitude of other new promising drugs are also in early clinical trials.

BIOLOGY
The Malignant Cell of Origin

The predominant cell type in the bone marrow of patients with multiple myeloma has the characteristics of a plasma cell (1). However, these cells have a low proliferative rate and have generally been unable to sustain tumor growth in vivo. These observations suggest that there are other myeloma precursor cells that are responsible for proliferation of the malignant popu-lation (2,3). The presence of such cells could also explain the observation that the malignant plasma cells appear to be restricted to the microenvironment of the bone marrow, although the disease is widely disseminated throughout the axial skeleton.

Because of the monoclonal nature of the immunoglobulin (Ig) synthesized by the malignant cells, the genes responsible for the production of this protein can be used as molecular markers. Furthermore, characteristic changes in these genes occur at different stages of B-cell differentiation, permitting identification of the cell types in this lineage that are part of the tumor clone (3–6). It has been proposed that the abnormal B-cells originate in the lymph nodes, and then migrate to the bone marrow, which provides a microenvironment that is conducive to terminal plasma-cell differentiation *(6,7)*.

The properties of the immunoglobulin genes permit determination of the stage of B-cell development during which malignant transformation to multiple myeloma occurs. Each antibody-producing B-cell produces a single type of antibody. Early in normal B-cell development, rearrangement of four gene segments results in development of the heavy-chain portion of a unique functional antibody. One gene segment encodes a constant region that determines the class of antibody (e.g., C-mu for IgM, C-gamma for IgG, and C-alpha for IgA). Three other gene segments encode the variable region of the heavy chain: variable (VH), diversity (D), and joining (JH). These three joined segments in the variable region constitute the specific antigen recognition site of the final antibody; the recombination of genes responsible for this region is unique to each antibody-producing cell.

The major portion of a specific heavy-chain variable region is derived from one of about 50 functional VH genes, 30 D genes, and six JH genes. Increased antibody specificity is accomplished by the addition of non-germline nucleotides (N segments) at the VHD and DJH joints. Once a functional heavy-chain rearrangement has occurred, the kappa—and if unsuccessful, the lambda light chain—undergoes a similar rearrangement of V, J, and C genes.

The specificity and avidity of the antibody for antigen is further increased by mutations of nucleotides within the sections of the variable region that bind antigen directly, known as complementarity-determining regions (CDRs). This process of somatic mutation occurs late in B-cell development in germinal centers, and ceases in terminally differentiated B-cells that secrete functional antibody.

A number of reports have suggested that malignant transformation in multiple myeloma occurs late in B-cell differentiation *(2,4–6)*. One study, for example, evaluated the Ig VH region sequence in 48 patients with multiple myeloma *(5)*. Sequence analysis of the expressed VH genes showed marked somatic mutation (median 8%), which only is found in the most differentiated B-cells after antigenic stimulation has occurred *(5)*. In more direct support of an antigenically driven process, there was a marked predilection for somatic mutations in the CDRs that bind antigen as compared to the other parts of the gene, which are primarily responsible for maintaining the structural integrity of the molecule, the so-called framework regions (FRs). The ratio of nucleotide substitutions that resulted in amino-acid replacement was significantly higher in the CDRs than in the FRs; this is the expected finding in antigenically driven cells. In addition, there was no clonal diversity in the VH genes and no clonal evolution during the course of the disease.

These observations are different from other B-cell tumors originating in germinal centers at earlier stages of B-cell differentiation. Another difference is that myeloma tumor cells show complete absence of the VH4.21 (VH4-34) gene *(8)*, which is rearranged with increased frequency in immature B-cells, other B-cell malignancies—particularly diffuse large B-cell lymphoma (which is derived from relatively immature B-cells) *(9)*—and in autoimmune diseases *(8)*. This gene encodes antibodies capable of recognizing self-antigens. Elimination of B-cells expressing this gene at least in part may explain the lack of autoimmune phenomena in multiple myeloma; it is also compatible with the final transforming event occurring at the stage of terminal B-cell differentiation. Although one study suggested involvement of cells at an earlier stage of B-cell differentiation *(3)*, most other studies are consistent with the findings of the malignant cell originating from a cell late in B-cell differentiation.

Immunophenotype

The presence of a unique molecular marker—the immunoglobulin gene expressed by the malignant clone—allows identification of the malignant cells, and, therefore, determination of the presence or absence of surface markers on the malignant clone.

CD34

CD34 is expressed on early hematopoietic precursors, including the pluripotent stem cell and some B-cells. This early hematopoietic antigen is not expressed on the malignant cells in multiple myeloma *(10)*; however, CD34-positive tumor cells have been described in some reports *(11)*. The general lack of expression of CD34 on the malignant cells may have clinical importance with autologous stem-cell transplantation. Selection of CD34-positive cells with an immunoadsorption column reduces tumor-cell contamination by 2.7 to more than 4.5 logs prior to autologous peripheral-blood progenitor cell transplantation *(12–14)*.

CD10

CD10, the common acute lymphoblastic leukemia antigen (CALLA), was originally described as a surface antigen present on the cells of some human acute lymphoblastic leukemias. CD10 is also expressed on a variety of hematopoietic cells, including B-cells at early and late stages of differentiation. The use of polymerase chain reaction (PCR) with patient-specific VH gene primers suggests that there is a small population of CD10-positive clonal cells in most, or all patients with multiple myeloma *(15)*. CD10 is expressed on germinal center B-cells with high proliferative activity; thus, the malignant subpopulation in myeloma may represent part of the clone that leads to disease progression. Consistent with this hypothesis is the anecdotal observation that CD10-expressing tumor cells appear in the circulation at the time of progression of myeloma *(16)*.

CD19 AND CD20

CD19 and CD20 are first expressed on precursor B-cells and are present on all mature B-cells. (See "B-cell development"). Malignant bone-marrow plasma cells from patients with multiple myeloma do not express these markers *(17)*, and there is reversible suppression of CD19-positive nonmalignant cells that correlates inversely with disease stage *(18,19)* Controversy exists regarding the presence of CD19 and CD20 on circulating malignant plasma cells. Some studies have found these markers on circulating cells *(20)*. However, these cells are likely to be mostly polyclonal rather than representing the tumor clone *(21,22)*.

Loss of CD19 expression may be pathogenetically important by contributing to the proliferation of malignant plasma cells. Consistent with this hypothesis are the observations that enforced CD19 expression in a myeloma cell line results in growth inhibition and reduced tumorigenicity *(23)*, and that higher CD19+ blood levels in patients were positively associated with improved survival*(24)*.

CD28

CD28 is an antigen present on T-cells that contributes to the costimulatory pathway of T-cell activation, by binding to its ligand CD80 (B7-1) and CD86 (B7-2) on antigen-presenting cells. CD28 is also present on some malignant plasma cells from patients with multiple myeloma *(25,26)*. Its expression on these cells is accompanied by expression of CD86 but not CD80, and is associated with disease progression and treatment failure *(26–28)*.

CD38

CD38 is acquired in the terminal differentiation stage of B-cells to plasma cells. There is also high expression of CD38 on malignant plasma cells in multiple myeloma *(29)*. If CD38 were expressed on all malignant cells, it may be possible to select for CD38-negative cells in autologous stem-cell transplantation and markedly reduce or eliminate tumor-cell contamination. However, there is a small population of CD38-negative cells in the myeloma clones *(29)*. These CD38-negative cells may represent less mature malignant cells with a greater capacity for proliferation.

CD56

The neural-cell adhesion molecule (NCAM) CD56 was originally detected on a variety of neural cells, but it is a member of the immunoglobulin superfamily. It is expressed on hematopoietic cells, particularly natural killer (NK) cells, and on the malignant plasma cells in the majority of patients with multiple myeloma *(25)*. Patients with plasma-cell leukemia are also often missing this adhesion molecule, and a subset of patients with myeloma in which CD56 is not or weakly expressed are more likely to develop a leukemic phase and have less osteolytic potential *(30,31)*. These observations suggest that CD56 expression helps to keep the malignant plasma cells in the bone-marrow microenvironment.

In comparison to the findings in multiple myeloma, CD56 is not expressed on the plasma cells from patients with monoclonal gammopathy of undetermined significance (MGUS) *(32)*. In addition, an elevated serum concentration of NCAM may help to differentiate multiple myeloma from MGUS *(33)*.

CD126

Interleukin (IL)-6 is essential for differentiation of normal B-cells into plasma cells, and is an essential survival factor for circulating plasma-cell precursors *(34,35)*. CD126, the IL-6-receptor alpha-chain, has been detected in activated B-cells, and circulating plasma-cell precursors in patients with reactive plasmacytoses *(36)*. In one study, CD126 was not detectable in normal plasma cells, but was expressed in malignant plasma cells in more than 80% of patients with multiple myeloma, plasmacytoma, or MGUS *(37)*. Of interest, in patients with MGUS and plasmacytoma, in whom normal and malignant plasma cells are known to co-exist, CD126 was expressed in neoplastic plasma cells, but not in phenotypically normal plasma cells.

CD138

Recent studies show that syndecan-1 (CD138) is frequently expressed on the surface of malignant cells from myeloma patients *(38,39)*. Syndecans are cell-surface proteoglycans that regulate a variety of cell behaviors by binding to the extracellular matrix and certain growth factors. In myeloma, syndecan-1 is targeted to uropods *(40)*, and seems to participate in the adhesion of the tumor cells to the bone-marrow extracellular matrix *(39)*. Interestingly, syndecan-1 shed from the tumor cells inhibits growth and induces apoptosis of malignant plasma cells, and inhibits osteoclast development *(41)*. A recent report suggests that serum syndecan-1 level may be a prognostic factor for myeloma, and that higher levels are associated with a worse outcome *(42)*.

Cytokines and Myeloma Growth and Bone Resorbing Factors

INTERLEUKIN-6

Interleukin-6 (IL-6) appears to function as an important growth and anti-apoptotic factor for multiple myeloma. This cytokine is produced in large amounts in the bone-marrow microenvironment, and has been reported to function as both an autocrine and paracrine growth factor, although the latter is likely to be more clinically predominant *(43–45)*. The bone-marrow stromal cells that comprise the microenvironment for the malignant plasma cells secrete large quantities of IL-6, and this production is enhanced by the adhesion of myeloma cells to stromal-cell cultures *(46)*. This synergism is evident in vitro, as the initiation of myeloma cell lines often requires the exogenous administration of IL-6 or adherence to bone-marrow stroma co-cultures *(47,48)*. The importance of this cytokine is also evident in vivo, as transgenic mice carrying an activated IL-6 gene develop polyclonal plasmacytosis *(49)*. Furthermore, elevated levels of IL-6 are often noted in patients with multiple myeloma and are associated with poor prognosis *(50,51)*. This cytokine appears to protect plasma cells from undergoing chemotherapy-induced apoptosis *(52–54)*. Finally, patients treated with anti-IL-6 monoclonal antibodies (MAbs) have responded to treatment, although presently this approach has been limited by the development of neutralizing human anti-mouse antibodies *(55,56)*. Clearly, given these findings, IL-6 plays an important role in the pathogenesis and acts as a potential target for the therapy of multiple myeloma.

INTERLEUKIN-1B

Interleukin-1β (IL-1β) is a potent bone-resorption factor, and can be produced by the myeloma cells directly *(57,58)*. By using *in situ* hybridization, IL-1β secretion was found to be increased in within bone-marrow aspirates derived from patients with MGUS, and MM when compared to normal controls *(59,60)*. Patients with lytic bone lesions were more likely to have elevated IL-1β transcripts. This factor can also induce IL-6 stromal-cell production, and thus can serve as a mediator of paracrine-induced myeloma-cell growth *(58)*.

TNF-α

Tumor necrosis factor alpha (TNF-α) has been found to protect myeloma cells from IL-6-deprived apoptosis, and can induce the growth of some myeloma cell lines *(58,61,62)*. TNF-α serum levels are often increased in patients with monoclonal gammopathies, and these levels may be predictive of transformation from MGUS to MM *(63,64)*. Intriguingly, the beneficial drug thalidomide may exert some of its beneficial effect by its inhibition of this cytokine.

VEGF

There is evidence for an increasing role of angiogenesis in the pathogenesis of multiple myeloma *(65,66)*. It is clear that vascular endothelial growth factor (VEGF) is produced by malignant plasma cells, and the receptors that bind this factor are expressed on bone-marrow stromal cells *(67)*. In fact, recent results show that VEGF increases IL-6 production by bone-marrow stromal cells from myeloma patients *(68)*. This may lead indirectly to increased bone loss in these patients. In addition to paracrine and autocrine effects on myeloma cells, VEGF may also play a role in myeloma bone disease. It is now clear that VEGF can replace M-CSF as a cause of early osteoclast development *(69)*.

RANK AND RANKL

Recent studies have also increased our understanding of the role of other specific proteins in the development of myeloma bone disease. A recently identified receptor for activation of nuclear factor (NF)-κB (RANK), a member of the TNF-receptor family, and its ligand, RANKL, have been shown to be key players in the development of osteoclasts *(70)*. Unlike other soluble bone-resorbing factors, the activity of these molecules requires direct cell-to-cell contact. It has been known for some time that osteoclastogenesis requires the direct interaction of osteoblasts or stromal cells with osteoclasts. The identification of RANK expressed on the surface of osteoclasts and RANKL on osteoblasts and stromal cells explains how this direct interaction leads to osteoclast development. TNF itself is capable of stimulating osteoblasts to increase expression of RANKL, although TNF may also stimulate osteoclast differentiation by a mechanism independent of the RANKL-RANK interaction *(71)*. Malignant plasma cells from myeloma patients have been recently shown to express RANKL *(72,73)*, so that it is possible that the tumor cells themselves may directly stimulate osteoclast development in the myeloma bone-marrow environment.

Importantly, a soluble decoy receptor called osteoprotegerin (OPG) exists, which binds RANKL and prevents the binding of the ligand to RANK *(74)*. In fact, animals that lack OPG show profound osteoporosis *(74)*. It is the delicate balance between soluble OPG and RANKL that determines the amount of bone loss. In two separate studies involving murine models, OPG prevented and reversed hypercalcemia of malignancy *(75)* and blocked cancer-induced bone destruction and bone pain without obvious toxicity *(76)*. Because of these promising preclinical results, OPG is now being evaluated in early clinical trials in myeloma and breast-cancer patients with bone metastases. Since myeloma tumor cells express RANKL, it is possible that blockage of the RANKL-RANK interaction may reduce osteoclast stimulation, and may also have inhibitory effects on the tumor cells themselves. Indeed, inhibition of the RANK-RANKL interaction by either RANK-Fc or OPG reduces bone loss in vitro *(77)*. Moreover, two recent studies show that either RANK-Fc or TR-Fc reduces both bone loss and tumor burden in SCID-Hu murine models of myeloma *(78,79)*.

Many of the proteins mentioned here activate the transcription-factor nuclear factor (NF)-κB. This transcription factor is known to bind to promoter regions and increase transcription of genes integral to myeloma pathogenesis, such as IL-6. The DNA-binding activity of NF-κB is determined by its association with a class of inhibitor proteins, known as IκB. When NF-κB is bound to IκB in the cytoplasm, it is rendered inactive. However, following cytokine signaling, degradation of the inhibitor occurs through a series of steps involving phosphorylation, ubiquitination, and proteasome-mediated degradation *(80–84)*. Tumor cells from myeloma patients contain increased activity of NF-κB *(85,86)*, and chemoresistant myeloma is associated with enhanced NF-κB DNA binding *(86)*. Reduction of NF-κB activity with inhibitors of proteasome function such as PS-341 has shown marked anti-myeloma effects in vitro *(86,87)* and in in vivo murine models of human myeloma *(88)*. Thus, this transcription factor represents a new potential target for myeloma treatment.

OTHER MYELOMA GROWTH FACTORS

Insulin-like growth factor (IGF) also appears to have a stimulatory role in myeloma cell growth *(89,90)*. This factor may increase the sensitivity of tumor cells to IL-6 *(91)* and inhibit dexamethasone-induced apoptosis *(92)*. IL-10 *(93)*, hepatocyte growth factor (HGF) *(94)*, granulocyte-macrophage colony-stimulating factor (GM-CSF) *(47,95)*, and, paradoxically, IFN-α have all been found in some in vitro and in vivo studies to stimulate myeloma cell growth. IFN-α can be both inhibitory *(96)* and stimulatory *(65)* in some myeloma-cell line models, which may explain the authors' experience with occasional patients who developed profound tumor-cell growth following its administration post-autologous transplantation.

OTHER MYELOMA BONE-RESORBING FACTORS

Recently, macrophage inflammatory protein-1α (MIP-1α) has been identified as an important factor involved in myeloma bone disease *(97)*. Levels of this cytokine are also elevated in the bone marrow of these patients. This chemokine is capable of inducing osteoclast formation in vitro, and antibodies to this protein block the induction of osteoclast formation by fresh bone-marrow plasma from myeloma patients. The importance of MIP-1α in inducing myeloma bone loss has been reinforced by a recent study showing that an anti-sense construct to this molecule reduces bone loss in severe combined immunodeficiency disease (SCID) mice containing a human myeloma cell line *(98)*. In addition, this chemokine attracts and activates monocytes, and is a potent inhibitor of early hematopoiesis.

M-CSF is present in increased amounts in the serum of myeloma patients and correlates with tumor load *(99,100)*. This cytokine is capable of attracting osteoclast precursors as well as enhancing survival of osteoclasts *(101–103)*. Although this factor along with RANKL are all that is required for osteoclastogenesis to occur in vitro, its role in myeloma bone disease remains unclear.

IL-11 stimulates osteoclastogenesis and inhibits bone formation *(104)*. It has been shown to be produced by osteoblasts, and is present in culture supernatants of bone-marrow cells from myeloma patients *(105)*. This cytokine stimulates RANKL expression through osteoblasts. In addition, recent studies have shown that HGF, which recently has been shown to be produced by malignant plasma cells *(106)*, may also induce IL-11 secretion by osteoblasts *(63)*. HGF is a potent stimulator of bone resorption *(107,108)*. Other cytokines such as IL-1 are capable of potentiating the effect of HGF on IL-11 secretion. High serum levels of HGF are associated with a poor prognosis in myeloma patients *(109)*.

Human Herpesvirus-8 (HHV-8) and Multiple Myeloma

Kaposi's sarcoma-associated herpesvirus, also known as HHV-8, is a member of the gamma herpesvirus family. HHV-8 was recently detected in the majority of bone-marrow stromal-cell cultures from myeloma patients and in a subset of cultures derived from patients with MGUS, yet only rarely in normal individuals *(110)*. *In situ* hybridization demonstrated that the virus was not within the plasma cell, but instead within the supporting dendritic cells in the bone-marrow microenvironment *(111)*. Although some groups have failed to corroborate these findings *(112,113)*, others have found similar evidence of HHV-8 in myeloma patient material *(114–117)*. Whether this viral infection is an epi-phenomenon or is important in myeloma pathogenesis remains uncertain. The recent finding that the strain of HHV-8 present within myeloma patients may be restricted and differ from that found in patients with Kaposi's sarcoma suggests the importance of HHV-8 in these patients' malignancy *(118)*. The observation that patients with active myeloma are more likely to exhibit HHV-8 infection than patients with inactive disease *(119,120)*, also argues against a mere epi-phenomenon.

Early serologic studies have failed to detect HHV-8 expression in myeloma patients *(121)*, but recent studies have successfully identified antibodies against HHV-8 in myeloma patients using a more sensitive technique *(122)*. The difficulty in documenting serologic evidence of HHV-8 in myeloma patients may reflect the relative immunodeficient state typically associated with the disease, or may indicate a specific immune defect preventing the generation of a serologic response to HHV-8. Alternatively, if a myeloma-specific HHV-8 strain exists, as our data suggest, this virus may have a different immunogenic profile compared to the HHV-8 strains commonly found in Kaposi's sarcoma.

Chromosomal and Genetic Abnormalities

Although numerous structural and numerical abnormalities have typically been found in myeloma cells, myeloma-associated cytogenetic abnormalities were not identified until recently. The study of cytogenetic abnormalities in myeloma has been hampered by the low proliferative rate of its malignant cells. Thus, conventional cytogenetics, which require cells in metaphase, were often unrewarding and underestimated the true prevalence of existing genetic abnormalities. The identification of karyotypic abnormalities in myeloma has recently improved significantly with the development of fluorescent *in situ* hybridization (FISH) and spectral karyotypic imaging studies. These techniques are capable of more discretely identifying existing abnormalities within malignant cells, and may allow subclassification of myeloma patients.

Virtually 100% of myeloma patients have chromosomal abnormalities in their plasma cells based on FISH *(123,124)*. FISH studies have demonstrated that 60–75% of myeloma patients have an illegitimate rearrangement involving the immunoglobulin heavy-chain gene at 14q32 *(125,126)*; the partner chromosomes often involve 11q, 4p, 16q, and 6p *(127–131)*. The identified genes include cyclin D and other growth factors (11q) *(132,133)*, the fibroblastic growth-factor receptor 3 (4p) *(129)*, the basic zipper C-MAF transcription factor (16q) *(128)*, and interferon (IFN) regulatory factor 4 (6p) *(130)*. A common mechanism by which these different genes may lead to malignant plasma-cell development has not been identified.

Other frequent chromosomal abnormalities involve loss of chromosome 13 and translocation of 1q *(134–137)*. In one study, 86% of patients with MM had abnormalities of chromosome 13. In addition, cytogenetic studies showed a significantly lower incidence of monosomy 13 in MGUS compared to myeloma and a significantly higher incidence of this deletion in post-MGUS myeloma compared to *de novo* myeloma *(138)*. These observations suggest that this chromosomal alteration may confer a growth or survival advantage to the malignant plasma cell, and may be involved in the transformation of MGUS to myeloma. The minimal region of deletion overlap identified in patients with myeloma is in the 13q14 region *(139)*. In a separate study, increased bone-marrow neovascularization was also significantly correlated with deletion of 13q14, but not with other cytogenetic, clinical, or laboratory parameters, providing a potential rationale for the use of anti-angiogenesis strategies (e.g., thalidomide) in the treatment of patients with high-risk cytogenetics *(140)*.

The loss of chromosome 13 or 11q translocation is associated with a poor prognosis *(134,136,141,142)*. In one report, for example, patients with abnormalities of both chromosomes 11 and 13 had a median overall survival of only 12 mo *(136)*. In a second report of 1000 consecutive patients receiving melphalan-based tandem high-dose therapy, the rate of 5-yr continuous complete remission (CR) was 35% and 0% for patients without and with chromosome 13 abnormalities, respectively ($p < 0.001$) *(142)*. Trisomies of 6, 9, and 17 have been associated with prolonged survival.

Cytogenetic changes have also been observed in patients with MGUS *(143)*. However, chromosomal abnormalities that may indicate a high rate of progression from MGUS to myeloma have not been identified, suggesting that additional events are required for malignant transformation.

In patients with multiple myeloma, other genetic abnormalities have been observed that are usually associated with more advanced disease. Ras mutations occur in a majority of patients *(144)*, and may be associated with more aggressive disease and a poor clinical outcome. In one series, for example, mutations in N-ras or K-ras were associated with a significantly lower survival than wild-type ras genes (2.1 vs 4 yr, $p = 0.01$) *(145)*. Abnormalities in the *p53* and retinoblastoma tumor-suppressor genes occur more frequently in patients with plasma-cell leukemia or more aggressive disease *(146)*. In addition to cyclin D overexpression in patients with 11q translocations, progression through the cell cycle can also result from loss of function of the cyclin D kinase inhibitors. Loss of some of these genes (*p15*, *p16*, and *p18*) occurs in occasional patients with multiple myeloma. However, methylation of these genes in malignant plasma cells may be more common and lead to loss of expression *(147,148)*, resulting in enhanced cyclin D activity. Fas (CD95) can induce apoptosis when bound to Fas ligand (FasL) *(149)*. Point mutations in Fas occur in some patients with multiple myeloma, and are associated with a lack of expression *(150)*. The role of these changes in the development or maintenance of myeloma remains unclear.

Angiogenesis

Although the importance of angiogenesis in solid tumors is well-established, its role in hematopoietic malignancies such as myeloma is just under exploration. Recent studies report a significant increase in bone-marrow microvessel density in patients with active myeloma compared to patients with inactive myeloma, MGUS patients, and normal subjects *(151–153)*. A recent abstract reported that a low level of angiogenesis is a major, favorable prognostic variable for event-free survival (EFS) as well as overall survival on multivariate analysis in myeloma patients *(154)*. The increased angiogenesis found in myeloma persists after autologous peripheral stem-cell transplantation, even in patients who achieve a complete response *(155)*, and this change may contribute to post-transplant relapse. Potential angiogenic factors mediating this increase in angio-genesis include basic fibroblast growth factor (BFGF) *(151)* in addition to vascular endothelial growth factor *(152)*.

TREATMENT
Therapy for Initial Disease

Patients with symptomatic myeloma should be treated as soon as the diagnosis is established. Because myeloma is an incurable disease with standard chemo-therapy except in rare cases *(156)*, this treatment is generally given for palliative purposes only. Despite the rarity of cure, however, responses to chemotherapy are high (50%–75%), and older studies show that treated patients have median survival times of 24–40 mo compared to less than 12 mo for untreated patients. Patients with asymptomatic and indolent disease do not require immediate therapy, since there is no difference in survival in patients treated at diagnosis vs those treated at time of disease progression *(157)*.

Many oncologists consider the combination of oral melphalan and prednisone (MP) optimal therapy, especially for the elderly and for patients with minimal disease. Response rates are usually around 40%, but very few patients achieve CR with this form of therapy.

Corticosteroids are the most important drug class in the treatment of myeloma. These agents directly induce the apoptotic death of myeloma cells. In addition, these drugs suppress production of growth-promoting and anti-apoptotic cytokines, and block their effects on myeloma cells. Monotherapy with high-dose steroids produces clinical response rates and progression and overall survival similar to more aggressive combination chemotherapy regimens *(158)*. An additional advantage of steroids without melphalan is the lack of bone-marrow toxicity with this form of therapy.

Several attempts have been made to improve the response rate and the overall survival benefit observed with MP therapy. The addition of vincristine, cyclophosphamide, and BCNU improves response rates *(159)* but has not changed overall survival, as confirmed in a recently published ECOG trial *(160)*.

The VAD protocol *(161)* was based on the original observation of Alexanian *(162)* that significant responses in refractory patients could be achieved with frequent pulses of high-dose prednisone. VAD employs doses of dexamethasone (40 mg/d × 4 d beginning on d 1, 9, and 17 of each 28- to 35-d cycle), which are the equivalent of a sixfold increase in prednisone, as initially used by Alexanian. In addition, continuous infusions of vincristine (0.4 mg/d × 4 d) and doxorubicin (9 mg/m^2/d × 4 d) are administered through an indwelling venous catheter, with the rationale that the slowly cycling tumor cells of myeloma are more likely to be injured by constant exposure to these agents. In the initial report *(161)*, 73% of relapsing and 43% of previously unresponsive patients responded to VAD. Responses were seen rapidly, usually within the first two cycles of therapy. Some patients may have been preselected for good prognosis, as evidenced by a low tumor burden (28% were stage I), and the fact that one-half the previously unresponsive patients who subsequently responded to VAD had demonstrated a stable tumor mass on initial chemotherapy. Nevertheless, the magnitude and frequency of the responses are impressive. With documented responses, the patients demonstrated clinical benefit with increased hemoglobin levels and performance status, and decreased bone pain and hypercalcemia. The major side effect was infection, documented in eight of 29 patients and causing unexplained fever in three others.

Several studies from other institutions confirm the promising results of the VAD protocol *(163,164)*. Response rates were similar to the initial report and toxicity was just as severe, with a 20–30% incidence of serious infection and occasional cases of steroid-induced psychosis or gastrointestinal toxicity. Some investigators administered prophylactic cimetidine and trimethoprim/sulfa during VAD therapy. Patients receiving VAD who develop steroid-induced psychosis may improve if the decadron is changed to prednisone 100 mg every other day *(165)*.

Used as initial therapy, VAD (infusional vincristine and doxorubicin with oral dexamethasone) produces faster and higher response rates than either dexamethasone or melphalan with prednisone, but has not been shown to improve overall survival. This regimen has the advantage that it does not produce permanent damage to stem cells, making it an ideal induction regimen for patients undergoing stem-cell collection in preparation for autologous transplantation.

Unfortunately, a recent meta-analysis examining 27 trials that randomized over 6500 patients with myeloma between combination chemotherapy and MP failed to demonstrate a significant survival advantage between the groups *(166)*.

Because IFN as a single agent has some activity and a different mechanism of anti-myeloma action than either chemotherapy or corticosteroids, natural IFN has been combined with MP *(167)* in a randomized study of stage II and III patients to assess response rate and overall survival. Although response rates were higher (68% vs 42%), especially in patients with IgA myeloma (85%), the addition of 7×10^6 IU/m^2/d of natural interferon-α (IFN-α); given d 1–5 and 22–26 of a 42-d cycle) did not increase overall survival. Two other randomized studies showed no benefit of adding IFN-α to MP with respect to response rates or survival *(168,169)*. One more recent study demonstrated improved progression-free (23 vs 16 mo) and overall survival times (39 vs 30 mo) for patients randomized to receive IFN-α in addition to VMCP, but these differences were not statistically significant *(170)*. In summary, IFN-α may improve response rates for patients with multiple myeloma, but at considerable expense and morbidity that does not translate into a meaningful prolongation in survival. Therefore, its use cannot be recommended in the initial management of most multiple myeloma patients.

High-Dose Chemotherapy

Because myeloma is sensitive to cytotoxic agents in most patients, dose-intensive chemotherapy with marrow transplantation has been evaluated in an attempt to induce complete remission and to improve disease-free survival. Initial trials focused on the use of allogeneic bone-marrow transplantation (Allo-BMT) in myeloma. This was only a viable option for myeloma patients less than 55 yr of age who had an HLA-identical sibling. As myeloma is a disease of the elderly, less than 5% of all patients are eligible for this procedure. Unfortunately, allogeneic transplantation was associated with a 40–50% treatment-related mortality (TRM) *(171,172)* although recent studies from the European Bone Marrow Transplant Registry suggest that the TRM has been reduced by nearly half *(173)*. This procedure has been shown to eliminate minimal residual disease in the bone marrow in some patients, whereas this was rarely observed following autologous transplantation *(174)*.

Another approach that can improve upon TRM and take advantage of a possible graft-vs-myeloma effect is the use of non-myeloablative chemotherapeutic regimens with allogeneic donor leukocytes *(175,176)*. Lokhorst and colleagues have shown this technique to be effective, even for patients who have relapsed after conventional allogeneic transplantation *(177)*. This procedure may become more acceptable, especially in light of its potential for achieving long-term survival with reduced toxicity.

For the few patients with an available identical twin, syngeneic transplantation in multiple myeloma appears to be the treatment of choice. Syngeneic transplantation was recently shown to confer a significantly better median overall survival time in myeloma patients as compared to matching myeloma patients who receive autologous or allogeneic transplants *(178)*. Progression-free survival time was also prolonged, and was comparable to that obtained for myeloma patients following allogeneic transplantation who survive the initial treatment.

Myeloablative chemotherapy with autologous transplantation is now widely performed for patients with myeloma, and has become part of the standard of care for those patients with advanced disease who are less than 65 yr of age. Several clinical trials have demonstrated the benefit of autologous transplantation in multiple myeloma *(179–182)*. A large phase III study was initiated in France comparing standard doses of chemotherapy to autologous transplantation *(183,184)*. Two hundred patients with stage II or stage III multiple myeloma received an initial 4 mo of VMCP alternating with VBAP. Patients were then randomized to receive an additional 8 mo of chemotherapy or 140 mg/m2 of melphalan + TBI followed by autologous bone-marrow transplantation. The study was analyzed on an intent-to-treat analysis, although only 74 of the 100 patients assigned to high-dose therapy actually received the autologous bone-marrow transplant. As may be expected, response rates were higher for the more aggressive approach (complete reimission [CR] = 22% vs 5%, partial remission [PR] + CR = 81% vs 57%, respectively). EFS was also prolonged in the patients randomized to transplantation (median EFS = 27 mo vs 18 mo). More intriguingly, overall survival was improved for these patients as well. Five-yr survival was only 12% for those patients who received standard chemotherapy, yet was 57% for those patients who were randomized to autologous transplantation. This difference was statistically significant, and was most pronounced in the subgroup of patients less than 60 yr of age. A more recent update of this study continues to demonstrate a doubling of overall survival after 5 yr. Despite this survival advantage, the majority of patients continue to relapse within 4 yr, with median survival times varying from 36–65 mo *(185-190)*.

Interestingly, it appears that the benefits of autologous transplantation are similar in patients undergoing this procedure at presentation (following some initial conventional chemotherapy) or at the time of first relapse *(191)*. However, although overall survival was similar between both groups, the quality of life was judged to be better for those patients who received early high-dose chemotherapy, probably because of the additional chemotherapy needed to re-attain remission following progressive disease. Elderly patients may also benefit from this more aggressive approach, but they tend to have slightly higher treatment-related mortality and more prolonged recovery times that may adversely impact their quality of life *(182,192)*.

Bone marrow was used as the hematologic support in early transplant studies but is rarely used today. Peripheral-blood progenitor cells are advantageous, because when used they offer patients a shorter duration of neutropenia and hospitalization, eliminate the need for an operating room for bone-marrow harvesting, and receive a reduced load of reinfused tumor cells following cytoreductive chemotherapy *(193–197)*. Our group compared multiple myeloma tumor burden in peripheral-blood progenitor cell (PBPC) and backup bone-marrow harvests from patients undergoing autologous transplantation. In almost every case, tumor burden was less in the PBPC product, translating into a median 14-fold reduction in contaminating tumor cells *(198)*.

In an attempt to improve upon these results, attempts have been made to eliminate contaminating tumor cells from the reinfused autograft products. We have previously demonstrated that the stem-cell antigen CD34 is not expressed by the malignant cells in patients with multiple myeloma *(199)*. Consequently, a phase III study was initiated comparing CD34-selected autografts to unmanipulated PBPC autografts for patients with multiple myeloma *(200)*. The CD34 selection procedure was safe, with equivalent neutrophil (median 12 d) and only a 2-d delay in platelet engraftment (median 11 vs 9 d). Infections were also comparable between the groups. In order to quantify tumor burden in the autografts, PCR amplification was performed with oligonucleotide primers derived from each patient's expressed Ig gene. The purging procedure resulted in a median 3.1 log reduction in autograft tumor burden; and, the majority of autografts were rendered tumor-free. Nevertheless, no improvement in progression-free or overall survival occurred in patients who received the purged autograft product *(201)*. Consequently, the study demonstrates that the re-infusion of malignant cells is not the main contributor to disease relapse in patients following autologous transplantation *(202)*.

Maintenance Therapy

Studies have shown that continued chemotherapy in patients who have achieved a stable remission offers no advantage in terms of duration of remission or survival. Subcutaneous IFN has been evaluated as maintenance therapy since the early 1990s *(203–208)*. Although there was initial enthusiasm for its efficacy based on an Italian study *(209)*, several recent randomized studies have shown at best only a modest increase in remission duration with no effect on overall survival *(210–214)*.

Two recent studies suggested that the combination of IFN and corticosteroids was effective as maintenance therapy *(215,216)*. However, it was unclear whether the benefit may be achieved with corticosteroids alone. In fact, a recently completed SWOG study showed that maintenance therapy with 50 mg of prednisone every other day following a >25% reduction to induction VAD-type chemotherapy improves progression-free survival as well as median overall survival time compared to patients receiving a physiologic dose (10 mg every other day) *(217)*. The treatment was well-tolerated, with no significant toxicity. This study suggests that patients who respond to induction chemotherapy should be treated with prednisone maintenance therapy to prolong the duration of remission and improved survival. Whether a similar benefit of prednisone maintenance therapy occurs following high-dose therapy remains unknown.

Therapy for Refractory Myeloma

Patients who relapse during therapy or within 6 mo of stopping maintenance, as well as primary resistant patients, have a very poor prognosis. Those with no evidence of progressive disease should be watched closely without therapy. Symptomatic patients may benefit from salvage therapy. Chemotherapy options for patients who are resistant to initial therapy or with relapsing disease are limited, but include: high-dose cyclophosphamide (3 g/m^2) and etoposide (900 mg/m^2) followed by GM-CSF *(218)*, EDAP *(219)*, or high-dose melphalan *(220)*.

Recently, Dr. Barlogie and his colleagues at the University of Arkansas conducted a phase II trial using single-agent thalidomide, and 32% of the patients achieved a response *(221)*. The drug was started at 200 mg/d and escalated every 2 wk to a maximum of 800 mg/d. A recent update of the initial report including 169 patients showed a 37% response rate *(222)*. Side effects were common, and consisted of sedation, constipation, and neuropathy. In addition to these side effects, recent studies show that a high rate of patients who received this drug developed thrombotic events, especially deep venous thrombosis *(223)*. Since this seminal publication, thalidomide has become a widely used agent in the treatment of multiple myeloma. In addition to thalidomide's anti-angiogenic effects that prompted its use in myeloma patients initially, the drug also suppresses TNF *(224)*. IL-12 *(225)* alters the expression of other cytokines as well. It has also been recently shown to augment NK cell cytotoxicity *(226)*, and markedly inhibit NF-κB activity by preventing phosphorylation of IκB *(227)*. It remains unclear which of these actions is most important in producing its anti-tumor effects in myeloma patients.

Smaller doses of thalidomide have been useful in patients, and we and others have found doses as low as 50 mg per d to be effective *(228)*. In our own experience, the combination of steroids and thalidomide seems particularly active. This has also been also shown by the MD Anderson group *(229)*. In fact, this combination has recently been evaluated as initial therapy in a small group of patients, and found to be highly effective with response rates in more than 75% of patients *(230)*. Unfortunately, the dose, schedule, and duration of thalidomide have not been clearly defined, but it is an effective agent for some myeloma patients. Newer anti-angiogenesis agents have been recently developed that will hopefully improve the activity and lessen some of the side effects associated with this medication. These drugs are currently in early phase I and II trials.

Inhibition of NF-κB activity with the proteasome inhibitor PS-341 produces anti-tumor effects in vitro and in vivo. Initial results from an ongoing multicenter phase II study have shown impressive responses in patients with highly resistant multiple myeloma *(231)*. However, the duration of these responses and the overall survival of these patients remain unknown. Interestingly, recent laboratory studies show that the concentration of chemotherapy required to produce cytotoxicity of chemoresistant myeloma cells in vitro can be reduced by 100,000–1,000,000-fold with the addition of noncytotoxic concentrations of PS-341 *(232)*. These effects are not observed on normal peripheral blood or bone-marrow stem cells.

Arsenic trioxide has shown to be cytotoxic to myeloma cells in vitro *(233,234)*, and emerging data indicate that this drug has anti-tumor activity for patients as well *(235)*. It is clear that arsenic trioxide can sensitize highly chemoresistant myeloma cell lines to chemotherapy at very low doses similar to PS-341 *(233)*. In fact, this drug inhibits NF-κB activity in myeloma cells *(233)*, and this may explain its anti-myeloma effects.

Bone Disease

At diagnosis, 60% of patients have lytic bone lesions, and another 20% have osteoporosis, pathologic fractures, or both *(236)*. Indeed, the major clinical manifestation of this malignancy is related to osteolytic bone destruction *(236,237)*. These patients often experience fractures, spinal-cord compression, bone pain, and hypercalcemia. Importantly, even patients who respond to chemotherapy may have progression of their skeletal disease *(238,239)*, and once the lytic bone lesion develops, recalcification and radiologic improvement are rare.

Many patients require radiotherapy and surgery to treat impending or actual fractures, or spinal-cord compression. Although radiotherapy may be effective, it should be used sparingly, because the irradiation of large areas of hematopoietically active bone marrow can make future chemotherapy intolerable or high-dose chemotherapy impossible.

Since complications related to bone disease are such an important part of the myeloma patient's life, efforts have been made to prevent these problems. Early randomized studies evaluating fluoride and calcium supplementation showed no clear benefit for these treatments *(240,241)*.

The bisphosphonates make up a new class of drugs that inhibit osteoclast function. Several pilot studies showed effective blocking of bone resorption in patients with myeloma, as evidenced by decreased bone pain, decreased serum calcium, and decreased calcium and hydroxypyroline excretion *(242,243)*. The initial studies completed in multiple myeloma used relatively weak agents such as etidronate and clodronate. In the Canadian study involving etidronate, 166 patients were randomized to etidronate (5 mg/kg) or placebo in addition to primary chemotherapy with melphalan and prednisone *(238)*. No significant difference in clinically meaningful events such as new fractures, hypercalcemic episodes, and bone pain were noted between the two arms.

Three large randomized trials have been published using oral clodronate in myeloma patients. In the Finnish trial, 336 newly diagnosed and previously untreated patients were randomized to receive either clodronate (2.4 g) or placebo daily for 2 yr *(244)*. All patients were also treated with intermittent oral melphalan and prednisolone. Patients treated with clodronate were less likely to have progression of lytic bone lesions (12%) compared to the placebo group (24%) ($p = 0.026$). However, the development of pathological fractures, hypercalcemia, analgesic use, and pain index scores did not differ significantly between the two arms.

Recently, the Medical Research Council published their results of a large randomized trial involving 549 patients with recently diagnosed myeloma *(247)*. Patients received either 1.6 g/d of oral clodronate or placebo in addition to alkylator-based chemotherapy. Treated patients developed less hypercalcemia and non-vertebral fractures ($p = 0.021$). Back pain and poor performance status were not significantly different between the two groups, except at one time point (24 mo), and the proportion of patients requiring radiotherapy was similar between the two arms. Overall, these three studies suggest that oral clodronate has a mild to modestly beneficial effect on bone pain and fracture development in multiple myeloma. Although there are advantages to oral administration, the poor and variable absorption (~1%), high cost, and gastrointestinal side effects make the clinical benefit marginal for these patients.

Pamidronate is 100-fold and 10-fold more potent in preventing bone resorption in vitro when compared with etidronate and clodronate, respectively. In multiple myeloma patients, results of open-label trials lasting up to 24 mo suggested that pamidronate disodium may be effective in reducing skeletal complications. Thus, a randomized, double-blind study was conducted to determine whether monthly 90-mg infusions of pamidronate compared to placebo reduced skeletal events in patients with Durie-Salmon stage III multiple myeloma with at least one lytic lesion who were receiving chemotherapy *(246)*. After the pre-planned initial time point of 9 mo, the proportion of myeloma patients with a skeletal event was 41% in patients receiving placebo, but only 24% in pamidronate-treated patients ($p < 0.001$). The patients randomized to receive pamidronate also had significant decreases in bone pain, and, in contrast to patients receiving the placebo, showed no deterioration in performance status or quality of life at the end of 9 mo. These benefits continued for the remaining 12 mo of the study. Although overall survival was not significantly different between the two treatment groups, the median survival time for the patients with more advanced disease (patients who had failed first-line chemotherapy) was 21 mo if they received pamidronate vs 14 mo for those on the placebo arm ($p = 0.04$) *(247)*.

All of the bisphosphonates are poorly absorbed orally (usually <1%). Similar to results with other oral bisphosphonates, (oral pamidronate (300 mg/d) does not have a beneficial effect on skeletal complications in myeloma patients *(248)*.

These drugs bind strongly to hydroxyapatite in bones and concentrate in areas where active bone remodeling occurs *(249)*. Once the drug becomes a part of the bone that is not remodeling, it is biologically inactive. As a result, continued administration of bisphosphonates is necessary to achieve the desired lasting inhibition of bone resorption, and we generally continue to administer these drugs to patients with multiple myeloma throughout their life. Bisphosphonates are actively excreted by the kidneys and can cause renal insufficiency. This process appears to be related to the dose and rate of infusion, and the newer more potent generation of agents are less likely to cause this toxicity because of the lower dosages required to achieve desirable clinical effects. Nevertheless, recently published results prove the safety of infusing pamidronate monthly to patients with severe renal impairment *(250)*.

Although when properly administered, renal dysfunction from intravenously administered pamidronate is very rare, recent studies have shown the potential for nephrotoxicity among patients who receive the drug at higher doses (>90 mg) *(251)*, infused too rapidly (in ≤2 h), or more frequently than every 3–4 wk. These patients initially develop albuminuria, and eventually may develop irreversible renal dysfunction. It is important to recognize that the presence of increasing proteinuria among myeloma patients who receive pamidronate is not necessarily indicative of progressive disease, and electrophoresis must be performed to determine the source of the urinary protein (Bence Jones protein or albumin).

Two more potent bisphosphonates have recently completed evaluation as part of larger randomized clinical trials and have been published in abstract form. In a randomized phase III trial, 198 MM patients who received monthly bolus injections of 2 mg of ibandronate did not have fewer skeletal events compared to patients who received a placebo. This poor result may be attributed to an inadequate study drug dose. Zoledronic acid appears to be the most potent bisphosphonate developed to date. It is at least 100 × as potent as pamidronate in mouse models, and was more effective at controlling hypercalcemia when compared to pamidronate in a recently published study *(252)*. The drug has been recently FDA-approved based on the results of the hypercalcemia study. In saddition, the drug has also been evaluated in the setting of bone metastases, including patients with multiple myeloma *(253,254)*. Two recently published randomized studies comparing pamidronate at a dose of 90 mg infused over 2 h compared to zoledronic acid infused over 15 min show that the newer bisphosphonate is as effective as pamidronate at preventing skeletal complications, but can be infused much more rapidly *(255,256)*. This drug has recently been FDA-approved for use in myeloma patients with lytic lesions. Whether higher doses of zoledronic acid can be shown to be more effective and safe will be evaluated in future clinical trials.

Recent in vitro studies demonstrate that the bisphosphonates may possess direct antitumor properties. These drugs particularly the more potent nitrogen-containing compounds can induce apoptosis of myeloma cells *(257)* and suppress the production of IL-6, an important myeloma growth factor, by bone-marrow stromal cells from myeloma patients *(258)*. In addition, the nitrogen-containing drugs have been recently shown to stimulate γδT-lymphocytes in order to produce anti-plasma-cell effects on tumor cells from myeloma patients in vitro *(259)*. The potential anti-myeloma effects of bisphosphonates may explain the prolonged survival seen in those salvage patients treated with intravenous (iv) monthly pamidronate in the randomized study.

Because of the promising preclinical results with OPG, an inhibitor of RANK signaling, a recent phase I study was conducted for patients with multiple myeloma metastatic to bone *(260)*. As a single dose, OPG effectively decreased bone resorption markers, although the effects of repetitive dosing are unknown at this time.

CONCLUSION

There have been major advances in our knowledge of the pathophysiology underlying multiple myeloma. For the first time, these new findings are having a clinical impact. Many new anti-myeloma drugs are now entering clinical trials for myeloma patients based on the promise from the laboratory, with early encouraging results. In addition, recent advances in our understanding of myeloma bone disease have led to new treatments with the potential to reduce the bony complications and treat the underlying disease as well.

REFERENCES

1. Vescio RA and Berenson JR. Myeloma, macroglobulinemia and amyloidosis. In: Haskell, CM, ed. *Cancer Treatment*, 5th ed., WB Saunders Company, Philadelphia, PA, pp. 1503–1539.
2. Billadeau D, Ahmann G, Greipp P, et al. The bone marrow of multiple myeloma patients contains B cell populations at different stages of differentiation that are clonally related to the malignant plasma cell. *J Exp Med* 1993; 178:1023.
3. Corradini P, Boccadoro M, Voena C, et al. Evidence for a bone marrow B cell transcribing malignant plasma cell VDJ joined to C mu sequence in immunoglobulin (IgG)- and IgA-secreting multiple myelomas. *J Exp Med* 1993; 178:1091.
4. Bakkus MH, Heirman C, Van Riet I, et al. Evidence that multiple myeloma Ig heavy chain VDJ genes contain somatic mutations but show no intraclonal variation. *Blood* 1992; 80:2326.
5. Vescio RA, Cao J, Hong CH, et al. Myeloma Ig heavy chain V region sequences reveal prior antigenic selection and marked somatic mutation but no intraclonal diversity. *J Immunol* 1995; 155:2487.
6. Pilarski LM, Jensen GS. Monoclonal circulating B cells in multiple myeloma: a continuously differentiating, possibly invasive, population as defined by expression of CD45 isoforms and adhesion molecules. *Hematol Oncol Clin N Am* 1992; 6:297.

7. Tricot G. New insights into role of microenvironment in multiple myeloma. *Lancet* 2000; 355:248.

8. Rettig MB, Vescio RA, Cao J, et al. VH gene usage is multiple myeloma: complete absence of the VH4.21 (VH4-34) gene. *Blood* 1996; 87:2846.

9. Hsu FJ, Levy R. Preferential use of the VH4 Ig gene family by diffuse large-cell lymphoma. *Blood* 1995; 86:3072.

10. Vescio RA, Hong CH, Cao J, et al. The hematopoietic stem cell antigen, CD34, is not expressed on the malignant cells in multiple myeloma. *Blood* 1994; 84:3283.

11. Szczepek AJ, Bergsagel PL, Axelsson L, et al. CD34+ cells in the blood of patients with multiple myeloma express CD19 and IgH mRNA and have patient-specific IgH VDJ gene rearrangements. *Blood* 1997; 89:1824.

12. Schiller G, Vescio R, Freytes C, et al. Transplantation of CD34+ peripheral blood progenitor cells after high-dose chemotherapy for patients with advanced multiple myeloma. *Blood* 1995; 86:390.

13. Vescio R, Schiller G, Stewart AK, et al. Multicenter phase III trial to evaluate CD34(+) selected versus unselected autologous peripheral blood progenitor cell transplantation in multiple myeloma. *Blood* 1999; 93:1858.

14. Lemoli RM, Martinelli G, Zamagni E, et al. Engraftment, clinical, and molecular follow-up of patients with multiple myeloma who were reinfused with highly purified CD34+ cells to support single or tandem high-dose chemotherapy. *Blood* 2000; 95:2234.

15. Cao J, Vescio RA, Rettig MB, et al. A CD10-positive subset of malignant cells is identified in multiple myeloma using PCR with patient-specific immunoglobulin gene primers. *Leukemia* 1995; 9:1948.

16. Ruiz-Arguelles GJ, Katzmann JA, Greipp PR, et al. Multiple myeloma: circulating lymphocytes that express plasma cell antigens. *Blood* 1984; 64:352.

17. Harada H, Kawano MM, Huang N, et al. Phenotypic difference of normal plasma cells from mature myeloma cells. *Blood* 1993; 81:2658.

18. Rawstron AC, Davies FE, Owen RG, et al. B-lymphocyte suppression in multiple myeloma is a reversible phenomenon specific to normal B-cell progenitors and plasma cell precursors. *Br J Haematol* 1998; 100:176.

19. Bergsagel PL, Smith AM, Szczepek A, et al. In multiple myeloma, clonotypic B lymphocytes are detectable among CD19+ peripheral blood cells expressing CD38, CD56, and monotypic Ig light chain [published erratum appears in *Blood* 1995 Jun 1;85(11):3365]. *Blood* 1995;85:436.

20. Rawstron AC, Owen RG, Davies FE, et al. Circulating plasma cells in multiple myeloma: characterization and correlation with disease stage. *Br J Haematol* 1997; 97:46.

21. Luque R, Brieva JA, Moreno A, et al. Normal and clonal B lineage cells can be distinguished by their differential expression of B cell antigens and adhesion molecules in peripheral blood from multiple myeloma (MM) patients—diagnostic and clinical implications. *Clin Exp Immunol* 1998; 112:410.

22. Zandecki M, Bernardi F, Genevieve F, et al. Involvement of peripheral blood cells in multiple myeloma: chromosome changes are the rule within circulating plasma cells but not within B lymphocytes. *Leukemia* 1997; 11:1034.

23. Mahmoud MS, Fujii R, Ishikawa H, Kawano MM. Enforced CD19 expression leads to growth inhibition and reduced tumorigenicity. *Blood* 1999; 94:3551.

24. Kay NE, Leong TL, Bone N, et al. Blood levels of immune cells predict survival in myeloma patients: results of an Eastern Cooperative Oncology Group phase 3 trial for newly diagnosed multiple myeloma patients. *Blood* 2001; 98:23.

25. Pellat-Deceunynck C, Bataille R, Robillard N, et al. Expression of CD28 and CD40 in human myeloma cells: a comparative study with normal plasma cells. *Blood* 1994; 84:2597.

26. Robillard N, Jego G, Pellat-Deceunynck C, et al. CD28, a marker associated with tumoral expansion in multiple myeloma. *Clin Cancer Res* 1998; 4:1521.

27. Pope B, Brown RD, Gibson J, et al. B7-2-positive myeloma: incidence, clinical characteristics, prognostic significance, and implications for tumor immunotherapy. *Blood* 2000; 96:1274.

28. Shapiro VS, Mollenauer MN, Weiss A. Endogenous CD28 expressed on myeloma cells up-regulates interleukin-8 production: implications for multiple myeloma progression. *Blood* 2001; 98:187.

29. Berenson JR, Vescio RA, Hong CH, et al. Multiple myeloma clones are derived from a cell late in B lymphoid development. *Curr Top Microbiol Immunol* 1995; 194:25.

30. Pellat-Deceunynck C, Barille S, Jego G, et al. The absence of CD56 (NCAM) on malignant plasma cells is a hallmark of plasma cell leukemia and of a special subset of multiple myeloma. *Leukemia* 1998; 12:1977.

31. Rawstron A, Barrans S, Blythe D, et al. Distribution of myeloma plasma cells in peripheral blood and bone marrow correlates with CD56 expression. *Br J Haematol* 1999; 104:138.

32. Sonneveld P, Durie BG, Lokhorst HM, et al. Analysis of multidrug-resistance (MDR-1) glycoprotein and CD56 expression to separate monoclonal gammapathy from multiple myeloma. *Br J Haematol* 1993; 83:63.

33. Ong F, Kaiser U, Seelen PJ, et al. Serum neural cell adhesion molecule differentiates multiple myeloma from paraproteinemias due to other causes. *Blood* 1996; 87:712.

34. Hirano T, Yasukawa K, Harada H, et al. Complementary DNA for a novel human interleukin (BSF-2) that induces B lymphocytes to produce immunoglobulin. *Nature* 1986; 324:73.

35. Kawano MM, Mihara K, Huang N, et al. Differentiation of early plasma cells on bone marrow stromal cells requires interleukin-6 for escaping from apoptosis. *Blood* 1995; 85:487.

36. Jego G, Robillard N, Puthier D, et al. Reactive plasmacytoses are expansions of plasmablasts retaining the capacity to differentiate into plasma cells. *Blood* 1999; 94:701.

37. Rawstron AC, Fenton JA, Ashcroft J, et al. The interleukin-6 receptor alpha-chain (CD126) is expressed by neoplastic but not normal plasma cells. *Blood* 2000; 96:3880.

38. Wijdenes J, Vooijs WC, Clement C, et al. A plasmocyte selective monoclonal antibody (B-B4) recognizes syndecan-1. *Br J Haematol* 1996; 94:318–323;

39. Ridley RC, Xiao H, Hata H, et al. Expression of syndecan regulates human myeloma plasma cell adhesion to type I collagen. *Blood* 1993; 81:767–774.

40. Borset M, Hjertner O, Yaccoby S, et al. Syndecan-1 is targeted to the uropods of polarized myeloma cells where it promotes adhesion and sequesters heparin-binding proteins. *Blood* 2000; 96:2528–2536.

41. Dhodapkar MV, Abe E, Theus E, et al. Syndecan-1 is a multifunctional regulator of myeloma pathobiology: control of tumor cell survival, growth, and bone cell differentiation. *Blood* 1998; 91:2679–2688.

42. Seidel C, Sundan A, Hjorth M, et al. Serum syndecan-1: a new independent prognostic marker in multiple myeloma. *Blood* 2000; 95:388–392.

43. Kawano M, Hirano T, Matsuda T, et al. Autocrine generation and requirement of BSF-2/IL-6 for human multiple myelomas. *Nature* 1988; 332:83–85.

44. Klein B, Zhang XG, Jourdan M, et al. Paracrine rather than autocrine regulation of myeloma-cell growth and differentiation by interleukin-6. *Blood* 1989; 73:517–526.

45. Klein B, Zhang XG, Lu ZY, et al. Interleukin-6 in human multiple myeloma. *Blood* 1995; 85:863–872.

46. Uchiyama H, Barut BA, Mohrbacher AF, et al. Adhesion of human myeloma-derived cell lines to bone marrow stromal cells stimulates interleukin-6 secretion. *Blood* 1993; 82: 3712–3720.

47. Zhang XG, Bataille R, Jourdan M, et al. Granulocyte-macrophage colony-stimulating factor synergizes with interleukin-6 in supporting the proliferation of human myeloma cells. *Blood* 1990; 76:2599–2605.

48. Jernberg H, Pettersson M, Kishimoto T, Nilsson K. Heterogeneity in response to interleukin 6 (IL-6), expression of IL-6 and IL-6 receptor mRNA in a panel of established human multiple myeloma cell lines [published erratum appears in *Leukemia* 1991 Jun;5(6):following 530]. *Leukemia* 1991; 5:255–265.

49. Suematsu S, Matsuda T, Aozasa K, et al. IgG1 plasmacytosis in interleukin 6 transgenic mice. *Proc Natl Acad Sci USA* 1989; 86:7547–7551.

50. Bataille R, Jourdan M, Zhang XG, et al. Serum levels of interleukin 6, a potent myeloma cell growth factor, as a reflect of disease severity in plasma cell dyscrasias. *J Clin Invest* 1989; 84:2008–2011.

51. Ludwig H, Nachbaur DM, Fritz E, et al. Interleukin-6 is a prognostic factor in multiple myeloma. *Blood* 1991; 77:2794–2795.

52. Lichtenstein A, Tu Y, Fady C, et al. Interleukin-6 inhibits apoptosis of malignant plasma cells. *Cell Immunol* 1995; 162:248–255.

53. Xu FH, Sharma S, Gardner A, et al. Interleukin-6-induced inhibition of multiple myeloma cell apoptosis: support for the hypothesis that protection is mediated via inhibition of the JNK/SAPK pathway. *Blood* 1998; 92:241–251.

54. Chauhan D, Pandey P, Ogata A, et al. Dexamethasone induces apoptosis of multiple myeloma cells in a JNK/SAP kinase independent mechanism. *Oncogene* 1997; 15:837–843.

55. Klein B, Wijdenes J, Zhang XG, et al. Murine anti-interleukin-6 monoclonal antibody therapy for a patient with plasma cell leukemia. *Blood* 1991; 78:1198–1204.

56. Bataille R, Barlogie B, Lu ZY, et al. Biologic effects of anti-interleukin-6 murine monoclonal antibody in advanced multiple myeloma. *Blood* 1995; 86:685–691.

57. Cozzolino F, Torcia M, Aldinucci D, et al. Production of interleukin-1 by bone marrow myeloma cells. *Blood* 1989; 74:380–387.

58. Carter A, Merchav S, Silvian-Draxler I, et al. The role of interleukin-1 and tumour necrosis factor-alpha in human multiple myeloma. *Br J Haematol* 1990; 74:424–431.

59. Donovan KA, Lacy MQ, Kline MP, et al. Contrast in cytokine expression between patients with monoclonal gammopathy of undetermined significance or multiple myeloma. *Leukemia* 1998; 12:593–600.

60. Lacy MQ, Donovan KA, Heimbach JK, et al. Comparison of interleukin-1 beta expression by in situ hybridization in monoclonal gammopathy of undetermined significance and multiple myeloma. *Blood* 1999; 93:300–305.

61. Jourdan M, Tarte K, Legouffe E, et al. Tumor necrosis factor is a survival and proliferation factor for human myeloma cells. *Eur Cytokine Netw* 1999; 10:65–70.

62. Borset M, Waage A, Brekke OL, et al. TNF and IL-6 are potent growth factors for OH-2, a novel human myeloma cell line. *Eur J Haematol* 1994; 53:31–37.

63. Filella X, Blade J, Montoto S, et al. Impaired production of interleukin 6 and tumour necrosis factor alpha in whole blood cell cultures of patients with multiple myeloma. *Cytokine* 1998; 10:993–996.

64. Filella X, Blade J, Guillermo AL, et al. Cytokines (IL-6, TNF-alpha, IL-1alpha) and soluble interleukin-2 receptor as serum tumor markers in multiple myeloma. *Cancer Detect Prev* 1996; 20:52–56.

65. Jourdan M, Zhang XG, Portier M, et al. IFN-alpha induces autocrine production of IL-6 in myeloma cell lines. *J Immunol* 1991; 147:4402–4407.

66. Vacca A, Ribatti D, Roncalli L, et al. Bone marrow angiogenesis and progression in multiple myeloma. *Br J Haematol* 1994; 87:505–508.

67. Bellamy WT, Richer L, Frutiger, et al. Expression of vascular endothelial growth factor and its receptors in hematopoietic malignancies. *Cancer Res* 1999; 59:728–733.

68. Dankbar B, Padro T, Leo R, et al. Vascular endothelial growth factor and interleukin-6 in paracrine tumor-stromal cell interactions in multiple myeloma. *Blood* 2000; 95:2630–2636.

69. Niida S, Kaku M, Amano H, et al. Vascular endothelial growth factor can substitute for macrophage colony-stimulating factor in the support of osteoclastic bone resorption. *J Exp Med* 1999; 190:293–298.

70. Hofbauer LC. Osteoprotegerin ligand and osteoprotegerin: novel implications for osteoclast biology and bone metabolism. *Soc Eur J Endocrinol* 1999; 141:195–210.

71. Kobayashi K, Takahashi N, Jimi E, et al. Tumor necrosis factor a stimulates osteoclast differentiation by a mechanism independent of the ODF/RANKL-RANK interaction. *J Exp Med* 2000; 191:275–285.

72. Altamirano CV, Ma HJ, Parker KM, et al. RANKL is expressed in malignant multiple myeloma (MM) cell lines. *Blood* 2000; 96:365a.

73. Shipman CM, Holen I, Lippitt JM, et al. Tumour cells isolated from patients with multiple myeloma express the critical osteoclastogenic factor, RANKL. *Blood* 2000; 96:360a.

74. Bucay N, Saroosi I, Dunstan CR, et al. Osteoprotegerin-deficient mice develop early onset osteoporosis and arterial calcification. *Genes Dev* 1998; 12:1260–1268

75. Capparelli C, Kostenuik PJ, Morony S, et al. Osteoprotegerin prevents and reverses hypercalcemia in a murine model of humoral hypecalcemia of malignancy. *Cancer Res* 2000; 60: 783–787.

76. Honore P, Luger NM, Sabino MAC, et al. Osteoprotegerin blocks bone cancer-induced skeletal destruction, skeletal pain and pain-related neurochemical reorganization of the spinal cord. *Nat Med* 2000; 6:521–528.

77. Altamirano CV, Neeser JA, Manyak S, et al. Malignant multiple myeloma cells expressing RANKL induce the formation or TRAP positive multinucleated cells. *Blood* 2001; 98:637a.

78. Yaccoby S, Pearse R, Epstein J, et al. Reciprocal relationship between myeloma-induced changes in the bone marrow microenvironment and myeloma cell growth. *Blood* 2000; 96:549a.

79. Pearse RN, Sordillo EM, Yaccoby S, et al. Administration of the TRANCE-antagonist TR-Fc limits myeloma-induced bone destruction. *Blood* 2000; 96:549a.

80. Beg AA, Baldwin AS, Jr: The I kappa B proteins: multifunctional regulators of Rel/NF-kappa B transcription factors. *Genes Dev* 1993; 7:2064–2070

81. Brown K, Park S, et al. Mutual regulation of the transcriptional activator NF-kappa B and its inhibitor, I kappa B-alpha. *Proc Natl Acad Sci USA* 1993; 90:2532–2536

82. Henkel T, et al. Rapid proteolysis of I kappa B-alpha is necessary for activation of transcription factor NF-kappa B. *Nature* 1993; 365:182–185.

83. Mellits KH, Hay RT, Goodbourn S. Proteolytic degradation of MAD3 (I kappa B alpha) and enhanced processing of the NF-kappa B precursor p105 are obligatory steps in the activation of NF-kappa B. *Nucleic Acids Res* 1993; 21:5059–5066

84. Palombella VJ, Rando OJ, Goldberg AL, et al. The ubiquitin-proteasome pathway is required for processing the NF- kappa B1 precursor protein and the activation of NF-kappa B. *Cell* 1994; 78:773–785.

85. Feinman R, et al. Role of NF-kappaB in the recue of multiple myeloma cells from glucocorticoid-induced apoptosis by bcl-2. *Blood* 1999; 93:3044–3052.

86. Ma H, Parker K, Manyak S, et al. The proteasome inhibitor enhances sensitivity of multiple myeloma tumor cells to chemotherapeutic agents. (Submitted.)

87. Hideshima T, et al. The proteasome inhibitor PS-341 inhibits growth, induces apoptosis, and overcomes drug resistance in human multiple myeloma cells. *Cancer Res* 2001; 61: 3071–3076.

88. LeBlanc R, Catley L, Hideshima T, et al. Proteasome inhibitor PS-341 inhibits multiple myeloma growth in a murine model. *Blood* 2001;98:774a.

89. Jelinek DF, Witzig TE, Arendt BK. A role for insulin-like growth factor in the regulation of IL-6-responsive human myeloma cell line growth. *J Immunol* 1997; 159:487–496.

90. Georgii-Hemming P, Wiklund HJ, Ljunggren O, Nilsson K. Insulin-like growth factor I is a growth and survival factor in human multiple myeloma cell lines. *Blood* 1996; 88:2250–2258.

91. Jelinek DF. Mechanisms of myeloma cell growth control. *Hematol Oncol Clin N Am* 1999; 13:1145–1157.

92. Xu F, Gardner A, Tu Y, Michl P, et al. Multiple myeloma cells are protected against dexamethasone-induced apoptosis by insulin-like growth factors. *Br J Haematol* 1997; 97:429–440.

93. Lu ZY, Zhang XG, Rodriguez C, et al. Interleukin-10 is a proliferation factor but not a differentiation factor for human myeloma cells. *Blood* 1995; 85:2521–2527.

94. Seidel C, Borset M, Turesson I, Abildgaard N, et al. Elevated serum concentrations of hepatocyte growth factor in patients with multiple myeloma. The Nordic Myeloma Study Group. *Blood* 1998; 91:806–812.

95. Celsing F, Hast R, Stenke L, Hansson H, Pisa P. Extramedullary progression of multiple myeloma following GM-CSF treatment—grounds for caution? *Eur J Haematol* 1992; 49:108.

96. Schwabe M, Brini AT, Bosco MC, et al. Disruption by interferon-alpha of an autocrine interleukin-6 growth loop in IL-6-dependent U266 myeloma cells by homologous and heterologous down-regulation of the IL-6 receptor alpha- and beta- chains. *J Clin Invest* 1994; 94:2317–2325.

97. Choi SJ, Cruz JC, Craig F, et al. Macrophage inflammatory protein 1-alpha is a potential osteoclast stimulatory factor in multiple myeloma. *Blood* 2000; 96:671–675.

98. Choi SJ, Alsina M, Oba Y, et al. Antisense construct to MIP-1-alpha blocks bone destruction in an in vivo model of myeloma. *Blood* 2000; 96:549a.

99. Nakamura M, Merchav S, Carter A, et al. Expression of a novel 3-5-kb macrophage colony-stimulating factor transcript in human myeloma cells. *J Immunol* 1989; 143:3543–3547.

100. Janowska-Wieczorek A, Belch AR, Jacobs A, et al. Increased circulating colony-stimulating factor-1 in patients with preleukemia, leukemia, and lymphoid malignancies. *Blood* 1991; 77:1796–1803.

101. MacDonald BR, Mundy GR, Clark S, et al. Effects of human recombinant CSF-GM and highly purified CSF-1 on the formation of multinucleated cells with osteoclast characteristics in long-term marrow cultures. *J Bone Mineral Res* 1986; 1:227–233.

102. Sarma U, Flanagan AM. Macrophage colony-stimulating factor induces substantial osteoclast generation and bone resorption in human bone marrow cultures. *Blood* 1996; 88:2531–2540.

103. Fuller K, Owens JM, Jagger CJ, et al. Macrophage colony-stimulating factor stimulates survival and chemotactic behaviour in isolated osteoclasts. *J Exp Med* 1993; 189:1733–1744.

104. Girasole G, Passeri G, Jilka RL, et al. Interleukin-11: a new cytokine critical for osteoclast development. *J Clin Invest* 1994; 93:1516.

105. Hjertner O, Torgersen ML, Seidel C, et al. Hepatocyte growth factor (HGF) induces interleukin-11 secretion from osteoblasts: a possible role for HGF in myeloma-associated osteolytic bone disease. *Blood* 1999; 94:3883–3888.

106. Borset M, Hjorth-Hansen H, Seidel et al. Hepatocyte growth factor and its receptor c-Met in multiple myeloma. *Blood* 1996; 88:3998–4004.

107. Fuller K, Owens J, Chambers TJ. The effect of hepatocyte growth factor on the behaviour of osteoclasts. *Biochem Biophys Res Comm* 1995; 212:334–340.

108. Grano M, Galimi F, Zambonin G, et al. Hepatocyte growth factor is a coupling factor for osteoclasts and osteoblasts in vitro. *Proc Natl Acad Sci USA* 1996; 93:7644–7648.

109. Seidel C, Borset M, Turesson I, Abildgaard N, et al. Elevated serum concentrations of hepatocyte growth factor in patients with multiple myeloma. *Blood* 1998; 91:806–812.

110. Rettig MB, Ma HJ, Vescio RA, et al. Kaposi's sarcoma-associated herpesvirus infection of bone marrow dendritic cells from multiple myeloma patients. *Science* 1997; 276:1851–1854.

111. Said JW, Rettig MR, Heppner K, et al. Localization of Kaposi's sarcoma-associated herpesvirus in bone marrow biopsy samples from patients with multiple myeloma. *Blood* 1997; 90:4278–4282.

112. Rask C, Kelsen J, Olesen G, et al. Danish patients with untreated multiple myeloma do not harbour human herpesvirus 8. *Br J Haematol* 2000; 108:96–98.

113. Bellos F, Goldschmidt H, Dorner M, et al. Bone marrow derived dendritic cells from patients with multiple myeloma cultured with three distinct protocols do not bear Kaposi's sarcoma associated herpesvirus DNA. *Ann Oncol* 1999; 10:323–327.

114. Chauhan D, Bharti A, Raje N, et al. Detection of Kaposi's sarcoma herpesvirus DNA sequences in multiple myeloma bone marrow stromal cells. *Blood* 1999; 93:1482–1486.

115. Brousset P, Meggetto F, Laharrague P, et al. Kaposi's sarcoma-associated herpesvirus (KSHV) in bone marrow biopsy from patients with multiple myeloma: PCR amplification of orf26 but not orf72 and orf75 sequences. *Br J Haematol* 2000; 108:197–198.

116. Raje N, Gong J, Chauhan D, et al. Bone marrow and peripheral blood dendritic cells from patients with multiple myeloma are phenotypically and functionally normal despite the detection of Kaposi's sarcoma herpesvirus gene sequences. *Blood* 1999; 93:1487–1495.

117. Belec L, Mohamed AS, Authier FJ, et al. Human herpesvirus 8 infection in patients with POEMS syndrome-associated multicentric Castleman's disease. *Blood* 1999; 93:3643–3653.

118. Ma HJ, Sjak-Shie NN, Vescio RA, et al. Human herpes virus 8 sequences from ORF26 and ORF65 in multiple myeloma patients show a disease specific pattern. *Clinical Cancer Res* 2000; 6:4226–4233.

119. Vescio RA, Wu CH, Zheng L, et al. Human herpesvirus 8 (KSHV) contamination of peripheral blood and autograft products from multiple myeloma patients. *Bone Marrow Transplant* 2000; 25:153–160.

120. Sjak-Shie NN, Vescio RA, Berenson JR. The role of human herpesvirus-8 in the pathogenesis of multiple myeloma. *Hematol Oncol Clin N Am* 1999; 13:1159–1167.

121. MacKenzie J, Sheldon J, Morgan G, et al. HHV-8 and multiple myeloma in the UK. *Lancet* 1997; 350:1144–1145.

122. Gao SJ, Alsina M, Deng JH, et al. Antibodies to Kaposi's sarcoma-associated herpesvirus (human herpesvirus 8) in patients with multiple myeloma. *J Infect Dis* 1998; 178:846–849.

123. Drach J, Schuster J, Nowotny H, et al. Multiple myeloma: high incidence of chromosomal aneuploidy as detected by interphase fluorescence in situ hybridization. *Cancer Res* 1995; 55:3854–3859.

124. Perez-Simon JA, Garcia-Sanz R, Tabernero MD, et al. Prognostic value of numerical chromosome aberrations in multiple myeloma: a FISH analysis of 15 different chromosomes. *Blood* 1998; 91:3366–3371.

125. Avet-Loiseau H, Li JY, Facon T, Brigaudeau C, et al. High incidence of translocations t(11;14)(q13;q32) and t(4;14)(p16;q32) in patients with plasma cell malignancies. *Cancer Res* 1998; 58:5640–5645.

126. Avet-Loiseau H, Brigaudeau C, Morineau N, et al. High incidence of cryptic translocations involving the Ig heavy chain gene in multiple myeloma, as shown by fluorescence in situ hybridization. *Genes Chromosomes Cancer* 1999; 24:9–15.

127. Bergsagel PL, Chesi M, Nardini E, et al. Promiscuous translocations into immunoglobulin heavy chain switch regions in multiple myeloma. *Proc Natl Acad Sci USA* 1996; 93:13,931.

128. Chesi M, Bergsagel PL, Shonukan OO, et al. Frequent dysregulation of the c-maf proto-oncogene at 16q23 by translocation to an Ig locus in multiple myeloma. *Blood* 1998; 91:4457.

129. Chesi M, Brents LA, Ely SA, et al. Activated fibroblast growth factor receptor 3 is an oncogene that contributes to tumor progression in multiple myeloma. *Blood* 2001; 97:729.

130. Iida S, Rao PH, Butler M, et al. Deregulation of MUM1/IRF4 by chromosomal translocation in multiple myeloma. *Nat Genet* 1997; 17:226.
131. Shaughnessy J Jr, Gabrea A, Qi Y, et al. Cyclin D3 at 6p21 is dysregulated by recurrent chromosomal translocations to immunoglobulin loci in multiple myeloma. *Blood* 2001; 98:217.
132. Ronchetti D, Finelli P, Richelda R, et al. Molecular analysis of 11q13 breakpoints in multiple myeloma. *Blood* 1999; 93:1330.
133. Janssen JW, Vaandrager JW, Heuser T, et al. Concurrent activation of a novel putative transforming gene, myeov, and cyclin D1 in a subset of multiple myeloma cell lines with t(11;14)(q13;q32). *Blood* 2000; 95:2691.
134. Cigudosa JC, Rao PH, Calasanz MJ, et al. Characterization of nonrandom chromosomal gains and losses in multiple myeloma by comparative genomic hybridization. *Blood* 1998; 91:3007.
135. Sawyer JR, Tricot G, Mattox S, et al. Jumping translocations of chromosome 1q in multiple myeloma: evidence for a mechanism involving decondensation of pericentromeric heterochromatin. *Blood* 1998; 91:1732.
136. Tricot G, Barlogie B, Jaganath S, et al. Poor prognosis in multiple myeloma is associated only with partial or complete deletions of chromosome 13 or abnormalities involving 11q and not other karyotype abnormalities. *Blood* 1995; 86:4250.
137. Avet-Louseau H, Daviet A, Sauner S, et al. Chromosome 13 abnormalities in multiple myeloma are mostly monosomy 13. *Br J Haematol* 2000; 111:1116.
138. Avet-Loiseau H, Li JY, Morineau N, et al. Monosomy 13 is associated with the transition of monoclonal gammopathy of undetermined significance to multiple myeloma. Intergroupe Francophone du Myelome. *Blood* 1999; 94:2583–2589.
139. Shaughnessy J, Tian E, Sawyer J, et al. High incidence of chromosome 13 deletion in multiple myeloma detected by multiprobe interphase FISH. *Blood* 2000; 96:1505.
140. Schreiber S, Ackermann J, Obermair A, et al. Multiple myeloma with deletion of chromosome 13q is characterized by increased bone marrow neovascularization. *Br J Haematol* 2000; 110:605.
141. Zojer N, Konigsberg R, Ackermann J, et al. Deletion of 13q14 remains an independent adverse prognostic variable in multiple myeloma despite its frequent detection by interphase fluorescence in situ hybridization. *Blood* 2000; 95:1925.
142. Desikan R, Barlogie B, Sawyer J, et al. Results of high-dose therapy for 1000 patients with multiple myeloma: durable complete remissions and superior survival in the absence of chromosome 13 abnormalities. *Blood* 2000; 95:4008.
143. Zandecki M, Lai JL, Genevieve F, et al. Several cytogenetic subclones may be identified within plasma cells from patients with monoclonal gammopathy of undetermined significance, both at diagnosis and during the indolent course of this condition. *Blood* 1997; 90:3682.
144. Kalakonda N, Rothwell DG, Scarffe JH, et al. Detection of N-Ras codon 61 mutations in subpopulations of tumor cells in multiple myeloma at presentation. *Blood* 2001; 98:1555.
145. Liu P, Leong T, Quam L, et al. Activating mutations of N- and K-ras in multiple myeloma show different clinical associations: Analysis of the Eastern Cooperative Oncology Group Phase III Trial. *Blood* 1996; 88:2699.
146. Corradini P, Inghirami G, Astolfi M, et al. Inactivation of tumor suppressor genes, p53 and Rb1, in plasma cell dyscrasias. *Leukemia* 1994; 8:758.
147. Tasaka T, Asou H, Munker R, et al. Methylation of the p16INK4A gene in multiple myeloma. *Br J Haematol* 1998; 101:558.
148. Guillerm G, Gyan E, Wolowiec D, et al. p16(INK4a) and p15(INK4b) gene methylations in plasma cells from monoclonal gammopathy of undetermined significance. *Blood* 2001; 98:244.

149. Silvestris F, Tucci M, Cafforio P, et al. Fas-L up-regulation by highly malignant myeloma plasma cells: role in the pathogenesis of anemia and disease progression. *Blood* 2001; 97:1155.

150. Landowski TH, Qu N, Buyuksal I, et al. Mutations in the fas antigen in patients with multiple myeloma. *Blood* 1997; 90:4266.

151. Vacca A, Ribatti D, Presta M, et al. Bone marrow neovascularization, plasma cell angiogenic potential, and matrix metalloproteinase-2 secretion parallel progression of human multiple myeloma. *Blood* 1999; 93:3064–3073.

152. Bellamy WT, Richter L, Frutiger Y, et al. Expression of vascular endothelial growth factor and its receptors in hematopoietic malignancies. *Cancer Res* 1999; 59:728–733.

153. Ribatti D, Vacca A, Nico B, et al. Bone marrow angiogenesis and mast cell density increase simultaneously with progression of human multiple myeloma. *Br J Cancer* 1999; 79:451–455.

154. Munshi N, Wilson CS, Penn J, et al. Angiogenesis in newly diagnosed multiple myeloma: poor prognosis with increased microvessel density (MVD) in bone marrow biopsies. *Blood* 1998; 92.

155. Rajkumar SV, Fonseca R, Witzig TE, et al. Bone marrow angiogenesis in patients achieving complete response after stem cell transplantation for multiple myeloma. *Leukemia* 1999; 13:469–472.

156. van Hoeven KH, Reed LJ, Factor SM. Autopsy-documented cure of multiple myeloma 14 years after M2 chemotherapy. *Cancer* 1990; 66:1472–1474.

157. Hjorth M, Hellquist L, Holmberg E, et al. Initial versus deferred melphalan-prednisone therapy for asymptomatic multiple myeloma stage I—a randomized study. Myeloma Group of Western Sweden. *Eur J Haematol* 1993; 50:95–102.

158. Alexanian R, Dimopoulos MA, Delasalle K, et al. Primary dexamethasone treatment in multiple myeloma. *Blood* 1992; 80:887–890.

159. Case DC, Jr., Lee DJ, Clarkson BD. Improved survival times in multiple myeloma treated with melphalan, prednisone, cyclophosphamide, vincristine and BCNU: M-2 protocol. *Am J Med* 1977; 63:897–903.

160. Oken MM, Harrington DP, Abramson N, et al. Comparison of melphalan and prednisone with vincristine, carmustine, melphalan, cyclophosphamide, and prednisone in the treatment of multiple myeloma: results of Eastern Cooperative Oncology Group Study E2479. *Cancer* 1997; 79:1561–1567.

161. Barlogie B, Smith L, Alexanian R. Effective treatment of advanced multiple myeloma refractory to alkylating agents. *N Engl J Med* 1984; 310:1353–1356.

162. Alexanian R, Yap BS, Bodey GP. Prednisone pulse therapy for refractory myeloma. *Blood* 1983; 62:572–577.

163. Monconduit M, Le Loet X, Bernard JF, et al. Combination chemotherapy with vincristine, doxorubicin, dexamethasone for refractory or relapsing multiple myeloma. *Br J Haematol* 1986; 63:599–601.

164. Sheehan T, Judge M, Parker AC. The efficacy and toxicity of VAD in the treatment of myeloma and related disorders. *Scand J Haematol* 1986; 37:425–428.

165. Buzaid AC, Durie BG. Management of refractory myeloma: a review. *J Clin Oncol* 1988; 6:889–905.

166. Combination chemotherapy versus melphalan plus prednisone as treatment for multiple myeloma: an overview of 6,633 patients from 27 randomized trials. Myeloma Trialists' Collaborative Group. *J Clin Oncol* 1998; 16:3832–3842.

167. Osterborg A, Bjorkholm M, Bjoreman M, et al. Natural interferon-alpha in combination with melphalan/prednisone versus melphalan/prednisone in the treatment of multiple myeloma stages II and III: a randomized study from the Myeloma Group of Central Sweden. *Blood* 1993; 81:1428–1434.

168. Cooper MR, Dear K, McIntyre OR, et al. A randomized clinical trial comparing melphalan/ prednisone with or without interferon alfa-2b in newly diagnosed patients with multiple myeloma: a Cancer and Leukemia Group B study. *J Clin Oncol* 1993; 11:155–160.

169. Musto P, Lombardi G, Matera R, et al. The expression of the multidrug transporter P-170 glycoprotein in remission phase is associated with early and resistant relapse in multiple myeloma. *Haematologica* 1991; 76:513–516.

170. Ludwig H, Cohen AM, Polliack A, et al. Interferon-alpha for induction and maintenance in multiple myeloma: results of two multicenter randomized trials and summary of other studies. *Ann Oncol* 1995; 6:467–476.

171. Tura S, Cavo M. Allogeneic bone marrow transplantation in multiple myeloma. *Hematol Oncol Clin N Am* 1992; 6:425–435.

172. Gahrton G. Allogeneic bone marrow transplantation in multiple myeloma. *Pathol Biol* (Paris) 1999, 47:188–191.

173. Gahrton G, Svensson H, Cavo, et al. Progress in allogeneic bone marrow and peripheral blood stem cell transplantation for multiple myeloma: a comparison between transplants performed 1983–1993 and 1994–1998 at European Group for Blood and Marrow Transplantation Centers. *Br J Haematol* 2001; 113:209–216.

174. Martinelli G, Terragna C, Zamagni E, et al. Molecular remission after allogeneic or autologous transplantation of hematopoietic stem cells for multiple myeloma. *J Clin Oncol* 2000; 18:2273–2281.

175. Slavin S, Nagler A, Naparstek E, et al. Nonmyeloablative stem cell transplantation and cell therapy as an alternative to conventional bone marrow transplantation with lethal cytoreduction for the treatment of malignant and nonmalignant hematologic diseases. *Blood* 1998; 91:756–763.

176. Badros A, Barlogie B, Morris C, et al. High response rate in refractory and poor-risk multiple myeloma after allotransplantation using a nonmyeloablative conditioning regimen and donor leukocyte infusions. *Blood* 2001; 98:2574–2579.

177. Lokhorst HM, Schattenberg A, Cornelissen JJ, et al. Donor lymphocyte infusions for relapsed multiple myeloma after allogeneic stem-cell transplantation: Predictive factors for response and long-term outcome. *J Clin Oncol* 2000; 18:3031–3037.

178. Gahrton G, Svensson H, Bjorkstrand B, et al. Syngeneic transplantation in multiple myeloma—a case-matched comparison with autologous and allogeneic transplantation. European Group for Blood and Marrow Transplantation. *Bone Marrow Transplant* 1999; 24:741–745.

179. Attal M, Harousseau JL, Stoppa AM, et al. A prospective, randomized trial of autologous bone marrow transplantation and chemotherapy in multiple myeloma. Intergroupe Francais du Myelome. *N Engl J Med* 1996; 335:91–97.

180. Harousseau JL, Attal M. The role of autologous hematopoietic stem cell transplantation in multiple myeloma. *Semin Hematolv* 1997; 34:61–66.

181. Lenhoff S, Hjorth M, Holmberg E, et al. Impact on survival of high-dose therapy with autologous stem cell support in patients younger than 60 years with newly diagnosed multiple myeloma: a population-based study. Nordic Myeloma Study Group. *Blood* 2000; 95:7–11.

182. Palumbo A, Triolo S, Argentino C, et al. Dose-intensive melphalan with stem cell support (MEL100) is superior to standard treatment in elderly myeloma patients. *Blood* 1999; 94: s1248–1253.

183. Attal M, Harousseau JL, Stoppa AM, et al. A prospective, randomized trial of autologous bone marrow transplantation and chemotherapy in multiple myeloma. Intergroupe Francais du Myelome. *N Engl J Med* 1996; 335:91–97.

184. Harousseau JL, Attal M. The role of autologous hematopoietic stem cell transplantation in multiple myeloma. *Semin Hematol* 1997; 34:61–66.

185. Bergsagel DE. Treatment of plasma cell myeloma. Annu Rev Med 1979; 30:431–443.
186. Jagannath S, Tricot G, Barlogie B. Autotransplants in multiple myeloma: Pushing the envelope. *Hematol Oncol Clin N Am* 1997; 11:363–381.
187. Goldschmidt H, Hegenbart U, Wallmeier M, et al. High-dose chemotherapy in multiple myeloma. *Leukemia* 1997; 11(Suppl 5):S27–31.
188. Vesole DH. Bone marrow and stem cell transplantation for multiple myeloma. *Cancer Treat Res* 1999; 99:171–94.
189. Fermand JP, Brechignac S. The role of autologous stem cell transplantation in the management of multiple myeloma. *Pathol Biol (Paris)* 1999; 47:199–202.
190. Tribalto M, Amadori S, Cudillo L, et al. Autologous peripheral blood stem cell transplantation as first line treatment of multiple myeloma: an Italian multicenter study. *Haematologica* 2000; 85:52–58.
191. Fermand JP, Ravaud P, Chevret S, et al. High-dose therapy and autologous peripheral blood stem cell transplantation in multiple myeloma: up-front or rescue treatment? Results of a multicenter sequential randomized clinical trial. *Blood* 1998; 92:3131–3136.
192. Siegel DS, Desikan KR, Mehta J, et al. Age is not a prognostic variable with autotransplants for multiple myeloma. *Blood* 1999; 93:51–54.
193. Reiffers J, Marit G, Boiron JM. Autologous blood stem cell transplantation in high-risk multiple myeloma. *Br J Haematol* 1989; 72:296–297.
194. Fermand JP, Chevret S, Ravaud P, et al. High-dose chemoradiotherapy and autologous blood stem cell transplantation in multiple myeloma: results of a phase II trial involving 63 patients. *Blood* 1993; 82:2005–2009.
195. Vesole DH, Jagannath S, Glenn L, et al. Autotransplantation in multiple myeloma. *Hematol Oncol Clin N Am* 1993; 7:613–630.
196. Cunningham D, Paz-Ares L, Gore ME, et al. High-dose melphalan for multiple myeloma: long-term follow-up data. *J Clin Oncol* 1994; 12:764–768.
197. Schiller G, Vescio R, Freytes C, et al. Autologous CD34-selected blood progenitor cell transplants for patients with advanced multiple myeloma. *Bone Marrow Transplant* 1998; 21:141–145.
198. Vescio RA, Han EJ, Schiller GJ, et al. Quantitative comparison of multiple myeloma tumor contamination in bone marrow harvest and leukapheresis autografts. *Bone Marrow Transplant* 1996; 18:103–110.
199. Vescio RA, Hong CH, Cao J, et al. The hematopoietic stem cell antigen, CD34, is not expressed on the malignant cells in multiple myeloma. *Blood* 1994; 84:3283–3290.
200. Vescio R, Schiller G, Stewart AK, et al. Multicenter phase III trial to evaluate CD34(+) selected versus unselected autologous peripheral blood progenitor cell transplantation in multiple myeloma. *Blood* 1999; 93:1858–1868.
201. Stewart K, Vescio R, Schiller G, et al. Purging of autologous peripheral blood stem cells using CD34 selection does not improve overall or progression-free survival after high-dose therapy: results of a multi-center randomized controlled trial. *J Clin Oncol* 2001; 19: 3771–3779.
202. Vescio R and Berenson J. Autologous transplantation. purging and the impact of minimal residual disease. *Hematol Oncol Clin N Am* 1999; 13:969–986.
203. Mandelli F, Avvisati G, Amadori S, et al. Maintenance treatment with recombinant interferon alfa-2b in patients with multiple myeloma responding to conventional induction chemotherapy. *N Engl J Med* 1990; 20:1430–1434.
204. Westin J, Rodjer S, Turesson I, et al. Interferon alfa-2b versus no maintenance therapy during the plateau phase in multiple myeloma: A randomised study. *Br J Haematol* 1995; 89: 561–568.
205. Browman GP, Bergsagel DE, Sicheri D, et al. Randomized trial of interferon maintenance in multiple myeloma: a study of the National Cancer Institute of Canada Clinical Trials Group. *J Clin Oncol* 1995; 13:2354–2360.

206. Ludwig H, Cohen AM, Polliack A, et al. Interferon-alpha for induction and maintenance in multiple myeloma: results of two multicenter randomized trials and summary of other studies. *Ann Oncol* 1995; 6:467–476.
207. Salmon SE, Crowley JJ, Grogan TM, et al. Combination chemotherapy, glucocorticoids, and interferon alfa in the treatment of multiple myeloma: A Southwest Oncology Group study. *J Clin Oncol* 1994; 12:2405–2414.
208. Peest D, Deicher H, Coldewey R, et al. A comparison of polychemotherapy and melphalan-prednisone for primary remission induction, and interferon-alpha for maintenance treatment, in multiple myeloma: a prospective trial of the German Myeloma Treatment Group. *Eur J Cancer* 1995; 31A:146–150.
209. Mandelli F, Avvisati G, Amadori S, et al. Maintenance treatment with recombinant interferon alfa-2b in patients with multiple myeloma responding to conventional induction chemotherapy. *N Engl J Med* 1990; 20:1430–1434.
210. Westin J, Rodjer S, Turesson I, et al. Interferon alfa-2b versus no maintenance therapy during the plateau phase in multiple myeloma: A randomised study. *Br J Haematol* 1995; 89: 561–568.
211. Browman GP, Bergsagel DE, Sicheri D, et al. Randomized trial of interferon maintenance in multiple myeloma: A study of the National Cancer Institute of Canada Clinical Trials Group. *J Clin Oncol* 1995; 13:2354–2360.
212. Ludwig H, Cohen AM, Polliack A, et al. Interferon-alpha for induction and maintenance in multiple myeloma: Results of two multicenter randomized trials and summary of other studies. *Ann Oncol* 1995; 6:467–476.
213. Salmon SE, Crowley JJ, Grogan TM, et al. Combination chemotherapy, glucocorticoids, and interferon alfa in the treatment of multiple myeloma: A Southwest Oncology Group study. *J Clin Oncol* 1994; 12:2405–2414.
214. Peest D, Deicher H, Coldewey R, et al. A comparison of polychemotherapy and melphalan-prednisone for primary remission induction, and interferon-alpha for maintenance treatment, in multiple myeloma: A prospective trial of the German Myeloma Treatment Group. *Eur J Cancer* 1995; 31A:146–150.
215. Palumbo A, Boccadoro M, Garino LA, et al. Interferon plus glucocorticoids as intensified maintenance therapy prolongs tumor control in relapsed myeloma. *Acta Haematol* 1993; 90:71–76.
216. Salmon SE, Crowley JJ, Balcerzak SP, et al. Interferon versus interferon plus prednisone remission maintenance therapy for multiple myeloma: A Southwest Oncology Group study. *J Clin Oncol* 1998; 16: 890–896.
217. Berenson JR, Crowley JJ, Grogan T, et al. Maintenance therapy with alternate-day prednisone improves survival in multiple myeloma patients. *Blood* 2002; 99:3163–3168.
218. Dimopoulos MA, Delasalle KB, Champlin R, et al. Cyclophosphamide and etoposide therapy with GM-CSF for VAD-resistant multiple myeloma. *Br J Haematol* 1993; 83:240–244.
219. Barlogie B, Vesole DH, Jagannath S. Salvage therapy for multiple myeloma: the University of Arkansas experience. *Mayo Clin Proc* 1994; 69:787–795.
220. Barlogie B, Jagannath S, Dixon DO, et al. High-dose melphalan and granulocyte-macrophage colony-stimulating factor for refractory multiple myeloma. *Blood* 1990; 76:677–680.
221. Singhal S, Mehta J, Desikan R, et al. Antitumor activity of thalidomide in refractory multiple myeloma. *N Engl J Med* 1999; 341:1565–1571.
222. Barlogie B, Desikan, Eddlemon, et al. Extended survival in advanced and refractory multiple myeloma after single-agent thalidomide; identification of prognostic factors in phase 2 study of 169 patients. *Blood* 2001; 98:492–494.
223. Zangari M, Anaissie E, et al. Increased risk of deep-venous thrombosis in patients with multiple myeloma receiving thalidomide and chemotherapy. *Bloodv* 2001:98:1614–1615.

224. Sastry PS. Inhibition of TNF-alpha synthesis with thalidomide for prevention of acute exacerbations and altering the natural history of multiple sclerosis. *Med Hypotheses* 1999; 53:76–77.

225. Moller DR, Wysocka M, Greenlee BM, et al. Inhibition of IL-12 production by thalidomide. *J Immunol* 1997; 159:5157–5161.

226. Davies FE, Raje N, Hideshima T, et al. Thalidomide and immunomodulatory derivatives augment natural killer cell cytotoxicity in multiple myeloma. *Blood* 2001; 98:210–216.

227. Keifer JA, Guttridge DC, Ashburner BP, et al. Inhibition of NF-kB activity by thalidomide through suppression of IkB kinase activity. *J Biol Chem* 2001; 276:22,382–22,387.

228. Larkin M. Low-dose thalidomide seems to be effective in multiple myeloma. *Lancet* 1999; 354:925.

229. Alexanian R. Thalidomide and prednisone in the treatment of multiple myeloma. *Blood* 1999; ASH 1999; 94:604a.

230. Rajkumar SV, Hayman S, Fonseca R, et al. Thalidomide plus dexamethasone (Thal/Dex) and thalidomide alone as first line therapy for newly diagnosed myeloma (MM). *Blood* 2000; 96:168a.

231. Richardson P, Berenson J, Irwin D, et al. Phase II study of PS-341, a novel proteasome inhibitor, alone or in combination with dexamethasone in patients with multiple myeloma who have relapsed following front-line therapy and are refractor to their most recent therapy. *Blood* 2001; 98:774a.

232. Ma MH, Parker KM, Manyak S, et al. Proteasome inhibitor PS-341 markedly enhances sensitivity of multiple myeloma cells to chemotherapeutic agents and overcomes chemo-resistance through inhibition of the NF-kB pathway. *Blood* 2001; 98:11:473a.

233. Ma MH, Borad MJ, Friedman J, et al. Arsenic trioxide-mediated growth inhibition of multiple myeloma cells correlated with inhibition of nuclear factor (NF)-kB activity. *Blood* 2001; 98:100a.

234. Grad JM, Bahlis NJ, Reis I, et al. Ascorbic acid enhances arsenic trioxide-induced cytotoxicity in multiple myeloma cells. *Blood* 2001; 98:805–813.

235. Hussein MA, Mason J, Ravandi F, et al. A phase II trial of arsenic trioxide (ATO) in patients (Pts) with relapsed or refractory multiple myeloma (MM): a preliminary report. *Blood* 2001; 98:378a.

236. Kyle RA. Multiple myeloma: review of 869 cases. Mayo Clin Proc 1975; 50:29–40.

237. Mundy GR, Bertolini DR. Bone destruction and hypercalcemia in plasma cell myeloma [published erratum appears in Semin Oncol 1986 Dec;13(4):lxiii]. *Semin Oncol* 1986; 13:291–299.

238. Belch AR, Bergsagel DE, Wilson K, et al. Effect of daily etidronate on the osteolysis of multiple myeloma. *J Clin Oncol* 1991; 9:1397–1402.

239. Kyle RA, Jowsey J, Kelly PJ, Taves DR. Multiple-myeloma bone disease. The comparative effect of sodium fluoride and calcium carbonate or placebo. *N Engl J Med* 1975; 293:1334–1338.

240. Harley JB, Schilling A, Glidewell O. Ineffectiveness of fluoride therapy in multiple myeloma. *N Engl J Med* 1972; 286:1283–1288.

241. Cohen HJ, Silberman HR, Tornyos K, Bartolucci AA. Comparison of two long-term chemotherapy regimens, with or without agents to modify skeletal repair, in multiple myeloma. *Blood* 1984; 63:639–648.

242. van Breukelen FJ, Bijvoet OL, van Oosterom AT. Inhibition of osteolytic bone lesions by (3-amino-1-hydroxypropylidene)-1, 1-bisphosphonate (A.P.D.). *Lancet* 1979; 1:803–805.

243. Siris ES, Sherman WH, Baquiran DC, et al. Effects of dichloromethylene diphosphonate on skeletal mobilization of calcium in multiple myeloma. *N Engl J Med* 1980; 302:310–315.

244. Lahtinen R, Laakso M, Palva I, et al. Randomised, placebo-controlled multicentre trial of clodronate in multiple myeloma. Finnish Leukaemia Group [published erratum appears in Lancet 1992 Dec 5;340(8832):1420]. *Lancet* 1992; 340:1049–1052.

245. McCloskey EV, MacLennan IC, Drayson MT, et al. A randomized trial of the effect of clodronate on skeletal morbidity in multiple myeloma. MRC Working Party on Leukaemia in Adults. *Br J Haematol* 1998; 100:317–325.

246. Berenson JR, Lichtenstein A, Porter L, et al. Efficacy of pamidronate in reducing skeletal events in patients with advanced multiple myeloma. Myeloma Aredia Study Group. *N Engl J Med* 1996; 334:488–493.

247. Berenson JR, Lichtenstein A, Porter L, et al. Long-term pamidronate treatment of advanced multiple myeloma patients reduces skeletal events. Myeloma Aredia Study Group. *J Clin Oncol* 1998; 16:593–602.

248. Brincker H, Westin J, Abildgaard N, et al. Failure of oral pamidronate to reduce skeletal morbidity in multiple myeloma: a double-blind placebo-controlled trial. Danish-Swedish co- operative study group. *Br J Haematol* 1998; 101:280–286.

249. Troehler U, Bonjour JP, Fleisch H. Renal secretion of diphosphonates in rats. *Kidney Int* 1975; 8:6–13.

250. Berenson JR, Rosen L, Vescio R, et al. Pharmacokinetics of pamidronate disodium in patients with cancer with normal or impaired renal function. *J Clin Pharmacol* 1997; 37:285–290.

251. Markowitz GS, Apel GB, Fine PL, et al. Collapsing focal segmental glomerulosclerosis following treatment with high-dose pamidronate. *J Am Soc Nephrol* 2000; 12:1164–1172.

252. Major PP, Lortholary A, Hon J, et al. Zoledronic acid is superior to pamidronate in the treatment of hypercalcemia of malignancy: a pooled analysis of two randomized, controlled clinical trials. *J Clin Oncol* 2001; 19:558–567.

253. Berenson JR, Vescio R, Henick K, et al. A Phase I, open label, dose ranging trial of intravenous bolus zoledronic acid, a novel bisphosphonate, in cancer patients with metastatic bone disease. *Cancer* 2001; 91:144–154.

254. Berenson JR, Vescio RA, Rosen LS, et al. A Phase I dose-ranging trial of monthly infusions of zoledronic acid for the treatment of osteolytic bone metastases. *Clin Can Res* 2001; 7:478–485.

255. Berenson JR, Rosen LS, Howell A, et al. Zoledronic acid reduces skeletal-related events in patients with osteolytic metastases. *Cancer* 2001; 91:1191–2000.

256. Rosen LS, Gordon D, Kaminski M, et al. Zoledronic acid versus pamidronate in the treatment of skeletal metastases in patients with breast cancer or osteolytic lesions of multiple myeloma: a phase III, double-blind, comparative trial. *Cancer J* 2001; 7:377–387.

257. Aparicio A, Gardner A, Tu Y, et al. In vitro cytoreductive effects on multiple myeloma cells induced by bisphosphonates. *Leukemia* 1998; 12:220–229.

258. Savage AD, Belson DJ, Vescio RA, et al. Pamidronate reduces IL-6 production by bone marrow stroma from multiple myeloma patients. *Blood* 1996; 88:105a.

259. Kunzmann V, Bauer E, Feurle, et al. Stimulation of γδ T cells by aminobisphosphonates and induction of antiplasma cell activity in multiple myeloma. *Blood* 2000; 96:384–392.

260. Greipp P, Facon T, Williams CD, et al. A single subcutaneous dose of an osteoprotegerin (OPG) construct (AMGN-0007) causes a profound and sustained decrease of bone resorption comparable to standard intravenous bisphosphonate in patients with multiple myeloma. *Blood* 2001; 98:775a.

10 Low-Grade Lymphoma

Christos Emmanouilides, MD

INTRODUCTION

Low-grade lymphoma is a term that encompasses diverse histologic lymphoma subtypes typically characterized by a slow proliferative rate, long natural history, and presumed incurability to conventional treatments when disseminated. This descriptive term was initially developed to describe the follicular small cleaved cell, the follicular mixed cell, and the small lymphocytic lymphoma of the Working Formulation (WF) *(1)*.

Although not formally recognized in later classification schemes, the concept of low-grade lymphoma has survived classification system changes, because it successfully conveys the notion of lymphomas of relatively low aggressiveness. Such lymphomas display a characteristic pattern of natural history with multiple remissions and relapses, are usually sensitive to various treatments, and become life-threatening only in the later stages of their course—usually several years after diagnosis. Thus, the term "low-grade lymphoma" is now synonymous to the term "indolent lymphoma." Although several new agents and innovative treatment modalities have been developed or are under investigation in recent years, the treatment of low-grade lymphoma continues to pose a challenge to clinicians and patients.

Low-grade lymphomas are increasing in frequency, as are other lymphoma subtypes *(2)*. It is expected that approximately one-third of new cases of NHL

From: *Current Clinical Oncology: Chronic Leukemias and Lymphomas:*
Biology, Pathophysiology, and Clinical Management
Edited by: G. J. Schiller © Humana Press Inc., Totowa, NJ

diagnosed—more than 56,000 per year—are low-grade lymphoma *(3)*. The increased incidence is not as impressive as that of certain types of aggressive NHL or extranodal lymphomas, and can be attributed to unknown environmental factors. The incidence of the disease increases with age. Epidemiological studies have shown an association with exposure to pesticides and herbicides or occupational exposure among construction workers *(3)*. None of those associations are as strong as the linkage of *H. pylori* infection of the stomach with gastric maltomas (MALT lymphomas) *(4,5)*. This association is supported by the finding of *H. pylori* in biopsy specimens of over 90% of the cases, the increased incidence of gastric maltoma along with prevalence of *H. pylori* in the population, and the frequent regression of the disease in response to antibiotic-mediated eradication of the infection. However, the etiology of the lymphoma cannot be determined in the vast majority of cases.

PATHOLOGY AND CLASSIFICATION

Several classification systems have been developed in the last decades, with various success in reproducibility and clinical usefulness. Separate "lymphoma schools" have often adopted different systems of classification, rendering communication among investigators difficult *(6–8)*. In the United States, the working formulation (WF) proposed in the early 80s, became widely acceptable because of its simplicity *(1)*. The categorization was based on morphologic appearance by routine microscopy as well as clinical behavior. The WF classification system introduced the clinically relevant categories of low-grade, intermediate-grade, and high-grade lymphomas, which usually predicted the expected clinical behavior of the entity. The success of this relatively simplistic and practical classification system was based on the fact that it appealed to clinicians, and it could satisfactory predict the clinical attributes of nearly two-thirds of all lymphomas that are either follicular or diffuse large B-cell. The WF could not encompass less common disease entities (such as types of T-cell lymphomas and mantle-cell lymphoma [MCL]), which became more distinguishable with the advent of immunophenotyping and molecular techniques. This weakness led to the development of the Revised European-American Classification of lymphoid neoplasms in 1994 *(9)*. This ambitious effort, spearheaded by expert pathologists, used evidence accumulated by routine histology, immunohistochemistry, molecular diagnostics, and lymphocyte biology, as well as clinical information to try to classify lymphomas according to their normal lymphocyte counterpart. Older entities were tested in reproducibility exercises, which led to the abandonment of certain WF categories as well as lumping together of others. For the most part, the contribution of the REAL classification was the recognition and characterization of the less common entities not previously recognized. The World Health Organization (WHO) adopted the REAL concept and with relatively minor modifications developed the WHO classification system, which is considered the current standard *(10)*. Further examination of some of the less common entities is still being proposed.

The WF recognizes three types of low-grade lymphoma. Small lymphocytic lymphoma (SLL) consists of mature and round small lymphocytes, which develop in diffuse and uniform pattern and efface the normal lymph-node architecture. Follicular small-cleaved-cell lymphoma (FSC) develops in a pseudo-follicular pattern, where more or less discrete nodularity is evident, often separated by fibrous bands. Nodules vary in size, whereas the majority of the cells have an irregular dense nucleus, are sometimes cleaved with coarse chromatin, and are small in size (centrocytes). Rarely, larger cells with open chromatin are also seen (centroblasts). In some areas of the node, a diffuse pattern of growth can be seen. Follicular, mixed small cleaved and large-cell (FM) has a similar pseudofollicular pattern of growth, but consists of a mixture of small cleaved and large-cell, whereas in large cells it is usually 20–50% *(11)*. If the proportion of large cells seen is >50%, the disease is classified as follicular large-cell lymphoma. Clearly, the distinction between the three subtypes of follicular lymphomas (FLs) cannot be exact, since they represent three segments of a continuous spectrum of increasing large-cell components. Other methods of differentiating between these entities have been proposed, as discussed here. The distinction between these entities is not always clinically significant, although follicular large-cell lymphomas are classified as intermediate-grade NHL by the WF, and are treated as aggressive lymphomas by most.

Because the REAL/WHO classification is based on the origin of the lymphocyte undergoing malignant transformation, helped by but not dependent on the microscopic appearance of the lymphoma, it recognizes the basic distinction between B-cell and T-cell lymphomas. Based on the same logic, all FLs are lumped together; a grading system of I, II, and III—which largely corresponds to the FSC, FM, and follicular large cell, respectively—is provided. The preferred way to assign the grading is by observing at least 20 high-power fields and estimate the average number of large cells seen (centroblasts): between 6 and 15 for grade II and below, or above that range for grades I and III, respectively *(12)*. Additionally, it recognizes the entities of marginal-zone lymphoma and mantle-cell lymphoma (MCL), which originate from B-cells of the marginal zone or the mantle zone, respectively. Marginal-zone lymphomas can be divided in extranodal (mucosa-associated lymphoid tissue—lymphomas, MALT-lymphoma, or maltoma) or nodal such as monocytoid and splenic lymphomas. REAL classifies Waldenströms' macroglobulinemia as lymphoplasmacytic lymphoma, based on the appearance and biologic features of the disease. The latter three lymphomas would be classified as SLL according to the WF, based solely on their similar morphology. In the REAL classification, the term "SLL" encompasses CLL, and is reserved for a particular small-cell indolent lymphoma consisting of CLL-like cells, usually expressing CD5 and CD23. The dual meaning of the SLL can be confusing, and physicians should always indicate whether they use it with the WF or REAL connotation.

As mentioned here, the category of low-grade lymphoma is abandoned in the REAL and WHO classifications. However, it is still used to describe indolent B-cell and often T-cell lymphomas with a natural history similar to WF-low-grade lymphomas. Thus, FLs grade I and II, marginal zone lymphomas, lymphoplasma-cytic lymphomas, and SLL can be described as low-grade lymphomas, consid-ering their indolent course, which resembles that of the prototype, FSC. Additionally, cutaneous T-cell lymphomas or large granular lymphocytic (LGL) leukemias can be characterized as low-grade lymphomas, but they are usually described separately.

BIOLOGY

All low-grade lymphomas B-cell lymphomas, with the exception of a subset of SLL/CLL, are derived from lymphocytes bearing rearranged and mutated immunoglobulin genes. Therefore, they can be characterized by their unique clonal immunoglobulin—known as idiotype—which is present on the surface of the cells. This characteristic can be used for proving the clonality of a B-cell population by detecting a preponderance of kappa or lamda light-chain immunohistochemically, or by performing PCR amplification of the IgH chro-mosomal region that would show prevalence of one band corresponding to the malignant clone among a random distribution of less intense polyclonal bands of the normal B-cells.

Virtually all FLs bear the t(14:18) chromosomal translocation *(13)*. This trans-location juxtaposes the bcl-2 oncogene to the transcriptionally active immuno-globulin heavy-chain locus on chromosome 14. Breakpoints occur at two well-defined regions of the bcl-2 gene, either the major breakpoint in the major-ity of the cases: MBR: t(14:18)(q32;q21) or the minor cluster region (mcr). Although in each lymphoma the junction sequence is unique, PCR techniques have been developed using primers for the MBR and mcr sequences that are already known and a consensus sequence of the immunoglobulin gene. Such PCR techniques enable the detection of minimal residual disease, with sensitiv-ity reaching one malignant cell in 100,000 *(14)*. As a result of the translocation, bcl-2 is overexpressed, with important implications for the biology of lympho-mas. Bcl-2 belongs to a family of anti-apoptotic factors that protect cells from apoptosis by neutralizing bax, stabilizing mitochondrial membrane, and pre-venting release of cytochrome C and possibly other mechanisms *(13,15)*. Cells expressing excessive bcl-2 are protected from apoptosis and thus gain a survival advantage, which is believed to make low-grade NHL incurable with chemo-therapy *(16)*. Because of the longevity of the lymphoma cells mediated by bcl-2, additional chromosomal abnormalities may occur over time, often resulting in the assumption of aggressive behavior and morphology, a phenomenon called transformation and often characterized by *p53* mutation. It should be noted that immunohistochemical detection of bcl-2 in tumor specimens is not always a result of translocation, since overexpression can occur during the dysregulation associated with oncogenesis in other non-follicular lymphomas as well as other tumors in the absence of t(11:14).

In maltoma, t(11:18) as well as mutation of *p53*, have been characterized *(17,18)*. This translocation may be associated with expression of *H. pylori*-associated lipopolysaccharides, and may partially explain the pathogenesis of the disease. In SLL/CLL trisomy of chromosome 12 in about one-third of the cases has been reported, as well as other translocations involving chromosome 11 and 14 *(19,20)*. In addition, a large subset of SLL/CLL patients display mutations of the V region, and express CD38, factors which are believed to be associated with exposure to the germinal center and confer a better prognosis *(21)*. Identifiation of possible oncogenes associated with the observed chromosomal abnormalities may lead to the discovery of important mechanisms of cell survival, and therefore may be of prognostic or therapeutic importance.

T-cell indolent lymphomas (Table 1), lymphoplasmacytic lymphoma including Waldenström's macroglobulinemia, chronic lymphocytic leukemia (CLL), and hairy cell leukemia (HCL) have unique features and are discussed separately. The discussion here applies mostly for the remainder of the B-cell low-grade lymphomas, and predominately for the FLs.

DIAGNOSIS AND STAGING

The typical patient with low-grade lymphoma is an older adult with painless adenopathy present for several months or years. Waxing and waning of the extent of adenopathy is a well-characterized phenomenon in FLs. Transient spontaneous regressions lasting for several months or years can also occur in a minority of patients. Systemic symptoms commonly characterized as B-symptoms, such as fatigue, night sweats, and weight loss, are usually absent, although the disease is already disseminated upon diagnosis in over 80% of the patients. LDH elevation is rare, whereas involvement of the bone marrow is frequently encountered. Mild splenomegaly and anemia can be seen upon presentation. Autoimmune cytopenia is rarely noted. Less often, a relatively small monoclonal gammopathy can be seen in protein electrophoresis, with the exception of lymphoplasmacytic lymphomas, in which a significant M component of IgM can be seen. Atypical presentations of FL include small-bowel obstruction or bleeding resulting from growth in Payer's patches, presentations as skin nodules, tonsilar growth, or even as breast nodules. Lymphocytosis is common in SLL, but it can also occur less often in other types of low-grade lymphomas such as the follicular types. Splenic marginal-zone lymphomas are often associated with profound splenomegaly—

Table 1
Indolent Lymphomas of the WHO/REAL Classification

B-CELL (CD20+):	
Small lymphocytic lymphoma/CLL	CD5+, CD23+, CD20 dim
Follicular lymphoma, grade I, II	CD10+, t(14:18)
Marginal zone lymphoma	CD10−, CD5−
Nodal	
Monocytoid	
Splenic	
Extranodal	
Maltoma	
Lymphoplasmacytic	IgM secretion, CD5±, CD23−, CD20 strong
Hairy cell leukemia	CD11c, CD103
T-CELL	
Cutaneous T-cell lymphoma	CD3+, CD4+
Mycosis Fungoides	
Sézary syndrome	
T-cell granular lymphocytic leukemia	CD56+
Anaplastic large-cell lymphoma of the skin	CD30+ (Ki-1)
Lymphomatoid papulomatosis	CD30+

with or without lymphocytosis and usually without adenopathy—and bone marrow may be involved.

By definition, extranodal marginal-zone lymphomas, such as maltomas, differ in their presentation. They usually occur in epithelial tissues such as the gastric mucosa and the GI tract in general, lacrimal glands, salivary glands, thyroid, breast, lungs, or the skin. In addition to the *H. pylori* infection, it appears that chronic autoimmune inflammation such as Sjogren's syndrome and Hashimoto thyroiditis may be associated with their development *(22)*. In most cases, patients present with stage I disease, and less often with regional node involvement. The endoscopic appearance of gastric maltoma may mimic peptic ulcer, although thickening of the gastric folds, nodularity, or nonspecific abnormalities of the gastric mucosa may be present.

NHL is classically staged based on the system used for Hodgkin's lymphoma, although the pattern of extension is not always the same, and the impact of advanced stage is blunted by the fact that most patients do present with stage III and IV disease. For instance, bone-marrow involvement is present in almost all patients with SLL or lymphoplasmacytic lymphoma because of the nature of the disease, yet this is not considered an adverse factor.

The diagnosis of lymphoma should be based on the morphologic review of an adequate tissue sample, usually an excised lymph node. Fine-needle aspirates may offer a useful initial assessment of the type of malignancy, substantially aided by flow-cytometry, but it often fails to provide the exact lymphoma subtype. Clearly the architecture of the growth of lymphoma is needed for the characterization of FLs. It is imperative that the first impression based on morphology is corroborated by the appropriate immunochemical studies; the expression of markers such as CD 19, CD20, CD5, CD23, bcl-2, bcl-1, and others as indicated by the case in question is assessed. For this reason, it is recommended that part of the tissue recovered from the biopsy is stored frozen so that additional studies can be performed if necessary to further delineate the lymphoma subtype.

The staging process intends to provide information that will be potentially useful in deciding therapeutic strategies and in assessing the prognosis. The extent of adenopathy can be determined by physical examination and CT scan imaging of the chest, abdomen, and pelvis. A PET scan may be useful to detect possible occult sites and to assess the nature of borderline nodes, although the intensity of uptake is on average less than that of aggressive lymphomas. Bone-marrow aspirate and biopsy are traditionally performed, especially when mild cytopenia is present. Routine laboratory tests may be supplemented by the assessment of albumin, LDH, b-2 microglobulin, and quantitative immunoglobulins. In patients with indolent presentation, some of those tests may be omitted, since they may be treated with expectant waiting, and thus the findings of the tests may not affect the therapeutic decision.

PROGNOSIS

In general, low-grade lymphomas respond well to chemotherapy, with periods of remissions that are progressively shorter following further retreatment. The median survival is approximately 8 yr and maybe up to 10 yr for SLL *(23,24)*. The overall survival does not seem to be favorably influenced by early treatment vs delayed initiation upon occurrence of symptoms. The expected survival has not changed for patients diagnosed in the last four decades, indicating that the utilization of newer chemotherapeutics may not have had a significant impact on overall survival. However, it is important to note that survival analysis requires a long follow-up period so that the impact of therapeutics introduced in the last decade cannot be fully assessed.

The risk factors identified for patients with aggressive lymphoma (age over 60 yr, stage III or IV, LDH elevation, more than one extranodal site, and depressed performance status) have been shown to apply for low-grade lymphoma as well *(25)*. The clinical usefulness of this system is limited by the fact that the majority of patients tend to aggregate in the low-risk groups and also most patients have stage IV disease; thus, the discriminatory value of the system is poor. Other risk stratification systems that incorporate tumor bulk, male sex, B symptoms, anemia, decreased albumin, and elevation of b2 microglobulin over 3 mg/L, have been proposed with success *(26,27)*. In particular, tumor bulk is defined by different criteria by various investigators (mass >5–7 cm, more than three masses > 4 cm, bone-marrow involvement >25%) and has been consistently associated with worse outcome, as opposed to aggressive lymphoma *(28,29)*. Not surprisingly, failure to achieve a complete response to first-line chemotherapy is associated with worse outcome and a median survival of approx 2 yr, whereas a life expectancy of 13 yr has been reported for complete responders; this observation is supported by most investigators *(26,30)*. In such patients, a complete response may merely be a marker of a more favorable lymphoma biology rather than a goal by itself that should be achieved by all means. Usually, the duration of the first remission is 1.5–3 yr.

Patients with low-grade lymphoma develop resistance to chemotherapy in the later stages of the disease, often accompanied by a change in the morphology, a particularly ominous event known as transformation. *(31)*. Transformed lymphoma appears as diffuse large-cell lymphoma, although a change from FSC to follicular large-cell lymphoma may also occur. Transformation occurs in nearly one-half of the patients with FL, especially during the latter stages of the disease, but it can be observed to a lesser extent in patients with other histologies *(32)*. A transformation can be associated with *p53* mutation, bcl-2 mutation, c-myc upregulation, or additional genetic abnormalities in the context of genetic instability *(33–36)*. A transformation can be suspected when the pattern of nodal growth accelerates or when systemic symptoms or an unusual pattern of metastasis occurs. It can be proved by excisional biopsy of a suspected lymph node, although sometimes fine-needle aspiration with appropriate immunostains and microscopy (Ki67 proliferation index, *p53* staining, or a preponderance of large transformed cells) may also be useful. A transformation may be a local event involving only one nodal region. In these cases, the disease may require only local treatment and yield a better outcome, but it is more commonly disseminated and conveys a median survival of less than 1 yr. In eligible patients, high-dose chemotherapy approaches can be used, often with success *(37,38)*.

TREATMENT

Our current understanding of the treatment of low-grade lymphomas includes the assumption that local disease may be potentially curable, whereas disseminated disease remains incurable with conventional therapies other than allogeneic bone-marrow transplant (Allo-BMT). It is also generally accepted that the survival of patients with disseminated disease is not influenced by deferring the onset of therapy. Therefore, in selected patients with stage I or II disease, treatment with curative intent may be implemented upon diagnosis. In the majority of patients who present with disseminated disease, a decision should be made whether to delay treatment until morbidity develops. Treatment initiation is often a difficult decision based on many factors, including the initial life expectancy of the patient, clinical parameters of the disease (such as tumor bulk, anemia, concern regarding transformation), comorbid conditions, availability of clinical trials or alternative, non-chemotherapeutic approaches, and, naturally, a patient's own preferences. Several studies have validated the watchful waiting approach, indicating that a delay in treatment does not compromise survival or the likelihood of response *(39)*. The median time from diagnosis until initiation of treatment can be 2–3 yr, whereas one-third of the patients may not have necessitated treatment for 5 yr *(40)*. The watch-and-wait approach requires frequent patient monitoring during the first several months to determine the pace of disease growth. Patient education and participation is important for the success of this approach. Less frequent visits should provide adequate follow-up for reliable patients who understand this concept.

There is no established first-line treatment for low-grade lymphomas, and no preferred sequence of therapeutic regimens upon retreatment. This makes the decision of choosing a particular regimen more difficult *(23,41)*. A typical low-grade lymphoma patient may receive up to 10 or more treatment courses during a lifetime. Regimens of proven efficacy tend to be used first, but in latter stages palliation can be achieved by non-standardized chemotherapy administration, often with spot irradiation, tailored to the individual patient's case and the type of toxicity one would prefer to avoid. As a general rule, regimens that have caused a remission of more than 6 mo are believed to be reasonably active if repeated. It is known that the duration of remission shortens upon subsequent treatment, and eventually the disease will become resistant and life-threatening, often in the context of transformation *(42)*.

When a treatment option is chosen, the goals should be clear and the benefits should be balanced against expected toxicity, with particular attention to long-term side effects that may adversely affect the survival of a patient who is expected to live many more years. Although patients who achieve a complete response to the initial treatment have a longer survival, use of aggressive regimens or even a high-dose chemotherapy approach to force a complete response has not been clearly shown to alter life expectancy. If chemotherapy is chosen early in the disease course, the treatment usually continues for up to two cycles beyond maximum response, if tolerated. The planned number of treatment cycles, dose intensity, and the duration of cycles should be flexible and modified when excessive myelotoxicity is noted, because the ultimate goal is palliation, unlike the case of aggressive lymphomas. Consideration should be given to dose reduction of renally excreted drugs such as fludarabine in older patients, who may have a reduced glomerular filtration rate, even with a serum creatinine level within the normal range. If corticosteroids are part of the regimen, monitoring of glucose levels or watching for opportunistic infections should be more rigorous in multiply treated or older patients. Indolent lymphomas may be associated with a state of immunosuppression, exacerbated by the extent and nature of previous chemotherapy.

In recent years, non-chemotherapeutic approaches have been developed for the treatment of lymphoma. The first monoclonal antibody (MAb) approved for the treatment of a malignancy was rituximab (Rituxan, Mabthera), an anti-CD20 chimeric antibody. Its launch in December of 1997 has forever changed our approach to the treatment of cancers. Several promising agents have followed since then. It is expected that the availability of such biologic or targeted modalities may finally alter the median overall survival of the disease, but support for this hypothesis will require follow-up of currently treated patients for several more years or decades.

Surgery

Surgery has limited therapeutic value in LGL. An excisional biopsy for a lymph node is usually required for diagnosis; subsequent lymph-node excisions may be required to exclude transformation. Splenectomy is often the sole diagnostic and therapeutic procedure in patients with splenic marginal-zone lymphoma. Generally, splenectomy may be performed in cases of splenomegaly, regardless of histology, both for symptomatic control of pain or for treatment of cytopenia, particularly when chemotherapy is anticipated. Surgery was once the treatment of choice for gastrointestinal lymphoma. Although it may still be the preferred strategy for solitary lymphoma of the small bowel in cases of obstruction, gastrectomy is no longer performed for gastric maltoma, because of the success of antibiotics and radiation therapy.

Radiation

Lymphomas are radiosensitive tumors. An involved area can usually be sterilized with radiation doses less than 45 Gy. The goals of external radiation therapy for low-grade as well as aggressive lymphomas are a cure for patients with localized disease, or palliation of a problematic or refractory mass when systemic treatment is ineffective or undesirable. Common indications include the presence of a bulky mass, organ dysfunction such as hydronephrosis or cord compression, painful bone lesions, disease in the orbits, or paraspinal.

Patients with stage I or II follicular or low-grade lymphoma are usually treated with involved field or extended-field radiation (43,44). A meticulous staging is indicated in such patients to rule out the presence of distant disease. Although in the majority of these patients the incidence of PCR positivity in the blood or bone marrow is very high (45), studies have indicated that a 10-yr disease-free survival can be achieved in at least one-third of the patients. It is unclear whether a combination with chemotherapy adds to this outcome, although nonrandomized phase II studies using cyclophosphamide, doxorubicin, vincristine, and prednisone

(CHOP)-based chemotherapy have resulted in nearly double 5-yr-disease-free survival *(46)*. Because it is considered counter-intuitive that chemotherapy may cure micrometastatic disease outside the radiation ports, combined modality therapy may delay relapses, and, although acceptable, has not become the treatment of choice in indolent lymphoma.

Localized maltomas, including *H. pylori*-associated gastric maltoma, can also be successfully treated with involved-field radiation therapy.

Older techniques of total lymphoid irradiation or other types of large fields have been abandoned for lack of proven superiority as well as the increased incidence of toxicity, including malignancy and bone-marrow suppression. Preferred radiation doses range from 30–40 cGy, as compared to earlier treatments that may have exceeded 50 cG. For the same reasons, radiation of intra-abdominal of pelvic disease in the early stages of lymphomas is generally avoided for fear of myelosuppression and toxicity, with the exception of gastric maltoma.

Chemotherapy

Chemotherapy remains the mainstay of treatment of low-grade lymphomas. Classically, alkylating agents have been used for over four decades with success. Chlorambucil (0.1 to 0.2 mg/kg/d) or cyclophosphamide (1.5 to 2.5 mg/kg/d) are the preferred oral single agents. Because of the fear of leukemogenesis with continuous exposure, chlorambucil can be given in pulses of 5 d monthly or once every 2 wk (16 mg/m2). Responses are slow and may take up to 1 yr to reach maximum benefit. Therapy can continue for up to 2 yr or for 2–3 mo beyond maximum response, but it can be repeated upon subsequent relapse, preferably when remission has lasted for more than 1 yr. There is no advantage of maintenance therapy. The obvious advantage of single agents are the convenience of oral administration, lack of hair loss, and lack of acute toxicity, such as nausea or immediate myelosuppression, whereas disadvantages include slow effectiveness and risk of leukemogenesis. For this reason, they are usually preferred for older patients in no need of an immediate response. Alternatively, CVP (cyclophosphamide 400 mg/m2 orally daily × 5 d, vincristine 2 mg, prednisone 100 mg/m2 daily × 5 d) is a combination given every 3 wk with a more rapid onset of action (median onset of CR 5 mo) and a higher expected response rate (90%) *(47,48)*. Alternative CVP-like regimens have developed using intravenous (iv) cyclophosphamide on d 1 (750 mg/m2 or 1 g/m2). Our experience indicates that the regimen using 750 mg/m2 may be somewhat less effective.

It is questionable whether adding doxorubicin to CVP (CHOP or CHOP-like regimens) increases efficacy in indolent lymphoma *(49)*. In a large SWOG study involving over 400 patients, the time to progression as well as the median survival (6.9 yr) were similar to those achieved with CVP, or chlorambucil, whereas toxicity was greater. As expected, there was no survival plateau *(50)*. Although doxorubicin-containing regimen (CHOP, or variants with reduced doxorubicin does) cannot be recommended as first-line treatment for low-grade lymphoma, they may be beneficial in patients with adverse presentations, systemic symptoms, or in any case where there is a need for rapid response or suspected transformation.

Purine analogs such as fludarabine and cladribine (2-CdA) have a documented response rate of approx 50% in relapsed low-grade lymphoma, which increases up to 90% when moved up to first-line *(51,52)*. Fludarabine is given at a dose of 25 mg/m^2 daily for 5 d every 4 wk, whereas cladribine can be given either as a continuous infusion of 0.1 mg/kg/d × 7 d, or as daily intermittent dosing of 0.14 mg/kg/d over 2 h for 5 d *(53)*. Both drugs are well-tolerated without nausea or hair loss, but immunosuppression, cytopenia, and rarely hemolytic reactions are concerns. More interesting—and perhaps more popular because of their apparent increased efficacy—are fludarabine-based combination regimens. In a MD Anderson study, the combination of fludarabine (25 mg/m^2 daily × 3 d) with mitoxantrone (10 mg/m^2 on d 1) and dexamethazone (20 mg daily × 5 d) produced a remarkable 94% response rate in relapsed or refractory low-grade lymphoma *(54)*. Because of the additional immunosuppression conferred by corticosteroids that predispose to opportunistic infections, prophylaxis against PCP is mandatory. Similar regimens that omit corticosteroids seem to be comparable in efficacy with reduced risk of infection *(55)*.

Combinations of nucleoside analogs with alkylating agents appear to be very effective, yet they pose a significant risk of acute toxicity, myelosuppression, and possibly secondary leukemias. Fludarabine at doses of 20 mg/m^2 daily for 5 d has been combined with escalating doses of cyclophosphamide (600–1000 mg/m^2) in an Eastern Cooperative Oncology Group (ECOG) study—produced a response in all treated patients with a 53% FFP at 5 yr *(56)*. With some variations, the combination has been tested by other groups as effective and significantly myelosuppressive *(57–61)*. In an American intergroup study comparing such a regimen to CVP, the fludarabine-cyclophosphamide arm was discontinued because of excess mortality. A combination using fludarabine at a dose of 25 mg/m^2 and cyclophosphamide at a dose of 250 mg/m^2 daily for 3 d may be better tolerated *(60)*. When such regimens are given, dose modification and the use of growth factors are frequently required, and careful monitoring for infections is necessary.

Several other chemotherapy agents can be used when the disease is refractory to the main two classes of agents described here. Etoposide as a single, often oral, agent or in combination with other drugs (in regimens such as ESHAP), natural or synthetic vinca alkaloids, such as navelbine, taxanes, methotrexate, and others can be used with palliative intent in eligible patients, often with rewarding results. Such patients are often appropriately directed toward investigational agents, or if eligible, may be referred for autologous or allogeneic transplants.

High-Dose Chemotherapy and Transplant

Transferring the successful experience from aggressive lymphomas, high-dose chemotherapy and autologous stem-cell transplant has been studied in patients with follicular or low-grade lymphomas. Obviously, this treatment can be applied in relatively younger patients, usually less than 65 yr old. Several conclusions have been derived from extensive studies in many centers *(62–64)*. It appears that there is no survival plateau after the autologous transplants with a constant rate of delayed relapse. The disease-free survival seems to be improved compared to the expected rate based on historical controls, but the overall survival is not clearly improved. The earlier the high-dose treatment is delivered, the better the outcome in terms of disease-free and overall survival. The feasibility of in vitro purging of the collected bone marrow may reflect a less resistant form of disease, and is associated with better disease-free survival, although it is very difficult to argue that the purging itself contributed to the improved outcome *(65)*. The lack of disease-free survival plateau, as well as the clinically important incidence of delayed myelosuppression, have tempered initial enthusiasm for this approach *(66)*. Despite the limitations described here and the lack of proof of survival advantage, high-dose chemotherapy is considered an acceptable—and possibly preferabe—treatment option for patients with high-risk disease with short remission and a rapid growth pace of the lymphoma. Obviously, maximum cytoreduction—if possible, a complete response—is preferred prior to stem-cell collection and stem-cell transplant *(67)*. In vitro purging is of uncertain value, but the advent of the monoclonal antibody (MAb) rituximab enables the use of in vivo purging, whereby the administration of the antibody several weeks prior to stem-cell collection may deplete circulating B-cells and thus render the stem-cell collection tumor-free, while at the same time assisting in the treatment of the lymphoma *(68,69)*.

Classical Allo-BMT is limited by donor availability and the age of the recipient, and is associated with significant treatment-related mortality. An international bone-marrow registry analysis involving 115 patients receiving Allo-BMT for advanced or refractory indolent lymphoma, has shown a 40% treatment-related mortality and a 49% 3-yr disease-free survival, with a plateau *(70)*. Currently, Allo-BMT is the only potentially curative treatment for advanced-stage disease, and proves the principle of a beneficial graft vs lymphoma (GVL) effect.

The advent of non-myeloablative, or reduced-intensity allogeneic stem-cell transplants (Allo-SCT) overcame the excessive treatment-related mortality (TRM), and may be particularly helpful in patients with indolent malignancies such as low-grade lymphoma *(71)*. Most regimens are based on fludarabine, and the purpose is to mediate sufficient immunosuppression to prevent rejection of donor cells, which will in turn mediate a GVL effect. The procedure is very promising, since the reduction of treatment-related morbidity increases the upper age limit of eligible patients. The procedure is characterized by slow conversion to full donor hematopoietic reconstitution, which is believed to protect from a severe acute GVHD reaction. Full donor chimerism is often facilitated by delayed donor lymphocyte infusion. It is now recognized that the risk of chronic GVHD is significant, probably because of the large number of T-cells in the peripheral stem-cell harvests, the currently preferred source of hematopoietic precursors, yet the procedure is expected to further evolve in the next few years and may become a very important therapeutic option for indolent lymphomas. At UCLA, all four patients with low-grade lymphoma (thus treated) are disease free, including one patient who received allogeneic cells, with the longest survivor at 3 yr since the transplant. An update of the MD Anderson experience involving 20 patients with indolent lymphoma undergoing related nonablative allogeneic transplant confirmed the excellent outcome (72). The median age of the patients was 51 yr (oldest: 67) and most were in complete remission (CR). Only one patient developed GVHD greater than 2. No relapses were seen after a median follow-up of 21 mo, whereas the 2-yr disease-free survival was 84%. Obviously, larger experience is needed to confirm these very encouraging results.

Biologic Agents

INTERFERON

Interferon (IFN) is an FDA-approved drug for the treatment of indolent lymphoma. Single-agent activity with a response rate of 30–70% range with a duration of months to well over 1 yr has been documented (40,73,74). A European study of untreated low-risk lymphoma patients using IFN for 18 mo (5 mU daily × 3 mo followed by tiw dosing) showed a 45% CR rate and a 70% overall respobnse rate (ORR) with a median time to progression of 35 mo (40). Most toxicities are dose-dependent and include malaise, cytopenia, and depression, and combined with the inconvenience of parenteral administration, often dissuade physicians and patients from its use.

The most important contribution of IFN may be in concurrent treatment with anthracycline-containing regimens for high-risk indolent lymphomas. Two randomized studies conducted by the ECOG as well by the Group D Etudes des Lymphomes de l' Adult (GELA) involving IFN at doses of 6 mu/m² for 5 d each cycle, or 5 mU tiw respectively, and involving regimens containing adriamycin that were less intense than CHOP, documented an overall survival advantage (75,76). In the ECOG study, the COPA group (cyclophosphamide, vincristine, prednisone, and adriamycin) had a survival of 5.7 yr, which was significantly prolonged to 7.8 yr in the IFN group (75). In the GELA study, the 5-yr survival was 56.4% in the CHVP group (cyclophosphamide, doxorubicin, VM-16, and prednisone), and increased to 70.5 with the addition of IFN (76). The survival advantage of IFN was not demonstrated in large cooperative group studies using

IFN as maintenance, although prolongation of disease-free survival is suggested *(77,78)*. The discrepancy may be related to the fact that these studies did not include anthracycline-containing regimens, the use of lower doses of IFN, the use as maintenance rather than concurrently with chemotherapy or combinations of these *(79)*.

MONOCLONAL ANTIBODIES (MABS)

MAbs have provided a significant advantage in the treatment of hematologic malignancies. The use of these antibodies offers higher tumor specificity than traditional systemic treatments. Recombinant technology allows the conversion of the original antibodies produced in laboratory animals to chimeric or primatized variants, which are less immunogenic and presumably interact better with Fc receptors on immune-effector cells or complement. CD20, a 35Kd surface-membrane phosphoprotein, has become a preferred target of MAbs immunotherapy in lymphoma. CD20 is expressed specifically within the B cell lineage from the early pre-B-cell stage to the mature B-cell stage, and disappears from the cell surface upon B-cell differentiation into Ig-secreting plasma cells. Although its function is still unclear, it is believed to play a role in B-cell proliferation and differentiation during lymphocyte development.

The chimeric mouse anti-human MAb, rituximab (IDEC-C2B8), is specific for the CD20 antigen *(80)*. The mechanisms by which rituximab induces its antitumor effect are not fully understood. Tumor regression by rituximab treatment in vivo is believed to involve complement-dependent cytotoxicity (CDC), antibody-dependent cell-mediated cytotoxicity (ADCC), and not well-defined direct effects *(81,82)*. Administration of rituxan in combination with chemotherapy presumes that rituxan may exert a direct action against lymphoma cells, beyond that of ADCC or complement activation; otherwise, combination with chemotherapy would be counterintuitive *(83–86)*. Laboratory experimentation has determined that the hyper-crosslinking of CD20 using rituximab on the surface of B-cell lymphoma cell lines leads to the induction of apoptosis through traditional caspase 3-mediated mechanisms *(84,85)*. Evidence also suggests that rituximab may be involved in the downregulation of autocrine IL-10 production and consequent bcl-2 downregulation, and may promote caspase activation *(87)*.

Rituximab is an attractive alternative to chemotherapy because of its lack of myelosuppression. In the rituxan pivotal study, a response rate was observed in approximately one-half of the patients with relapsed or refractory low-grade lymphoma treated with four weekly infusions of rituximab at the dose of 375 mg/ m2, with a median duration of response of 13 mo *(88)*. This observation has been confirmed by additional studies, some involving previously untreated patients *(89–91)*. It became apparent that the response rate in patients with SLL may be lower, which correlates with the lesser density of CD20 antigen on the cell surface. Although somewhat lower responses were noted, remarkable efficacy was noted in refractory, multiply pretreated patients or those with bulky disease *(92)*. Because of its long terminal half-life, which after repeated dosing becomes similar to that of native IgG, and its unique mechanism of action (MOA), responses may continue to occur well after the last infusion. Rituximab infusion is associated with frequent infusion-related reactions such as fevers, chills, hypotension, and less commonly bronchospasm, cutaneous reactions, which are believed to be partially mediated through complement activation *(93–96)*. In rare cases, death occurs—typically in patients with circulating lymphoma, and occasionally caused by tumor lysis. The reaction is less intense with subsequent infusions and seems to be markedly blunted when given after chemotherapy pretreatment *(97)*. Delayed, unusual complications may include autoimmune phenomena such as uveitis or vasculitis *(98)*. Retreatment with rituximab can induce a new response in about 40% of previously responded patients *(99)*. Although somewhat controversial, the duration of the reported subsequent remission seems to be longer. Multiple retreatments are possible, since it appears that there is no cumulative toxicity and that despite sustained depletion of normal B-cells, there is no increase in infectious risks. A non-comparison study involving 37 patients who received eight weekly doses of rituxan suggested that although the overall response rate does not increase dramatically, the duration of remission may be longer by as much as 50% *(100)*. An administration schedule of eight weekly doses has been approved by the FDA, although the decision whether to use four or eight rituximab infusions cannot be made based on medical evidence. Customarily, the eight-weekly regimen is preferred for patients with small lymphocytic histology or relatively bulky disease. As expected, rituximab is active as first-line treatment, especially in patients with low-risk disease, with a surprisingly similar response rate to that observed in relapsed patients *(101,102)*. Maintenance treatment with rituximab every 6 mo has been proposed, with encouraging results and an observed 1-yr FFP of 77% *(103)*. The concept is undergoing randomized investigation by cooperative group studies. However, considering the relatively satisfactory retreatment results, the most important question is which strategy—i.e., retreatment upon relapse or rituximab maintenance until disease progression—will delay the inevitable emergence of resistance. The question remains unanswered at this point, and the apparent prolongation of time to progression in the maintenance studies should be seen critically.

The use of rituxan in conjunction with chemotherapy is feasible because of non-overlapping toxicities, although it is possible that it may slightly increase neutropenia *(104)*. There is a theoretical question regarding the sequence between rituximab and chemotherapy. Laboratory evidence indicates that there may be synergy between rituximab and most chemotherapeutics, and in some instances pretreatment with rituximab is required for synergy or sensitization to chemotherapy to occur *(86,105)*. The design of most clinical trials has incorporated the concept of pretreatment by one day to several weeks. However, the randomized study of CHOP vs CHOP-rituximab in patients with aggressive lymphoma by GGLA has documented a response rate and survival benefit of the chemoimmuno-therapy arm, despite concurrent administration on the same day with chemotherapy and following dexamethazone premedication *(104)*. Theoretical concerns about the use of corticosteroids, which are supposed to mediate a state of immunosuppression that may oppose ADCC-mediated rituximab efficacy, have not prevented the clinical practice of combining rituximab with corticosteroid-containing regimens such as CHOP or FND. The success of rituximab given with chemotherapy may be the result of the direct action of rituximab on cell survival pathways—thus rendering cells more susceptible to apoptosis independent of ADCC, which may in fact be synergistic with corticosteroids.

In a study of 40 mostly untreated patients with low-grade lymphoma who received a CHOP and rituximab combination, a 100% rate of CR was noted *(106)*. Most remarkably, the median time to progression was not reached after a median follow-up of over 4 yr. In this study, rituximab was given weekly twice before chemotherapy, then every other cycle while on CHOP and subsequently twice more as consolidation. As explained prevously, it has not been determined whether this is the best method to combine rituximab with chemotherapy. Other trials use rituximab with each cycle 1–2 d before chemotherapy, as well as on the same date with chemotherapy. Practical considerations—and particularly the reactions of the first infusion that may require frequent infusion halts and resumption at lower rate— often dictate the timing of the administration. Rituximab has been combined with FND, fludarabine monotherapy, CVP, IFN, IL-2, or other regimens with encouraging preliminary results *(107–110)*. In particular, the combination with IFN has been associated with prolonged duration of response by approx 50% *(111)*. In a study in which rituxan is initiated following two cycles of cyclophosphamide and mitoxantrone, the problem of first infusion reaction was not apparent, suggesting a possible alternative method of administration beginning at the third cycle of the treatment if severe infusion-related reactions are a concern *(97)*. In some trial designs, rituximab is administered as consolidation immediately following the end of chemotherapy. However, based on the in vitro evidence of synergy or sensitization between the antibody and chemotherapy, concurrent rather than sequential administration may be preferable. This is supported by a randomized study in which a higher response rate was noted in CLL patients with concurrent rather than sequential administration. In general, given its alternative nature, rituximab seems to be readily combined with all types of other modalities, including high-dose chemotherapy, radiation, or even other antibodies. Considering its ability to render blood PCR-negative for evidence of circulating lymphoma, even if this may be a compartment phenomenon, it has been used prior to stem-cell transplant in patients with B-cell lymphoma *(68,69,112)*.

Campath-1H is a chimeric antibody approved for the treatment of refractory CLL. The expected response rate in fludarabine-refractory CLL is 30–40%, with a median time to progression of 7 mo *(113,114)*. The responses are usually significantly higher in untreated patients *(115)*. Campath seems to be more active against circulating cells, which are cleared in most patients, and less so for nodal disease. The response rate in lymphomas is in the 10–20% range, although significantly higher efficacy is noted in cutaneous T-cell lymphoma such as Sézary and Mycosis fungoides (MF), as well as in prolymphocytic leukemia *(116–119)*. The target of campath is CD52 and is expressed in both B- and T- lymphocytes as well as in monocytes. Therefore, a more profound transient immunosuppression is caused by its use, resulting in higher risk for conventional as well as opportunistic infections. The established dose of campath is 30 mg IV over a period of 2 h 3× weekly for up to 12 wk. A dose-escalation phase is required with a starting dose of 2 mg and escalating to 10 mg and finally 30 mg on consecutive days if no infusion-reactions greater than grade II are noted. Prophylaxis for pneumocystis carinii and herpes simplex is necessary. There is no experience in combining campath with chemotherapy, but since campath administration is often associated with cytopenia, co-administration with chemotherapy may not be as simple as with rituximab.

Other MAbs against lymphoma are currently under investigation. Epratuzumab, an anti-CD22 antibody, has been shown to produce a response in about one-half of low-grade lymphoma patients in early studies, and is currently studied alone and in combination with rituximab *(120)*. Anti-CD22 antibodies cause internalization of the complex, which can lead to effective immunotoxins *(120)*. Antibodies against surface targets such as CD80, CD114, HLA-class II, and other antigens are currently under investigation *(121)*.

RADIOIMMUNOTHERAPY

Targeted radioimmunotherapy is feasible and effective in patients with B-cell lymphoma. Several studies have been completed involving a large number of patients with low-grade or transformed lymphoma. The most advanced approaches employ an anti-CD20 antibody. Zevalin uses the murine antibody IDEC-2B8, which is the precursor of rituximab and Y-90, a high-energy beta-emitter, as the radioactive isotope of choice. Bexxar is based on the B1 antiCD20 antibody conjugated with I-131, both a beta- and gamma-ray emitter. Both antibodies are delivered as a short iv injection preceded by an infusion of the plain antibody to optimize the distribution of radioactivity. The Zevalin dose is calculated based on radioactivity content of 0.3 to 0.4 mCi/kg, and Bexxar is given at an individualized dose calculated after dosimetry with total body counts following injection of a test dose to account for the variability of I-131 elimination, so that a total body exposure of 65–75 cGy is delivered; thyroid protection with potassium iodine is necessary *(122,123)*. The observed response rate in patients with relapsed or refractory low-grade lymphoma for both products are in the 80% range, with a median duration of response of approx 1 yr *(124–126)*. A randomized study comparing rituximab vs radioimmunotherapy with Zevalin demonstrated the higher response rate achieved by the radioactive compound, without a difference in time to progression *(127)*. The dose-limiting toxicity of radioimmunotherapy is cytopenia, and the degree depends on the amount of bone-marrow involvement by the disease. Patients with more than 25% involvement have been excluded from the studies and cannot tolerate the doses described here. Regimens tailored to such patients, often with repeated doses of smaller amounts of radiotherapy, are under development. The kinetics of bone-marrow suppression are different from the usual chemotherapy myelosuppression: the nadir of blood counts usually occurs 6–8 wk after treatment, and a gradual recovery may last several weeks or months *(128)*. Radioimmunotherapy may be useful in inducing responses in chemotherapy-refractory patients with satisfactory marrow reserves, in patients who want to avoid repetitive chemotherapy cycles and would prefer a single treatment, and in patients who are refractory to rituximab. The use of radioimmunotherapy supported by stem-cell transplant has been proposed *(129)*. Ongoing studies are investigating possible applications as consolidation following induction chemotherapy with CHOP. However, caution is needed when the treatment is administered early in the course of the disease in patients with long expected survival, until the long-term toxicity and possible role in increasing delayed myelodysplasia or leukemia are further elucidated. Zavalin was approved for the treatment of low grade, follicular or transformed B-cell NHL, in February of 2002.

Experimental Approaches

Vaccines have been proposed for the treatment of patients with FL during the past several decades. Preliminary work at Stanford with idiotype vaccines has indicated that patients capable of mounting an immune response to idiotype vaccination during remission tend to have much improved disease-free survival compared to those who do not *(130,131)*. At NCI, investigators were able to eliminate minimal residual disease in patients after idiotype vaccination *(132)*. However, the development of large quantities of idiotype is a laborious effort, significantly alleviated by techniques using PCR amplification and transduction methods, rather than the older and more cumbersome method of growing hybridomas. This promising hypothesis is currently being tested in large randomized studies, in which idiotype protein conjugated with KLH is injected subcutaneously and supported by GM-CSF administration. Methods using idiotype-pulsed dendritic cells have had remarkable results in a limited number of patients *(133)*.

Anti-sense oligonucleotides in the thioate form are relatively more stable, and are being tested in a variety of tumor types. In a study involving anti-sense for bcl-2 continuous infusion in patients with FL, in vivo downregulation of bcl-2 protein was demonstrated in about one-half of the tested patients, whereas one response among 21 patients was noted *(134)*. The apparently modest clinical efficacy of this trial is not discouraging *per se*, because bcl-2 is a rather defensive factor acting through prevention of apoptosis, so that it may facilitate chemotherapy-induced cell death. Randomized studies are currently underway, and are anxiously awaited. Protein kinase C has been another target for experimental anti-sense targeting in NHL *(135)*. Proteosome inhibitors have shown activity in multiple myeloma and excellent activity in vivo against lymphoma. The clinical activity in lymphoma is unknown, and is currently under investigation.

The development of the hybridization and gene expression analysis by microchips is expected to lead to the discovery of certain important gene targets that may lead to rational therapeutics. It is hoped that a combined multifaceted approach attacking several pathways at the same time, possibly in conjunction with apoptosis-inducing as well as immune system recruiting agents, will lead to the development of a therapeutic approach, in which low-grade lymphoma cells will be chronically suppressed, if not completely eliminated.

REFERENCES

1. National Cancer Institute sponsored study of classifications of non-Hodgkin's lymphomas: summary and description of a working formulation for clinical usage. The Non-Hodgkin's Lymphoma Pathologic Classification Project. *Cancer* 1982; 49(10):2112–2135.
2. Ries LAG, Bea MBH. SEER Cancer Statistics Review. NIH Publication No: 94–2789, Bethesda MD, US Dept of HHS, 1994.
3. Landis SH, Murray T, Bolden S, Wingo PA. Cancer statistics, 1999. *CA Cancer J Clin* 1999; 49(1):8–31, 1.
4. Isaacson PG. Gastric lymphoma and Helicobacter pylori. *N Engl J Med* 1994; 330(18): 1310–1311.
5. Cavalli F, Isaacson PG, Gascoyne RD, Zucca E. MALT Lymphomas. *Hematology* (Am Soc Hematol Educ Program) 2001;241–258.
6. Lukes RJ, Collins RD. Immunologic characterization of human malignant lymphomas. *Cancer* 1974; 34(4 Suppl):Suppl-503.
7. Nathwani BN, Kim H, Rappaport H, Solomon J, Fox M. Non-Hodgkin's lymphomas: a clinicopathologic study comparing two classifications. *Cancer* 1978; 41(1):303–325.
8. Lennert K, Stein H, Kaiserling E. Cytological and functional criteria for the classification of malignant lymphomata. *Br J Cancer* 1975; 31(Suppl 2):29–43.
9. Harris NL, Jaffe ES, Stein H, Banks PM, Chan JK, Cleary ML, et al. A revised European-American classification of lymphoid neoplasms: a proposal from the International Lymphoma Study Group. *Blood* 1994; 84(5):1361–1392.
10. Harris NL, Jaffe ES, Diebold J, Flandrin G, Muller-Hermelink HK, Vardiman J, et al. The World Health Organization classification of neoplastic diseases of the hematopoietic and lymphoid tissues. Report of the Clinical Advisory Committee meeting, Airlie House, Virginia, November, 1997. *Ann Oncol* 1999; 10(12):1419–1432.
11. Warnke RA, Kim H, Fuks Z, Dorfman RF. The coexistence of nodular and diffuse patterns in nodular non-Hodgkin's lymphomas: significance and clinicopathologic correlation. *Cancer* 1977; 40(3):1229–1233.

12. Mann RB, Berard CW. Criteria for the cytologic subclassification of follicular lymphomas: a proposed alternative method. *Hematol Oncol* 1983; 1(2):187–192.
13. Tsujimoto Y, Cossman J, Jaffe E, Croce CM. Involvement of the bcl-2 gene in human follicular lymphoma. *Science* 1985; 228(4706):1440–1443.
14. Telatar M, Grody WW, Emmanouilides C. Detection of bcl-2/IgH rearrangements by quantitative-competitive PCR and capillary electrophoresis. *Mol Diagn* 2001; 6(3):161–168.
15. Strasser A, O'Connor L, Huang DC, O'Reilly LA, Stanley ML, Bath ML, et al. Lessons from bcl-2 transgenic mice for immunology, cancer biology and cell death research. *Behring Inst Mitt* 1996;(97):101–117.
16. Reed JC. Bcl-2: prevention of apoptosis as a mechanism of drug resistance. *Hematol Oncol Clin N Am* 1995; 9(2):451–473.
17. Liu H, Ye H, Dogan A, Ranaldi R, Hamoudi RA, Bearzi I, et al. T(11;18)(q21;q21) is associated with advanced mucosa-associated lymphoid tissue lymphoma that expresses nuclear BCL10. *Blood* 2001; 98(4):1182–1187.
18. Liu H, Ruskon-Fourmestraux A, Lavergne-Slove A, Ye H, Molina T, Bouhnik Y, et al. Resistance of t(11;18) positive gastric mucosa-associated lymphoid tissue lymphoma to Helicobacter pylori eradication therapy. *Lancet* 2001; 357(9249):39–40.
19. Knuutila S, Elonen E, Teerenhovi L, Rossi L, Leskinen R, Bloomfield CD, et al. Trisomy 12 in B cells of patients with B-cell chronic lymphocytic leukemia. *N Engl J Med* 1986; 314(14):865–869.
20. Tsujimoto Y, Yunis J, Onorato-Showe L, Erikson J, Nowell PC, Croce CM. Molecular cloning of the chromosomal breakpoint of B-cell lymphomas and leukemias with the t(11;14) chromosome translocation. *Science* 1984; 224(4656):1403–1406.
21. Damle RN, Wasil T, Fais F, Ghiotto F, Valetto A, Allen SL, et al. Ig V gene mutation status and CD38 expression as novel prognostic indicators in chronic lymphocytic leukemia. *Blood* 1999; 94(6):1840–1847.
22. Royer B, Cazals-Hatem D, Sibilia J, Agbalika F, Cayuela JM, Soussi T, et al. Lymphomas in patients with Sjogren's syndrome are marginal zone B-cell neoplasms, arise in diverse extranodal and nodal sites, and are not associated with viruses. *Blood* 1997; 90(2):766–775.
23. Horning SJ. Low-grade lymphoma 1993: state of the art. *Ann Oncol* 1994; 5 (Suppl 2):23–27.
24. Morrison WH, Hoppe RT, Weiss LM, Picozzi VJ, Jr., Horning SJ. Small lymphocytic lymphoma. *J Clin Oncol* 1989; 7(5):598–606.
25. Foussard C, Desablens B, Sensebe L, Francois S, Milpied N, Deconinck E, et al. Is the International Prognostic Index for aggressive lymphomas useful for low-grade lymphoma patients? Applicability to stage III-IV patients. The GOELAMS Group, France. *Ann Oncol* 1997; 8(Suppl 1):49–52.
26. Davidge-Pitts M, Dansey R, Bezwoda WR. Prolonged survival in follicular non Hodgkins lymphoma is predicted by achievement of complete remission with initial treatment: results of a long-term study with multivariate analysis of prognostic factors. *Leuk Lymphoma* 1996; 24(1–2):131–140.
27. Denham JW, Denham E, Dear KB, Hudson GV. The follicular non-Hodgkin's lymphomas— II. Prognostic factors: what do they mean? *Eur J Cancer* 1996; 32A(3):480–490.
28. Ersboll J, Schultz HB, Pedersen-Bjergaard J, Nissen NI. Follicular low-grade non-Hodgkin's lymphoma: long-term outcome with or without tumor progression. *Eur J Haematol* 1989; 42(2):155–163.
29. Lopez-Guillermo A, Montserrat E, Bosch F, Escoda L, Terol MJ, Marin P, et al. Low-grade lymphoma: clinical and prognostic studies in a series of 143 patients from a single institution. *Leuk Lymphoma* 1994; 15(1-2):159–165.
30. Longo DL, Young RC, Hubbard SM, Wesley M, Fisher RI, Jaffe E, et al. Prolonged initial remission in patients with nodular mixed lymphoma. *Ann Intern Med* 1984; 100(5):651–656.
31. Acker B, Hoppe RT, Colby TV, Cox RS, Kaplan HS, Rosenberg SA. Histologic conversion in the non-Hodgkin's lymphomas. *J Clin Oncol* 1983; 1(1):11–16.

32. Camacho FI, Mollejo M, Mateo MS, Algara P, Navas C, Hernandez JM, et al. Progression to large B-cell lymphoma in splenic marginal zone lymphoma: a description of a series of 12 cases. *Am J Surg Pathol* 2001; 25(10):1268–1276.

33. Matolcsy A, Warnke RA, Knowles DM. Somatic mutations of the translocated bcl-2 gene are associated with morphologic transformation of follicular lymphoma to diffuse large-cell lymphoma. *Ann Oncol* 1997; 8(Suppl 2):119–122.

34. Takimoto Y, Takafuta T, Imanaka F, Kuramoto A, Sasaki N, Nanba K. Histological progression of follicular lymphoma associated with p53 mutation and rearrangement of the C-MYC gene. *Hiroshima J Med Sci* 1996; 45(2):69–73.

35. Arcinas M, Heckman CA, Mehew JW, Boxer LM. Molecular mechanisms of transcriptional control of bcl-2 and c-myc in follicular and transformed lymphoma. *Cancer Res* 2001; 61(13):5202–5206.

36. Nagy M, Balazs M, Adam Z, Petko Z, Timar B, Szereday Z, et al. Genetic instability is associated with histological transformation of follicle center lymphoma. *Leukemia* 2000; 14(12):2142–2148.

37. Chen CI, Crump M, Tsang R, Stewart AK, Keating A. Autotransplants for histologically transformed follicular non-Hodgkin's lymphoma. *Br J Haematol* 2001; 113(1):202–208.

38. Apostolidis J, Foran JM, Johnson PW, Norton A, Amess J, Matthews J, et al. Patterns of outcome following recurrence after myeloablative therapy with autologous bone marrow transplantation for follicular lymphoma. *J Clin Oncol* 1999; 17(1):216–221.

39. Portlock CS, Rosenberg SA. No initial therapy for stage III and IV non-Hodgkin's lymphomas of favorable histologic types. *Ann Intern Med* 1979; 90(1):10–13.

40. Brice P, Bastion Y, Lepage E, Brousse N, Haioun C, Moreau P, et al. Comparison in low-tumor-burden follicular lymphomas between an initial no-treatment policy, prednimustine, or interferon alfa: a randomized study from the Groupe d'Etude des Lymphomes Folliculaires. Groupe d'Etude des Lymphomes de l'Adulte. *J Clin Oncol* 1997; 15(3):1110–1117.

41. Cabanillas F, Horning S, Kaminski M, Champlin R. Managing Indolent Lymphomas in Relapse: Working Our Way Through a Plethora of Options. *Hematology* (Am Soc Hematol Educ Program) 2000;166–179.

42. Romaguera JE, McLaughlin P, North L, Dixon D, Silvermintz KB, Garnsey LA, et al. Multivariate analysis of prognostic factors in stage IV follicular low-grade lymphoma: a risk model. *J Clin Oncol* 1991; 9(5):762–769.

43. Mac Manus MP, Hoppe RT. Is radiotherapy curative for stage I and II low-grade follicular lymphoma? Results of a long-term follow-up study of patients treated at Stanford University. *J Clin Oncol* 1996; 14(4):1282-1290.

44. Wilder RB, Jones D, Tucker SL, Fuller LM, Ha CS, McLaughlin P, et al. Long-term results with radiotherapy for Stage I-II follicular lymphomas. *Int J Radiat Oncol Biol Phys* 2001; 51(5):1219–1227.

45. Lopez-Guillermo A, Cabanillas F, McDonnell TI, McLaughlin P, Smith T, Pugh W, et al. Correlation of bcl-2 rearrangement with clinical characteristics and outcome in indolent follicular lymphoma. *Blood* 1999; 93(9):3081–3087.

46. McLaughlin P, Fuller L, Redman J, Hagemeister F, Durr E, Allen P, et al. Stage I-II low-grade lymphomas: a prospective trial of combination chemotherapy and radiotherapy. *Ann Oncol* 1991; 2(Suppl 2):137–140.

47. Hoppe RT, Kushlan P, Kaplan HS, Rosenberg SA, Brown BW. The treatment of advanced stage favorable histology non-Hodgkin's lymphoma: a preliminary report of a randomized trial comparing single agent chemotherapy, combination chemotherapy, and whole body irradiation. *Blood* 1981; 58(3):592–598.

48. Portlock CS, Rosenberg SA. Combination chemotherapy with cyclophosphamide, vincristine, and prednisone in advanced non-Hodgkin's lymphomas. *Cancer* 1976; 37(3): 1275–1282.

49. Bishop JF, Wiernik PH, Wesley MN, Kaplan RS, Diggs CH, Barcos MP, et al. A randomized trial of high dose cyclophosphamide, vincristine, and prednisone plus or minus doxorubicin (CVP versus CAVP) with long-term follow-up in advanced non-Hodgkin's lymphoma. *Leukemia* 1987; 1(6):508–513.

50. Dana BW, Dahlberg S, Nathwani BN, Chase E, Coltman C, Miller TP, et al. Long-term follow-up of patients with low-grade malignant lymphomas treated with doxorubicin-based chemotherapy or chemoimmunotherapy. *J Clin Oncol* 1993; 11(4):644–651.

51. Redman JR, Cabanillas F, Velasquez WS, McLaughlin P, Hagemeister FB, Swan F, Jr., et al. Phase II trial of fludarabine phosphate in lymphoma: an effective new agent in low-grade lymphoma. *J Clin Oncol* 1992; 10(5):790–794.

52. Castaigne S. 2-Chlorodeoxyadenosine in haematological malignancies. *Nouv Rev Fr Hematol* 1993; 35(1):13–14.

53. Morton J, Taylor K, Bunce I, Eliadis P, Rentoul A, Moore D, et al. High response rates with short infusional 2-chlorodeoxyadenosine in de novo and relapsed low-grade lymphoma. Australian and New Zealand Lymphoma Study Group. *Br J Haematol* 1996; 95(1): 110–115.

54. Keating MJ, McLaughlin P, Cabanillas F. Low-grade non-Hodgkin's lymphoma—development of a new effective combination regimen (fludarabine, mitoxantrone and dexamethasone; FND). *Eur J Cancer Care* (Engl) 1997; 6(4 Suppl):21–26.

55. Emmanouilides C. Treatment of indolent lymphoma with fludarabine/mitoxantrone combination: a phase II trial. *Hematol Oncol* 1998 Sep 1916;107–116.

56. Hochster HS, Oken MM, Winter JN, Gordon LI, Raphael BG, Bennett JM, et al. Phase I study of fludarabine plus cyclophosphamide in patients with previously untreated low-grade lymphoma: results and long-term follow-up—a report from the Eastern Cooperative Oncology Group. *J Clin Oncol* 2000; 18(5):987–994.

57. Santini G, Nati S, Spriano M, Gallamini A, Pierluigi D, Congiu AM, et al. Fludarabine in combination with cyclophosphamide or with cyclophosphamide plus mitoxantrone for relapsed or refractory low-grade non-Hodgkin's lymphoma. *Haematologica* 2001; 86(3): 282–286.

58. Flinn IW, Byrd JC, Morrison C, Jamison J, Diehl LF, Murphy T, et al. Fludarabine and cyclophosphamide with filgrastim support in patients with previously untreated indolent lymphoid malignancies. *Blood* 2000; 96(1):71–75.

59. Lossos IS, Paltiel O, Polliack A. Salvage chemotherapy using a combination of fludarabine and cyclophosphamide for refractory or relapsing indolent and aggressive non-Hodgkin's lymphomas. *Leuk Lymphoma* 1999; 33(1-2):155–160.

60. Frewin R, Turner D, Tighe M, Davies S, Rule S, Johnson S. Combination therapy with fludarabine and cyclophosphamide as salvage treatment in lymphoproliferative disorders. *Br J Haematol* 1999; 104(3):612–613.

61. Lazzarino M, Orlandi E, Montillo M, Tedeschi A, Pagnucco G, Astori C, et al. Fludarabine, cyclophosphamide, and dexamethasone (FluCyD) combination is effective in pretreated low-grade non-Hodgkin's lymphoma. *Ann Oncol* 1999; 10(1):59–64.

62. Foran JM, Apostolidis J, Papamichael D, Norton AJ, Matthews J, Amess JA, et al. High-dose therapy with autologous haematopoietic support in patients with transformed follicular lymphoma: a study of 27 patients from a single centre. *Ann Oncol* 1998; 9(8):865–869.

63. Cao TM, Horning S, Negrin RS, Hu WW, Johnston LJ, Taylor TL, et al. High-dose therapy and autologous hematopoietic-cell transplantation for follicular lymphoma beyond first remission: the Stanford University experience. *Biol Blood Marrow Transplant* 2001; 7(5):294–301.

64. Horning SJ, Negrin RS, Hoppe RT, Rosenberg SA, Chao NJ, Long GD, et al. High-dose therapy and autologous bone marrow transplantation for follicular lymphoma in first complete or partial remission: results of a phase II clinical trial. *Blood* 2001; 97(2):404–409.

65. Gribben JG, Freedman AS, Neuberg D, Roy DC, Blake KW, Woo SD, et al. Immunologic purging of marrow assessed by PCR before autologous bone marrow transplantation for B-cell lymphoma. *N Engl J Med* 1991; 325(22):1525–1533.

66. Gribben JG. Stem-cell transplantation for indolent lymphoma. *Semin Hematol* 1999; 36(4 Suppl 5):18-25.

67. Freedman AS, Gribben JG, Neuberg D, Mauch P, Soiffer RJ, Anderson KC, et al. High-dose therapy and autologous bone marrow transplantation in patients with follicular lymphoma during first remission. *Blood* 1996; 88(7):2780–2786.

68. Emmanouilides C, Lill M, Rosenfelt F, Abdelkedous S, Telatar M, Grody M, et al. MINE-Rituxan Purging and In Vivo Purging in Patietns With Lymphoma. *Blood* 2001; 98(11), a3077:11–16.

69. Magni M, Di Nicola M, Devizzi L, Matteucci P, Lombardi F, Gandola L, et al. Successful in vivo purging of CD34-containing peripheral blood harvests in mantle cell and indolent lymphoma: evidence for a role of both chemotherapy and rituximab infusion. *Blood* 2000; 96(3):864–869.

70. van Besien K, Sobocinski KA, Rowlings PA, Murphy SC, Armitage JO, Bishop MR, et al. Allogeneic bone marrow transplantation for low-grade lymphoma. *Blood* 1998; 92(5):1832–1836.

71. Khouri IF, Keating M, Korbling M, Przepiorka D, Anderlini P, O'Brien S, et al. Transplant-lite: induction of graft-versus-malignancy using fludarabine- based nonablative chemotherapy and allogeneic blood progenitor-cell transplantation as treatment for lymphoid malignancies. *J Clin Oncol* 1998; 16(8):2817–2824.

72. Khouri IF, Saliba RM, Giralt SA, Lee MS, Okoroji G-J, Hagemeister FB, et al. Nonablative allogeneic hemtopoetic transplantatin as adoptive immunotherapy for indolent lymphoma: low incidence of toxicity, acute graft versus host disease, and treatment related mortality. *Blood* 2001; 98(13):3595–3599.

73. Horning SJ, Merigan TC, Krown SE, Gutterman JU, Louie A, Gallagher J, et al. Human interferon alpha in malignant lymphoma and Hodgkin's disease. Results of the American Cancer Society trial. *Cancer* 1985; 56(6):1305–1310.

74. Horning SJ. Follicular lymphoma: have we made any progress? Ann Oncol 2000; 11(Suppl 1):23–27.

75. Smalley RV, Weller E, Hawkins MJ, Oken MM, O'Connell MJ, Haase-Statz S, et al. Final analysis of the ECOG I-COPA trial (E6484) in patients with non-Hodgkin's lymphoma treated with interferon alfa (IFN-alpha2a) plus an anthracycline-based induction regimen. *Leukemia* 2001; 15(7):1118–1122.

76. Solal-Celigny P, Lepage E, Brousse N, Tendler CL, Brice P, Haioun C, et al. Doxorubicin-containing regimen with or without interferon alfa-2b for advanced follicular lymphomas: final analysis of survival and toxicity in the Groupe d'Etude des Lymphomes Folliculaires 86 *Trial. J Clin Oncol* 1998; 16(7):2332–2338.

77. Fisher RI, Dana BW, LeBlanc M, Kjeldsberg C, Forman JD, Unger JM, et al. Interferon alpha consolidation after intensive chemotherapy does not prolong the progression-free survival of patients with low-grade non-Hodgkin's lymphoma: results of the Southwest Oncology Group randomized phase III study 8809. *J Clin Oncol* 2000; 18(10):2010–2016.

78. Arranz R, Garcia-Alfonso P, Sobrino P, Zamora P, Carrion R, Garcia-Larana J, et al. Role of interferon alfa-2b in the induction and maintenance treatment of low-grade non-Hodgkin's lymphoma: results from a prospective, multicenter trial with double randomization. *J Clin Oncol* 1998; 16(4):1538–1546.

79. Allen IE, Ross SD, Borden SP, Monroe MW, Kupelnick B, Connelly JE, et al. Meta-analysis to assess the efficacy of interferon-alpha in patients with follicular non-Hodgkin's lymphoma. *J Immunother* 2001; 24(1):58–65.

80. Reff ME, Carner K, Chambers KS, Chinn PC, Leonard JE, Raab R, et al. Depletion of B cells in vivo by a chimeric mouse human monoclonal antibody to CD20. *Blood* 1994; 83(2):435–445.

81. Harjunpaa A, Junnikkala S, Meri S. Rituximab (anti-CD20) therapy of B-cell lymphomas: direct complement killing is superior to cellular effector mechanisms. *Scand J Immunol* 2000; 1951:634–641.

82. Anderson DR, Grillo-Lopez A, Varns C, Chambers KS, Hanna N. Targeted anti-cancer therapy using rituximab, a chimaeric anti-CD20 antibody (IDEC-C2B8) in the treatment of non-Hodgkin's B-cell lymphoma. *Biochem Soc Trans* 1997; 25(2):705–708.

83. Alas S, Bonavida B, Emmanouilides C. Potentiation of fludarabine cytotoxicity on non-Hodgkin's lymphoma by pentoxifylline and rituximab [In Process Citation]. *Anticancer Res* 2000; Sept–Oct 1920:2961–2966.

84. Shan D, Ledbetter JA, Press OW. Signaling events involved in anti-CD20-induced apoptosis of malignant human B cells. *Cancer Immunol Immunother* 2000; 1948:673–683.

85. Hofmeister JK, Cooney D, Coggeshall KM. Clustered CD20 induced apoptosis: src-family kinase, the proximal regulator of tyrosine phosphorylation, calcium influx, and caspase 3-dependent apoptosis. *Blood Cells Mol Dis* 2000; 1926:133–143.

86. Demidem A, Lam T, Alas S, Hariharan K, Hanna N, Bonavida B. Chimeric anti-CD20 (IDEC-C2B8) monoclonal antibody sensitizes a B cell lymphoma cell line to cell killing by cytotoxic drugs. *Cancer Biother Radiopharm* 1997; 12(3):177–186.

87. Alas S, Emmanouilides C, Bonavida B. Inhibition of interleukin 10 by rituximab results in down-regulation of bcl-2 and sensitization of B-cell non-Hodgkin's lymphoma to apoptosis. *Clin Cancer Res* 2001; 7(3):709–723.

88. McLaughlin P, Grillo-Lopez AJ, Link BK, Levy R, Czuczman MS, Williams ME, et al. Rituximab chimeric anti-CD20 monoclonal antibody therapy for relapsed indolent lymphoma: half of patients respond to a four-dose treatment program. *J Clin Oncol* 1998; 1916:2825–2833.

89. Feuring-Buske M, Kneba M, Unterhalt M, Engert A, Gramatzki M, Hiller E, et al. IDEC-C2B8 (Rituximab) anti-CD20 antibody treatment in relapsed advanced-stage follicular lymphomas: results of a phase-II study of the German Low-Grade Lymphoma Study Group. *Ann Hematol* 2000; 1979:493–500.

90. Foran JM, Gupta RK, Cunningham D, Popescu RA, Goldstone AH, Sweetenham JW, et al. A UK multicentre phase II study of rituximab (chimaeric anti-CD20 monoclonal antibody) in patients with follicular lymphoma, with PCR monitoring of molecular response. *Br J Haematol* 2000; 109:81–88.

91. Tobinai K, Kobayashi Y, Narabayashi M, Ogura M, Kagami Y, Morishima Y, et al. Feasibility and pharmacokinetic study of a chimeric anti-CD20 monoclonal antibody (IDEC-C2B8, rituximab) in relapsed B-cell lymphoma. The IDEC-C2B8 Study Group. *Ann Oncol* 1998; 1909:527–534.

92. Davis TA, White CA, Grillo-Lopez AJ, Velasquez WS, Link B, Maloney DG, et al. Single-agent monoclonal antibody efficacy in bulky non-Hodgkin's lymphoma: results of a phase II trial of rituximab. *J Clin Oncol* 1999; 1917:1851–1857.

93. Tobinai K, Kobayashi Y, Narabayashi M, Ogura M, Kagami Y, Morishima Y, et al. Feasibility and pharmacokinetic study of a chimeric anti-CD20 monoclonal antibody (IDEC-C2B8, rituximab) in relapsed B-cell lymphoma. The IDEC-C2B8 Study Group. *Ann Oncol* 1998; 9(5):527–534.

94. Dillman RO. Infusion reactions associated with the therapeutic use of monoclonal antibodies in the treatment of malignancy. *Cancer Metastasis Rev* 1999 1918;465–471.

95. Maloney DG, Liles TM, Czerwinski DK, Waldichuk C, Rosenberg J, Grillo-Lopez A, et al. Phase I clinical trial using escalating single-dose infusion of chimeric anti-CD20 monoclonal antibody (IDEC-C2B8) in patients with recurrent B-cell lymphoma. *Blood* 1994; 84(8):2457–2466.

96. Byrd JC, Waselenko JK, Maneatis TJ, Murphy T, Ward FT, Monahan BP, et al. Rituximab therapy in hematologic malignancy patients with circulating blood tumor cells: association with increased infusion-related side effects and rapid blood tumor clearance. *J Clin Oncol* 1999; 17(3):791–795.

97. Emmanouilides C, Rosen P, Telatar M, Malone R, Bosserman L, Menco H, et al. Excellent tolerance of rituximab when given after mitoxantrone/cyclophosphamide: an effective and safe combination for indolent non-Hodgkin's lymphoma. *Clin Lymphoma* 2000; 1(2): 146–151.

98. Estalilla OC, Koo CH, Brynes RK, Medeiros LJ. Intravascular large B-cell lymphoma. A report of five cases initially diagnosed by bone marrow biopsy. *Am J Clin Pathol* 1999; 112(2):248–255.

99. Davis TA, Grillo-Lopez AJ, White CA, McLaughlin P, Czuczman MS, Link BK, et al. Rituximab anti-CD20 monoclonal antibody therapy in non-Hodgkin's lymphoma: safety and efficacy of re-treatment. *J Clin Oncol* 2000; 18(17):3135–3143.

100. Piro LD, White CA, Grillo-Lopez AJ, Janakiraman N, Saven A, Beck TM, et al. Extended Rituximab (anti-CD20 monoclonal antibody) therapy for relapsed or refractory low-grade or follicular non-Hodgkin's lymphoma. *Ann Oncol* 1999; 10(6):655–661.

101. Hainsworth JD, Burris HA, III, Morrissey LH, Litchy S, Scullin DC, Jr., Bearden JD, III, et al. Rituximab monoclonal antibody as initial systemic therapy for patients with low-grade non-Hodgkin lymphoma. *Blood* 2000; 95:3052–3056.

102. Colombat P, Salles G, Brousse N, Eftekhari P, Soubeyran P, Delwail V, et al. Rituximab (anti-CD20 monoclonal antibody) as single first-line therapy for patients with follicular lymphoma with a low tumor burden: clinical and molecular evaluation. *Blood* 2001; 97:101–106.

103. Hainsworth JD. Rituximab as first-line systemic therapy for patients with low-grade lymphoma. *Semin Oncol* 2000; 27(6 Suppl 12):25–29.

104. Coiffier B, Ferme C, Hermine O, Haioun C, Baumelou E, Solal-Celigny P, et al. Rituximab plus CHOP in the treatment of elderly patietns with diffuse large B-cell lymphoma. *Blood* 2001;98(11) a3025:11–16.

105. Alas SB. Potentiation of fludarabine cytotoxicity on non-Hodgkin's lymphoma by pentoxifylline and rituximab. *Anticancer Res* 2000; 20;2961–2966.

106. Czuczman MS, Grillo-Lopez AJ, White CA, Saleh M, Gordon L, LoBuglio AF, et al. Treatment of patients with low-grade B-cell lymphoma with the combination of chimeric anti-CD20 monoclonal antibody and CHOP chemotherapy. *J Clin Oncol* 1999; 17:268–276.

107. Maloney GD. Monoclonal antibodies in lymphoid neoplasia: principles for optimal combined therapy.[In Process Citation]. *Semin Hematol* 2000; 37:17–26.

108. Cheson BD. New chemotherapeutics strategies for the treatment of indolent lymphoid malignancies. *Semin Hematol* 1999; 36:26–33.

109. McLaughlin P, Hagemeister FB, Rodriguez MA, Sarris AH, Pate O, Younes A, et al. Safety of fludarabine, mitoxantrone, and dexamethasone combined with rituximab in the treatment of stage IV indolent lymphoma. *Semin Oncol* 2000; 27(6 Suppl 12):37–41.

110. Horning JS. Investigation of monoclonal antibody therapy with conventional and high-dose treatment: current clinical trials. *Semin Hematol* 2000; 37(4 Suppl 7):27–33.

111. Sacchi S, Federico M, Vitolo U, Boccomini C, Vallisa D, Baldini L, et al. Clinical activity and safety of combination immunotherapy with IFN- alpha 2a and Rituximab in patients with relapsed low grade non-Hodgkin's lymphoma. *Haematologica* 2001; 86(9):951–958.

112. Voso MT, Pantel G, Weis M, Schmidt P, Martin S, Moos M, et al. In vivo depletion of B cells using a combination of high-dose cytosine arabinoside/mitoxantrone and rituximab for autografting in patients with non-Hodgkin's lymphoma. *Br J Haematol* 2000; 109(4): 729–735.

113. Osterborg A, Dyer MJ, Bunjes D, Pangalis GA, Bastion Y, Catovsky D, et al. Phase II multicenter study of human CD52 antibody in previously treated chronic lymphocytic leukemia. European Study Group of CAMPATH-1H Treatment in Chronic Lymphocytic Leukemia. *J Clin Oncol* 1997; 15(4):1567–1574.

114. Keating MJ. Progress in CLL, chemotherapy, antibodies and transplantation. *Biomed Pharmacother* 2001; 55(9-10):524–528.

115. Pangalis GA, Dimopoulou MN, Angelopoulou MK, Tsekouras C, Vassilakopoulos TP, Vaiopoulos G, et al. Campath-1H (anti-CD52) monoclonal antibody therapy in lymphoproliferative disorders. *Med Oncol* 2001; 18(2):99–107.

116. Lundin J, Osterborg A, Brittinger G, Crowther D, Dombret H, Engert A, et al. CAMPATH-1H monoclonal antibody in therapy for previously treated low-grade non-Hodgkin's lymphomas: a phase II multicenter study. European Study Group of CAMPATH-1H Treatment in Low-Grade Non-Hodgkin's Lymphoma. *J Clin Oncol* 1998; 16(10):3257–3263.

117. Dyer MJ. The role of CAMPATH-1 antibodies in the treatment of lymphoid malignancies. *Semin Oncol* 1999; 26(5 Suppl 14):52–57.

118. Khorana A, Bunn P, McLaughlin P, Vose J, Stewart C, Czuczman MS. A phase II multicenter study of CAMPATH-1H antibody in previously treated patients with nonbulky non-Hodgkin's lymphoma. *Leuk Lymphoma* 2001; 41(1–2):77–87.

119. Keating MJ, Cazin B, Coutre S, Birhiray R, Kovacsovics T, Langer W, et al. Campath-1H treatment of t-cell prolymphocytic leukemia in patients for whom at least one prior chemotherapy regimen has failed. *J Clin Oncol* 2002; 20(1):205–213.

120. D'Orazio AI. 37th Annual American Society of Clinical Oncology Meeting. San Francisco, CA. May 12-15, 2001. *Clin Lymphoma* 2001; 2(1):11–17.

121. Press OW, Leonard JP, Coiffier B, Levy R, Timmerman J. Immunotherapy of Non-Hodgkin's Lymphomas. *Hematology* (Am Soc Hematol Educ Program) 2001;221–240.

122. Kaminski MS, Zasadny KR, Francis IR, Fenner MC, Ross CW, Milik AW, et al. Iodine-131-anti-B1 radioimmunotherapy for B-cell lymphoma. *J Clin Oncol* 1996; 14(7):1974–1981.

123. Witzig TE, White CA, Wiseman GA, et al. Phase I/II trial of IDEC-Y2B8 radioimmunotherapy for treatment of relapsed or refractory CD20(+) B-cell non-Hodgkin's lymphoma. *J Clin Oncol* 1999; 17:3793–3803.

124. Press OW. Radiolabeled antibody therapy of B-cell lymphomas. *Semin Oncol* 1999; 26(5 Suppl 14):58–65.

125. Witzig TE. Radioimmunotherapy for patients with relapsed B-cell non-Hodgkin lymphoma. *Cancer Chemother Pharmacol* 2001; 48(Suppl 1):S91–S95.

126. Kaminski MS, Estes J, Zasadny KR, Francis IR, Ross CW, Tuck M, et al. Radioimmunotherapy with iodine (131)I tositumomab for relapsed or refractory B-cell non-Hodgkin lymphoma: updated results and long-term follow-up of the University of Michigan experience. *Blood* 2000; 96(4):1259–1266.

127. Witzig TE, Gordon LI, Cabariellas F, et al. Randomized controlled trial of Yttrium-90-labeled Ibritumomab tiuxetan radioimmunotherapy vs rituximab immunotherapy for patients with relapsed or refractory low-grade follicular or transformed B-cell non-Hodgkins lymphoma. *J Clin Oncol* 2002; 20(10):2453–2463.

128. Wiseman GA, White CA, Witzig TE, Gordon LI, Emmanouilides C, Raubitschek A, et al. Radioimmunotherapy of relapsed non-Hodgkin's lymphoma with zevalin, a 90Y-labeled anti-CD20 monoclonal antibody. *Clin Cancer Res* 1999; 5(10 Suppl):3281s–3286s.

129. Press OW, Eary JF, Gooley T, Gopal AK, Liu S, Rajendran JG, et al. A phase I/II trial of iodine-131-tositumomab (anti-CD20), etoposide, cyclophosphamide, and autologous stem cell transplantation for relapsed B-cell lymphomas. *Blood* 2000; 96(9):2934–2942.

130. Hsu FJ, Caspar CB, Czerwinski D, Kwak LW, Liles TM, Syrengelas A, et al. Tumor-specific idiotype vaccines in the treatment of patients with B-cell lymphoma—long-term results of a clinical trial. *Blood* 1997; 89(9):3129–3135.

131. Levy R. Karnofsky Lecture: immunotherapy of lymphoma. *J Clin Oncol* 1999; 17(11 Suppl):7–12.

132. Bendandi M, Gocke CD, Kobrin CB, Benko FA, Sternas LA, Pennington R, et al. Complete molecular remissions induced by patient-specific vaccination plus granulocyte-monocyte colony-stimulating factor against lymphoma. *Nat Med* 1999; 5(10):1171–1177.

133. Timmerman JM, Levy R. Dendritic cell vaccines for cancer immunotherapy. *Annu Rev Med* 1999; 50:507–529.

134. Waters JS, Webb A, Cunningham D, Clarke PA, Raynaud F, di Stefano F, et al. Phase I clinical and pharmacokinetic study of bcl-2 antisense oligonucleotide therapy in patients with non-Hodgkin's lymphoma. *J Clin Oncol* 2000; 18(9):1812–1823.

135. Emmanouilides C, Saleh A, Laufman L, et al. Phase II trial of the efficacy and afety of 151 5 3521/LY 900003, an antisense inbibitor of PKC-alpha, in patients with low grade, non-Hodgkins lymphoma. *ASCO* 2002; abstract.

11 Aggressive Large-Cell Lymphomas

R. Gregory Bociek, MD
and James O. Armitage, MD

INTRODUCTION

Aggressive large-cell lymphomas (diffuse large B-cell lymphoma, peripheral T-cell lymphoma, and systemic anaplastic large-cell lymphoma) account for approximately 30%, 6%, and 2% of newly diagnosed non-Hodgkin's lymphomas, respectively *(1)*. Although they are clearly different diseases biologically, these illnesses share a number of clinical characteristics. The epidemiology, pathogenesis/biology, diagnosis, and treatment of these disorders is discussed in this chapter.

TRENDS IN THE INCIDENCE/EPIDEMIOLOGY
OF NON-HODGKIN'S LYMPHOMAS

Non-Hodgkin's lymphomas collectively remain the sixth and fifth most common malignancy in men and women respectively *(2)*, with a projected incidence

From: *Current Clinical Oncology: Chronic Leukemias and Lymphomas:*
Biology, Pathophysiology, and Clinical Management
Edited by: G. J. Schiller © Humana Press Inc., Totowa, NJ

Table 1
Factors Associated with the Development of Non-Hodgkin's Lymphomas

Immunodeficiency states
    Congenital
        Severe combined immunodeficiency
        Common variable immunodeficiency
        Wiskott-Aldrich syndrome
        Ataxia-telangiectasia
    Acquired
        HIV infection
        Solid organ transplantation
        High-dose chemotherapy with stem-cell transplantation
Infectious agents
    Helicobacter pylori
    Human T-Cell leukemia virus-1 (HTLV-1)
    Epstein-Barr virus
Physical/chemical agents
    Prior chemotherapy exposure
    Prior radiotherapy exposure
    Herbicides

of roughly 61,000 new cases in 2002. Non-Hodgkin's lymphoma also remains the fifth leading cause of cancer death in males of all ages, and in females over the age of 80 *(2)*. Age-adjusted incidence rates for this illness have clearly been on the rise for the last three decades *(2,3)*, for reasons largely unexplained, since lymphomas related to Human Immunodeficiency Virus (HIV) infection *(4)* and those associated with post-transplant immunosuppressive states *(5,6)* appear to account for only a small proportion of the increased number of cases. Recent 5-yr overall survival rates appear to be slightly better when compared to the 1970s *(2)*.

Diffuse large B-cell lymphoma is the most common form of non-Hodgkin's lymphoma diagnosed in the United States, accounting for approximately one-third of cases *(7)*. Like most forms of non-Hodgkin's lymphoma, its age-adjusted incidence rate has climbed steadily, and nearly doubled from 2.8 cases per 100,000 in 1980 to 4.9 cases per 100,000 in 1997 *(7)*. Long-term trends in anaplastic large-cell lymphoma and peripheral T-cell lymphoma have not been documented, because both illnesses are comparatively rare and are more newly recognized entities. It is likely that anaplastic large-cell lymphoma will become diagnosed more frequently over time as its features become more widely recognized.

ETIOLOGIC FACTORS IN NON-HODGKIN'S LYMPHOMAS

Factors that have long been implicated in the pathogenesis of non-Hodgkin's lymphomas are shown in Table 1 and include congenital or acquired immuno-deficiency states, exposure to certain physical agents or ionizing radiation, and certain infectious agents. Infection with human T-lymphotropic virus 1 (HTLV-1) appears to be the cause of the adult T-cell leukemia/lymphoma that is endemic to parts of Japan and the Caribbean. Viral infection (and reactivation), particularly with Epstein-Barr virus (EBV), remains a possible cofactor in the development of *de novo* non-Hodgkin's lymphomas in immunocompetent individuals, although its has been most fully studied and elucidated in endemic Burkitt's lymphoma *(8)* and in post-transplant-associated lymphoproliferative disorders *(9,10)*. Recent observations on human herpesvirus-8 (HHV-8) add further strength to virally mediated hypotheses. HHV-8 was initially found in Kaposi's sarcoma tissue of patients with HIV infection *(11)*, but has more recently been identified in primary body-cavity lymphomas, generally in patients who also have HIV infection. In one study, HHV-8 was present in 15 of 19 cases, (all male), and 13 of those 15 were also infected with HIV *(4)*. The presence of HHV-8 has also been associated with multicentric Castleman's disease in both HIV-positive and HIV-negative patients, although the association between HHV-8 and multicentric Castleman's disease appears to be stronger for individuals infected with HIV *(12)*. A functional role for HHV-8 in the pathogenesis of these illnesses has not yet been demonstrated. It is possible that viruses act as stimulatory cofactors, which cause excess lymphocytic stimulation and proliferation and eventually lead to an oncogenic mutational event and subsequent uncontrolled growth of a single cell.

PATHOLOGIC CLASSIFICATION OF NON-HODGKIN'S LYMPHOMAS

The classification of non-Hodgkin's lymphoma continues to evolve and change over time. Previous classification schemes have included the Rapaport, Lukes-Collins, and Working Formulation (WF) classifications *(13–15)*. The Rapaport classification separated entities on the basis of a nodular or diffuse lymph-node architecture, and on the appearance of the individual malignant cells (well-differentiated vs poorly differentiated). The WF classification of non-Hodgkin's lymphomas was developed by the National Cancer Institute (NCI) in 1982 in an attempt to further standardize terminology and derive prognostic information in non-Hodgkin's lymphomas. In this classification scheme, lymphomas were classified principally on the basis of the architecture of the growth pattern within malignant nodes (i.e., a follicular vs diffuse pattern), and on the size of the predominant malignant cell (small cleaved vs large non-cleaved vs mixed populations). By its very nature, this classification scheme was subject to a certain degree of inter- and intra-observer variability *(16)*, but was both relatively simple and clinically functional because it relied solely on morphologic characteristics, was reproducible, and identified three reasonably distinct groups of lymphomas (low-grade, intermediate-grade, and high-grade) based on their biology and natural history. Treatment patterns were largely based on stage and biologic grade (based on the three subgroups), recognizing that within each group the illnesses were still distinct entities to some degree.

The illness now known as diffuse, large B-cell lymphoma in the World Health Organization/Revised European/American Lymphoma (REAL/WHO) Classifications *(17,18)* incorporates certain Working Formula entities (e.g., immunoblastic lymphoma, diffuse mixed small- and large-cell lymphoma), which are no longer part of present-day classification schemes.

The discovery of unique subtypes of non-Hodgkin's lymphoma that were not part of earlier classification schemes (e.g., mantle cell lymphoma [MCL], anaplastic large-cell lymphoma, peripheral T-cell lymphoma) in part drove the need for a revised lymphoma classification. Present-day schemes have shifted from the use of purely morphologic criteria such as those used by the Rapaport system *(13)* or the NCI's Working Formulation (WF) *(15)* to those that reflect an increase in present-day technological capabilities as well as the understanding of more subtle aspects of lymphocyte ontogeny and biology. This includes the use of cytogenetic testing to detect the presence or absence of characteristic chromosomal abnormalities, polymerase chain reaction (PCR) to detect the presence of characteristic gene rearrangements, and the ability to accurately determine the presence of both clonality and the immunophenotype of malignant lymphocytes using techniques such as flow cytometry.

PATHOLOGY OF DIFFUSE LARGE B-CELL LYMPHOMA, PERIPHERAL T-CELL LYMPHOMA, AND ANAPLASTIC LARGE-CELL LYMPHOMA

Diffuse Large B-Cell Lymphoma

Diffuse large B-cell lymphomas are characteristically composed of large cells that morphologically resemble centroblasts or immunoblasts. The cells have vesicular nuclei, prominent nucleoli, and a moderate-to-high proliferation fraction *(18)*. Other cells seen in association with the large cells may include large cleaved cells *(19)*, and anaplastic large cells identical to those seen in anaplastic large-cell lymphoma*(18)* This lymphoma may also occasionally resemble lymphocyte-predominant Hodgkin's disease morphologically. The cells often express surface immunoglobulin, and common B-cell antigens (e.g., CD19, 20, 22, CD45), and are usually CD5- and CD10-negative *(18)*. Diffuse large B-cell lymphoma lacks a unifying cytogenetic abnormality, although the t(14;18) bcl-2 gene rearrangement is seen in a proportion of cases *(20)*. Molecular rearrangements for bcl-6 and the c-myc/immunoglobulin heavy-chain fusion gene have also been reported in this subtype of non-Hodgkin's lymphoma *(21)*.

Anaplastic Large-Cell Lymphoma

Anaplastic large-cell lymphoma was not a recognized histologic entity in the WF classification, although morphologically it would have fallen under the subtype of immunoblastic lymphoma. It was first described as regressing atypical histiocytosis in 1982 by Flynn and colleagues *(22)*. Since this tumor stained with the antibody for the Hodgkin's associated antigen Ki-1 (for Kiel-1, now known as CD30), other terms associated with this malignancy included Ki-1 lymphoma, lymphocyte-depleted Hodgkin's disease, and Hodgkin's sarcoma. This illness is notable because it is often misdiagnosed as an anaplastic carcinoma or undifferentiated neoplasm as a result of its morphologic appearance and the expression of epithelial membrane antigen *(23)*. Although a number of lymphomas stain positive for CD30 *(24)*, only anaplastic large-cell lymphoma has the characteristic anaplastic large cells, and associated t(2;5) chromosomal abnormality *(25)*. Histologically, the tumor is composed of large anaplastic cells with pleomorphic nuclei, which may be horseshoe-shaped. Generally, the cells are larger than those seen in diffuse large B-cell lymphoma, and may contain multiple nuclei and often multiple nucleoli. Multinucleated cells may appear similar to the Hodgkin's-Reed-Sternberg cell. The majority of cells display T-cell surface antigens; however, some express B-cell antigens, and some do not express B- nor T-associated antigens (the so-called null-cell phenotype) *(18)*. Immunopheno-typically, the cells usually express CD30, and are variably positive for CD45, CD25, CD15, CD3, and other T-cell antigens *(18)*. Fifty to sixty percent of cases display T-cell receptor gene rearrangement, and the remainder show no evidence of T-cell-receptor or immunoglobulin gene rearrangements *(26,27)*.

The (2;5) translocation seen in anaplastic large-cell lymphoma results in the fusion of part of the nucleophosmin gene (NPM) on chromosome 5 with the anaplastic lymphoma kinase (ALK) gene, a receptor tyrosine kinase gene on chromosome 2. The resulting fusion protein is known as the NPM-ALK protein. Normal lymphoid cells do not express ALK protein, and as a result, the demonstration of an immunohistochemical reaction to the ALK protein is highly specific for the (2;5) translocation. The introduction of the NPM-ALK gene into murine hematopoietic cells leads to the development of a transplantable large-cell lymphoma *(28)*, suggesting that the translocation may be functionally associated with the development of this lymphoma in humans as well.

A review of 123 cases of lymphomas expressing the ALK protein, CD30, epithelial-membrane antigen, and lacking B-cell markers described by Benharroch et al. *(23)* revealed that ALK-positive lymphomas display a broad spectrum of morphologic features, ranging from small-cell tumors to those with the classic anaplastic large-cell description. All cases examined contained a particular cell with an eccentrically placed horseshoe- or kidney-shaped nucleus, and this was considered to be the unifying feature of all ALK-positive tumors in this series. Slightly more than 50% expressed T-cell lineage, but none expressed B-cell lineage. Immunophenotypic data from a study of 33 anaplastic large-cell lymphomas by Krenacs and colleagues *(29)* suggests that more than 50% of these tumors originate from lymphocytes with cytotoxic potential.

At the present time, a single gold standard pathologic definition for this disease does not exist. The WHO classification has proposed that the diagnosis requires consideration of both morphology and immunophenotype. Present recommendations are to use this term for cases with typical morphology and immunophenotype, classifying them further as ALK-positive or negative.

Peripheral T-Cell Lymphoma

This illness is referred to as peripheral T-cell lymphoma, unspecified in the REAL classification and as peripheral T-cell lymphoma, not otherwise characterized in the WHO classification. In the WF, this entity would most likely have been classified as either diffuse small cleaved cell, diffuse mixed small cleaved and large-cell, or large-cell immunoblastic lymphoma. As this is still a relatively rare subtype of non-Hodgkin's lymphoma, it remains difficult to fully understand and classify. The proposed WHO classification has not subclassified this disease, since there do not appear to be clearly defined patterns of immunophenotype or T-cell-receptor rearrangements that would assist in further subclassification. Clinical syndromes (e.g., nodal vs extranodal presentations) may be essential to further subclassification of this entity in future studies. This illness is characterized pathologically by a heterogeneous morphology, with mixed populations of small and large cells. The neoplastic cells often have irregular nuclei, and occasionally very large cells resembling Hodgkin's/Reed-Sternberg cells may be seen *(18)*. The immunophenotype is variable, but cells may be positive for CD2, CD3, CD5, and CD7. They may be CD4- and CD8-positive or -negative. B-cell antigens are absent. T-cell-receptor genes are usually rearranged *(18)*. The postulated normal counterpart to this malignancy is the T-cell in various stages of maturation. Cytogenetic analysis has demonstrated that chromosomal abnormalities are quite frequent in this illness *(30)*, although no characteristic abnormality has been described with any frequency.

CLINICAL FEATURES OF LARGE-CELL LYMPHOMAS

Clinical Features of Diffuse Large B-Cell Lymphoma

Patients with diffuse large B-cell lymphoma generally present with either superficial lymph-node masses, symptoms caused by local lymphadenopathy (e.g., abdominal pain, dysphagia, dyspnea) or constitutional symptoms such as fever, weight loss, or night sweats. Lymph-node masses are generally characterized by patients as having a fairly rapid growth rate, and extranodal involvement may be observed in organs such as bone/bone marrow, stomach, liver, spleen, testes, thyroid, and kidney.

The entity known as primary mediastinal (thymic) large B-cell lymphoma usually involves the thymus at diagnosis, and thymic B-lymphocytes are the presumed normal counterpart to the malignant cells. This clinical presentation appears to be somewhat more common in young females, and symptoms and signs are likely to be related to the presence of a large, bulky anterior mediastinal mass (e.g., superior vena cava obstruction or cardiac tamponade). Patients may have associated B symptoms, and may occasionally present with associated pleural/pericardial effusions (31). A case of primary mediastinal large B-cell lymphoma in a young male has been reported with aberrant expression of β-HCG (32). Although likely rare, the obvious implication is the possible mis-diagnosis of a germ-cell tumor in this clinical situation. This tumor may be associated with extranodal involvement at sites other than bone marrow, including the central nervous system (CNS) (33) and intra-abdominal organs (31). The International Prognostic Index (34) has been demonstrated to have predictive significance for this illness, similar to that of diffuse large B-cell lymphoma (35). Two retrospective analyses comparing clinical outcomes in primary mediastinal large B-cell lymphoma with diffuse large B-cell lymphoma have been conducted. The first, conducted by the Groupe d'Etude des Lymphomes de l'Adulte (GELA) (36) reviewed 141 cases of primary mediastinal large B-cell lymphoma, and compared outcomes with 916 cases of nonmediastinal diffuse large B-cell lymphoma. Although there were some differences in patterns of extranodal involvement, a stratified analysis using the International Prognostic Index demonstrated no difference in disease-free or overall survival between the two groups. A smaller comparative study by the Nebraska Lymphoma Study Group (35) similarly demonstrated similar outcomes between mediastinal and nonmediastinal presentations with respect to failure-free and overall survival.

In summary, although primary mediastinal large B-cell lymphoma is a recognizably distinct clinicopathologic entity, its clinical behavior appears to be the same as that of nonmediastinal large B-cell lymphomas, and thus should be treated with the same underlying therapeutic principles as those for nonmediastinal presentations of diffuse large B-cell lymphoma.

Clinical Features of Anaplastic Large-Cell Lymphoma

Anaplastic large-cell lymphoma shares many features in common with diffuse large B-cell lymphoma. This illness generally presents with nodal involvement, although reported extranodal sites of involvement have included skin, bone, bone marrow, meninges, pleura, and muscle (37,38). Primary CNS involvement in this disease is extremely rare (39). A series describing 96 cases of anaplastic large-cell lymphoma by Falini et al. *(40)* observed that the tumor appears to be more common in the first three decades of life, with a male:female ratio of 3:1. Seventy-two percent of patients presented with advanced disease, and 75% had constitutional symptoms (fever/weight loss) at diagnosis. Sixty percent of patients had extranodal disease, and skin, bone, bone marrow, and soft tissue were the most common sites. On average, ALK-negative cases appeared to be older and had fewer extranodal sites of disease. ALK-positive patients had a higher complete remission (CR) rate (77% vs 56%) and better overall survival compared to ALK-negative cases (71% vs 15% at 9 yr, $p = 0.0007$). In the ALK-positive cases, use of the age-adjusted International Prognostic Index identified a group of patients with an extremely good prognosis (0–1 risk factors; 5-yr overall survival 94%) as compared with cases with ≥ 2 risk factors (5-yr overall survival 41%). Multivariate analysis identified both ALK positivity and International Prognostic Index age-adjusted score as having independent predictive value for survival.

Clinical Features of Peripheral T-Cell Lymphoma

Peripheral T-cell lymphomas are relatively rare in the United States, accounting for only 6% of all non-Hodgkin's lymphoma in one series *(1)*. The illness often presents with constitutional symptoms, elevated LDH, and sites of bulky disease *(1)*. Extranodal sites of disease are common, and unusual sites such as the prostate *(41)* and testicles *(42)*, have been reported. This disease often presents in an advanced stage at diagnosis *(1,43)* and a report by Ansell et al. suggests that the International Prognostic Index has significant prognostic value in this illness *(44)*. At least two retrospective analyses have compared outcomes in patients with peripheral T-cell lymphomas, as compared with aggressive B-cell lymphomas. A report from MD Anderson *(45)* evaluated six trials of front-line chemotherapy for aggressive lymphomas conducted between 1984 and 1995, examining the relative prognostic effects of immunophenotype. A total of 492 cases had immunophenotyping data available. Sixty-eight cases met the histopathologic criteria for peripheral T-cell lymphoma. As compared with patients with B-cell immunophenotype demonstrated inferior outcomes for patients independent of both International Prognostic Index and MD Anderson prognostic tumor score. A subset of T-cell lymphoma patients ($n = 10$) with anaplastic large-cell lymphoma appeared to demonstrate a trend toward superior overall survival relative to the other subtypes of T-cell lymphoma. Similarly, a report from the GELA *(46)* compared outcomes of 288 patients with peripheral T-cell lymphomas to 1595 patients with aggressive B-cell lymphomas. Unadjusted CR rates, 5-yr overall, and event-free survival (EFS) were all superior in the subset of patients with B-cell immunophenotype. Five-year overall survival was superior in the subset of T-cell lymphoma patients with anaplastic large-cell lymphoma (64%) as compared with both other peripheral T-cell subtypes (35%) and diffuse large B-cell lymphoma (53%). Finally, multivariate analysis demonstrated that non-anaplastic T-cell immunophenotype had a poorer 5-yr survival compared with diffuse large B-cell lymphoma, independent of International Prognostic Index scores. Therefore, although this disease appears to be curable in a proportion of patients, its prognosis appears to be poorer in comparison with diffuse large B-cell lymphoma independent of the presence or absence of other known prognostic factors.

STAGING AND PROGNOSTIC FACTORS

Staging for these illnesses should employ the usual tests used to stage most patients with non-Hodgkin's lymphoma. A complete history and physical exam should be performed, including an evaluation of possible risk factors (including risk factors for HIV infection), concentrating especially on symptoms and signs that could alter subsequent investigations or management (e.g., pain in a weight-bearing bone, GI symptomatology, or neurologic manifestations). The history and physical exam should be complemented with a complete blood count, serum chemistries (renal and hepatic function panels) including lactate dehydrogenase (LDH). Imaging studies should include posteroanterior chest radiographs or CT scan of the chest, as well as CT scans of the abdomen and pelvis. Bone-marrow aspiration and biopsy should be performed in virtually all patients to complete staging. Patients with involvement of Waldeyer's ring should have additional GI imaging studies performed. Patients with involvement of the nasopharynx, paranasal sr®uses, orbit, paraspinal masses, or testicular lymphoma should undergo diagnostic lumbar puncture to rule out CNS involvement, and consideration should be given to the use of CNS prophylaxis in these patients *(47,48)*. Sites of disease not detectable by physical examination should be re-imaged partly through treatment to ensure an appropriate response to therapy, and all areas of known disease (including bone marrow if positive at diagnosis) should be re-evaluated at the completion of therapy to ensure the patient has achieved a CR. Clinicians should also become familiar with the new international response criteria for evaluating non-Hodgkin's lymphoma, published recently by Cheson et al. *(49)* (Table 2).

The use of prognostic factors in aggressive lymphomas is principally to help identify those patients likely to be cured with conventional therapy, and conversely, to help identify patients who are unlikely to be cured with front-line conventional therapy, in whom strong consideration for enrollment in novel clinical trials should be given. The most popular internally validated study of prognostic factors was published by the International Non-Hodgkin's Lymphoma Prognostic Factors Project in 1993 *(34)*. This study examined clinical presentations and prognostic factors in 3273 patients diagnosed with aggressive non-Hodgkin's lymphomas (WF classifications F-H). Seven prognostic factors were chosen as likely to be most relevant, based on previous studies of prognostic factors. From among 1872 cases in whom complete information on all of these

Table 2
Response Criteria for Non-Hodgkin's Lymphoma

Complete Response (CR)

1. Complete disappearance of all detectable clinical and radiographic evidence of disease, disappearance of all disease-related symptoms if present before therapy, and normalization of any biochemical abnormalities definitely assignable to lymphoma.
2. All lymph nodes and nodal masses ≤1.5 cm in greatest transverse diameter for nodes greater than 1.5 cm before therapy. Previously involved nodes that were 1.1–1.5 cm in their greatest transverse diameter before treatment must be ≤1 cm in their greatest transverse diameter after treatment, or have decreased by more than 75% using the sum of the products of their greatest diameters (SPD).
3. The spleen or any other organ considered to be enlarged before therapy because of the involvement of lymphoma must have decreased in size and must not be palpable on physical examination. Any macroscopic nodules detected in any organs on imaging techniques should no longer be present.
4. The bone-marrow biopsy and aspirate must be negative for disease if involved at study entry.

Complete Response/Unconfirmed (CRu)

This includes patients who fulfill criteria 1 and 3 of the complete response, but with one or more of the following features:
1. A residual lymph node mass >1.5 cm in greatest transverse diameter that has regressed by more than 75% in the SPD. Individual nodes that were previously confluent must have regressed by more than 75% in their SPD compared with the size of the original mass.
2. Indeterminate bone marrow (increase number or size of aggregates without cytologic or architectural atypia).

Partial Response (PR)

1. A decrease in SPD of ≥50% for the six largest dominant nodes or nodal masses.
2. No increase in the size of the other nodes, liver, or spleen.
3. Splenic and hepatic nodules must regress by at least 50% in the SPD.
4. With the exception of splenic and hepatic nodules, involvement of other organs is considered assessable and not measurable disease.
5. No new sites of disease.

Stable Disease (SD)

This is defined as less than a PR but not progressive disease.

Relapsed Disease (RD)

1. Appearance of any new lesion or increase of ≥50% in the size of the previously involved sites (only applies to patients that achieve a CR or CRu). The new lesion must be >1.5 cm by radiographic evaluation or >1 cm by physical examination.
2. An increase ≥50% in greatest diameter of any previously identified node greater than 1 cm in its shortest axis or in the SPD of more than one node.

Progressive Disease (PD)

1. An increase of ≥25% from nadir in the SPD of any previously identified abnormal node for PRs or nonresponders.
2. The appearance of any new lesion during or at the end of therapy that is >1.5 cm by radiographic evaluation or >1 cm by physical examination.

seven prognostic factors was available, a larger training sample and smaller validation sample were randomly chosen. A step-down regression analysis was performed first on the training sample, and subsequently the validation sample. The analysis identified five dichotomous factors as having independent prognostic significance. These were age ($\leq$60 yr vs >60 yr), Ann Arbor stage (I or II vs III or IV), number of extranodal sites ($\leq$1 vs >1), performance status (0–1 vs $\geq$2), and serum LDH level ($\leq$ normal vs >normal). Each of these factors was associated with an approximately twofold increase in risk of death, and as such it was believed that a cumulative score could be devised to estimate the probability of survival for an individual patient based on the number of risk factors. Five risk groups were identified, referred to as low-risk (0–1 risk factors), low intermediate risk (two risk factors), high intermediate risk (3 risk factors), and high-risk (4 or 5 risk factors). The 5-yr probability of survival for each of these four risk groups was 73%, 51%, 43%, and 26%, respectively. An age-adjusted index was also developed for patients $\leq$60 yr of age, using stage, LDH level, and performance status to identify four risk groups based on 0–3 adverse risk factors. These subgroups had 5-yr survival rates of 83%, 69%, 46%, and 32%, respectively. The major use of this prognostic index presently should be for the identification of high-risk patients unlikely to be cured with anthracycline-based chemotherapy alone, in whom a search for novel clinical trials should be carried out.

TREATMENT OF LARGE-CELL LYMPHOMAS

Primary Therapy

EARLY-STAGE DISEASE

Prior to the advent of modern-day combination chemotherapy regimens, patients with early-stage disease (stage I and II) were treated with radiotherapy alone. The outcomes for these patients depended in part on the accuracy and extent of staging. A restrospective analysis by Kaminski and colleagues (50) looking at outcomes in patients treated with radiotherapy for Ann Arbor stage I and II large-cell lymphoma observed a 25% 5-yr probability of freedom from relapse for patients who received radiotherapy to one side of the diaphragm. For patients who received radiotherapy to both sides of the diaphragm, the probability of freedom from relapse was 67%. A study from the University of Chicago reported on 36 patients with pathologically staged diffuse aggressive lymphoma between 1970 and 1986 (51). Therapy consisted of extended-field radiation in 27 patients and involved field in nine patients. The median tumor dose was 50 gy. Actuarial 10-yr relapse-free survival was 91% and 35% for stage I and stage II patients, respectively. Sites of failure were commonly outside of treatment fields or in sites of bulky disease. The outcome of patients with early-stage disease treated solely with radiotherapy thus appears to depend on the determination of staging (i.e., laparotomy staged vs clinically staged), the presence of adverse risk factors such as bulky disease, and the size of the radiation field (involved field vs extended field vs total nodal irradiation).

The discovery and development of cytotoxic drugs led to the design of what would eventually become several "generations" of combination chemotherapy regimens designed to treat non-Hodgkin's lymphomas. The recognition of high failure rates for radiotherapy in patients with bulky disease and the availability of systemic therapy plus the potential morbidity of staging laparotomies led investigators to begin using clinical staging procedures and to treat patients with combined modality regimens. Chemotherapy regimens were generally designed to take advantage of additive/synergistic anticancer effects of multiple active drugs, while attempting to maintain safe non-overlapping toxicity profiles between agents.

A publication from Longo et al. at the National Cancer Institute (NCI) reported on the use of four cycles of combination chemotherapy followed by 40 gy involved-field radiation therapy in 47 clinically staged patients with aggressive non-Hodgkin's lymphoma (52). Systemic therapy consisted of the ProMACE-MOPP regimen (prednisone, methotrexate, doxorubicin, cyclophosphamide, etoposide, nitrogen mustard, vincristine, and procarbazine) (53). There was no treatment-related mortality (TRM), and complete remissions were seen in 45 patients (96%). With a median follow-up duration of 42 mo, no complete responders had relapsed at the time of publication. A similar study by Jones et al. (54) looked retrospectively at the outcome of treatment with CHOP (cyclophosphamide, doxorubicin, vincristine, and prednisone) (55) with or without the use of involved-field radiotherapy after chemotherapy in 142 patients with diffuse large-cell lymphoma treated on protocols at the University of Arizona and University of British Columbia. The number of cycles of CHOP varied between two and eight. Patients who received radiotherapy were treated with doses ranging from 30 to 60 gy. One hundred forty patients achieved complete remission (99%), and actuarial relapse-free survival at 5 yr was 82%. There was no TRM, and no late toxicity with respect to acute leukemias or cardiac events. Relapse-free survival was not statistically significantly different comparing chemotherapy only (34 patients) with combined modality therapy (108 patients, $p = 0.2$), although the lack of randomization, lack of multivariate analysis, and small number of chemotherapy-only patients may have hindered any ability to demonstrate a difference between these two treatment approaches.

A randomized trial by Nissen (56) compared extended-field radiotherapy alone to radiotherapy plus adjuvant chemotherapy in 73 patients with clinical stage I or II non-Hodgkin's lymphoma. Chemotherapy consisted of vincristine, streptonigrin, cyclophosphamide, and prednisone. With a median follow-up of 5 yr, only 10% of patients in the combined modality arm had relapsed compared with 54% of patients randomized to receive radiotherapy only ($p < 0.01$). No difference in overall survival was seen; however, a trend toward improved survival was noted in favor of the combined modality arm.

A more recently published randomized trial by Miller et al. *(57)* clearly demonstrated an advantage for combined-modality therapy in early-stage disease. In this trial, 401 patients with clinical stage I, IE, or non-bulky stage II or II E disease (defined as no tumor masses ≥10 cm) were randomized to either eight cycles of CHOP or to three cycles of CHOP followed by involved-field radiotherapy (with doses in the range of 40 to 55 gy). The median age was 59 yr, and 75% of patients had diffuse large-cell lymphoma. Patients were well-balanced for prognostic factors. Two-thirds of patients had stage I disease. Patients randomized to receive combined modality therapy had superior 5-yr progression-free survival (77% vs 64%, $p = 0.03$) and overall survival (82% vs 72%, $p = 0.02$). Based on results from randomized trials such as these, combined modality therapy has become the accepted standard of care for patients with clinical stage I or non-bulky clinical stage II disease.

Advanced-Stage Disease

Similarly, treatment of advanced stage (III and IV) aggressive non-Hodgkin's lymphoma has seen an evolution of treatment regimens over time. So-called first-"generation" chemotherapy regimens included combinations such as CHOP *(55)*, BACOP (bleomycin, doxorubicin, cyclophosphamide, vincristine, prednisone) *(58)*, and CAP-BOP (cyclophosphamide, doxorubicin, procarbazine, bleomycin, vincristine, and prednisone) *(59)*. Regimens such as BACOP and CAP-BOP were designed to prevent recurrence by continuing therapy with nonmyelosuppressive agents (bleomycin or prednisone) during myeloid recovery. Subequently, second-generation regimens were generally designed to maximize exposure to multiple drugs active in non-Hodgkin's lymphoma using alternating schedules of non-crossresistant drugs. This included regimens such as ProMACE-MOPP *(53)* and M-BACOD (methotrexate, bleomycin, doxorubicin, cyclophosphamide, vincristine, dexamethasone) *(60)*. Finally, the third generation of non-Hodgkin's lymphoma included regimens such as MACOP-B (methotrexate, doxorubicin, cyclophosphamide, vincristine, prednisone, bleomycin) *(61)*, which was designed to be an intensive, short 12-wk program, and another intense alternating non-crossresistant regimen known as ProMACE-CytaBOM (prednisone, methotrexate, doxorubicin, cyclophosphamide, etoposide, cytarabine, bleomycin, and vincristine) *(62)*. Usual difficulties with selection bias in phase II trials led investigators to believe that second- and third-generation regimens represented an improvement in outcome relative to earlier regimens such as CHOP. However, these regimens were usually more difficult to administer as a result of toxicity resulting from increased dose-intensity, and the use of high doses of drugs such as methotrexate. Also, in some cases, with longer duration of follow-up than were included in the initial studies, recurrence rates began to look more similar to earlier regimens such as CHOP. Any uncertainty or bias regarding the best treatment regimen was finally put to rest by the results of a large randomized phase III trial conducted by the Southwest Oncology Group and published in 1993 *(63)*. This large and highly statistically powered study randomized 1138 patients with bulky stage II-stage IV aggressive non-Hodgkin's lymphoma to one of four combination chemotherapy regimens: CHOP, m-BACOD, MACOP-B, or ProMACE-CytaBOM. Patients were stratified on five pretreatment disease characteristics (the presence of an abnormal LDH, marrow involvement, bulky disease, age ≥65, and WF histology). Unfortunately, many patients were excluded from the study after randomization (239 patients were deemed ineligible after randomization, mainly for ineligible histology), and the analysis was performed only on 899 eligible patients (i.e., not by intent-to-treat). The study demonstrated no significant difference in complete response rates, disease-free survival, or overall survival. A trend in favor of lower treatment related mortality in favor of CHOP was observed ($p = 0.09$). Based largely on the outcome of this trial, CHOP has become what is considered standard therapy for patients with newly diagnosed aggressive non-Hodgkin's lymphoma.

This trial was obviously considered to be a major success in clarifying the role of CHOP as a standard therapy for this illness. Although the subset of patients with low-risk disease have approximately a 70% probability of cure with modern therapy *(34)*, greater more than 50% of patients present with advanced disease or other poor prognostic features, and less than one-half of these patients can expect to be cured with conventional chemotherapy alone. This observation should be seen as a challenge to develop and study novel treatment strategies, which could offer improvement in outcomes for patients with high-risk disease.

NEW APPROACHES FOR PATIENTS WITH ADVANCED/HIGH-RISK DISEASE

Attempts to improve the cure rate with front-line therapy for patients with advanced disease have included testing the role of consolidative or early high-dose therapy/autologous hematopoietic stem-cell transplantation *(64–66)* and the addition of monoclonal antibody (MAb) therapy to chemotherapy regimens *(67)*. A recently reported trial comparing CHOP to CHOP/rituximab in elderly patients with stage II–IV diffuse large B-cell lymphoma has demonstrated improved disease-free and overall survival for patients randomized to CHOP/rituximab *(68)*. A similar trial (with a second randomization to maintenance rituximab vs no further therapy) has recently been completed by the Eastern Cooperative Oncology Group, though no results have yet been published for this trial. Pilot studies are also ongoing to evaluate the potential role of post-chemotherapy idiotype vaccine strategies.

Early/Consolidative High-Dose Therapy/Autologous Stem-Cell Transplantation. A number of randomized trials have examined the effect of adding high-dose therapy/autologous stem-cell transplantation as an early or consolidative up-front treatment for newly diagnosed aggressive lymphomas. Difficulties in the evaluation/interpretation of these studies are encountered largely because of power/sample size issues, plus the observation that many of the trials were designed to test hypotheses which differed from one another in subtle ways, making such trials difficult to compare directly.

Based on the observation that patients with slow responses to CHOP have a lower probability of achieving complete remissions (CR) *(69)*, Verdonck et al. *(64)* conducted a randomized trial designed to compare eight cycles of standard CHOP to four cycles of CHOP followed by high-dose chemotherapy/autologous bone-marrow transplantation. Sixty-nine patients considered to be slow responders (defined as having attained a partial remission (PR) but no bone-marrow involvement after three cycles of CHOP) were randomized. There was no significant difference in complete response rates, disease-free, event-free, or overall survival between the two groups. Also, interestingly, the disease-free survival of fast responders (who were not randomized) was not different than that of either study group. The small sample size of this trial, however, would have made the trial highly underpowered and thus unable to detect anything other than an extremely large treatment difference between the two randomized groups.

Gianni et al. *(65)* randomized 98 patients with newly diagnosed or progressive diffuse large B-cell non-Hodgkin's lymphoma to receive either 12 wk of MACOP-B or to a dose-intense sequential induction regimen (consisting of doxorubicin, prednisone, vincristine, cyclophosphamide, high-dose methotrexate/leukovorin, and etoposide delivered over 8-9 planned weeks), followed by high-dose chemotherapy/bone-marrow transplantation. Complete responses were higher in the sequential therapy arm (96% vs 70%) and at a median follow-up of 55 mo, the probability of freedom from progression (84% vs 49%, $p < 0.001$), freedom from relapse (88% vs 70%, $p = 0.055$), and EFS (76% vs 49%, $p = 0.004$) were all clearly superior in the sequential therapy/autologous transplant group. A trend toward improved survival for the high-dose group (81% vs 55%, $p = 0.09$) was observed for this group as well.

Finally, a large prospective trial from France (LNH87-2) enrolled 1043 patients with newly diagnosed aggressive non-Hodgkin's lymphoma and at least one adverse prognostic factor (poor performance status, two or more extra-nodal sites, tumor burden ≥10 cm, bone-marrow or CNS involvement, Burkitt's or lymphoblastic lymphoma) to a sequential therapy protocol. Patients were initially randomized to one of two anthracycline-containing regimens (doxorubicin, cyclophosphamide, vindesine, bleomycin, predinisone vs mitoxantrone cyclophosphamide, vindesine, bleomycin, and predinisone). Five hundred forty-one complete responders were further randomized to receive consolidative therapy with either high-dose methotrexate, ifosfamide, etoposide, and asparaginase, plus cytarabine, or to high-dose cyclophosphamide, and carmustine, plus etoposide with autologous bone marrow. Although no difference in overall survival was demonstrated for all randomized intent-to-treat patients, a retrospective analysis of randomized patients who had two or more risk factors by the International Prognostic Index *(34)* and underwent bone-marrow transplantation experienced improved disease-free survival (59% vs 39%) and overall survival (65% vs 52%) at 5 yr compared with patients receiving the non-transplant consolidative therapy *(66)*. A recently reported update with a median follow-up of 8 yr continues to confirm superior 8-yr disease-free survival (55% vs 39%) and overall survival (64% vs 49%) for high-risk patients *(70)*.

A recent randomized trial reported by Santini et al. observed a similar trend toward improved outcomes for patients with intermediate-high and high-risk indices by the International Prognostic Index who received consolidative high-dose chemotherapy/bone-marrow transplantation *(71)*. Other randomized trials presently reported only in abstract form have not confirmed the advantage of high-dose chemotherapy/autologous stem-cell transplantation as a consolidative approach to high-risk patients.

In summary, despite differences in therapies, and hypotheses being tested, some trials support the notion that patients with high-risk disease may experience prolonged disease-free or EFS with early consolidative stem-cell transplantation, but the ability to definitively improve survival in this group of patients remains unclear. It also apprears that the strategy of short, intensive induction regimens may be the most likely way of obtaining benefit if one uses this strategy.

Salvage Therapy

Patients who fail to attain complete remission with induction therapy, or who relapse after initial complete remission, have a poor prognosis with further conventional chemotherapy. A number of pilot/phase II trials of high-dose therapy/ autologous stem-cell transplantation for patients with relapsed aggressive non-Hodgkin's lymphoma conducted in the late 1980s, and early 1990s *(72–74)* suggested the possibility of improved outcomes with this modality compared with concurrent controls or historical results of conventional salvage therapy, and ultimately led to the development of a randomized trial known as the Parma trial for this patient population *(75)*. In this trial, 215 patients aged 18–60 yr in first or second relapse with aggressive non-Hodgkin's lymphomas received two cycles of dexamethasone, cytarabine, and cisplatin (DHAP) followed by an assessment of response. One hundred nine patients attained at least a partial remission and were randomized to either four additional courses of DHAP given 3–4 wk apart or to high-dose chemotherapy with carmustine, etoposide, cytarabine, and cyclophosphamide (BEAC) followed by autologous bone marrow transplantation. Patients with tumor masses ≥5 cm at relapse underwent involved-field radiotherapy, which was delivered after the second cycle of DHAP in the experimental arm, and at completion of chemotherapy in the conventional treatment arm. This trial was able to conclusively demonstrate a significant improvement in EFS (46%

vs 12%, $p = 0.001$) and overall survival (53% vs 32%, $p = 0.038$) at 5 yr for patients randomized to the experimental arm, and as such defined the present-day standard of care for patients with relapsed chemosensitive aggressive non-Hodgkin's lymphomas. Further data from this trial published by Blay and colleagues examined the applicability of the International Prognostic Index to these patients *(76)*. Although limited by sample size and the potential biases associated with subset analyses, this study suggests that there is probably no significant difference in outcome after transplantation for patients with 0, 1, 2, or three risk factors at relapse. Also, interestingly, patients with no adverse risk factors by the International Prognostic Index had a similar probability of survival at 5 yr, regardless of whether they received conventional therapy or transplantation.

Clinical trials attempting to improve on the outcome in patients with relapsed or chemorefractory disease have included the use of both labeled *(77)* and unlabeled *(78)* MAbs, both as single agents, and in combination with autologous stem-cell transplantation. However no randomized comparisons of these therapies currently exist, and as such, high-dose chemotherapy/autologous stem-cell transplantation with involved-field radiotherapy for large tumor masses remains the standard of care for patients with chemosensitive relapses. Patients with chemorefractory disease at relapse have a low probability of obtaining prolonged disease-free survival with conventional autologous stem-cell transplantation, and should be considered for accrual to clinical trials.

Finally, although allogeneic transplantation has become a fairly standard indication for diseases such as acute and chronic myelogenous leukemia, its role in patients with relapsed/refractory aggressive lymphomas remains poorly defined. Although observational data comparing autologous transplantation to allogeneic transplantation suggests a lower probability of relapse for patients who receive allografts *(79)*, this type of study design cannot exclude the possibility that at least some of the difference in outcome results from a lack of tumor-cell infusion in allogeneic grafts. However, in patients with aggressive lymphomas who have relapsed after allogeneic transplantation, attempts to induce graft-vs-host disease through either the withdrawal of immunosuppression, or by using donor leukocyte infusions, have led to tumor regression and durable remissions *(80)*, suggesting the presence of a true immunologic graft-vs-lymphoma (GVL) effect. Unfortunately, the apparent decrease in relapse appears to be offset by complications of graft-vs-host disease and infection, so that no improvement in overall survival is evident in patients who receive allografts for aggressive lymphomas.

CONCLUSIONS

Ongoing changes in our understanding of the biology, prognostic factors, and treatment of aggressive subtypes of non-Hodgkin's lymphomas have helped clinicians to understand which patients are most likely to benefit from standard therapy, and conversely, which patients require consideration of novel therapies. Continued efforts aimed at identifying newer therapies and the best roles for present available therapies will undoubtedly continue to improve long-term outcomes for all patients diagnosed with aggressive forms of non-Hodgkin's lymphomas.

REFERENCES

1. Armitage JO, Weisenburger DD for the Non-Hodgkin's Lymphoma Classification Project. New approach to classifying non-Hodgkin's lymphomas: Clinical features of the major histologic subtypes. *J Clin Oncol* 1998;16:2780–2795.
2. Jemel A, Thomas A, Murray T, Thun M. Cancer Statistics. 2002. CA-A *Cancer J Clin* 2002;52:23–47.
3. Greiner TC, Medeiros LJ, Jaffe ES. Non-Hodgkin's lymphoma. *Cancer* 1995;75:370–380.
4. Nador RG, Cesarman E, Dawson DB, Ansari MQ, Said J, Knowles DM. Primary effusion lymphoma: a distinct clinicopathologic entity associated with the Kaposi's sarcoma-associated Herpes virus. *Blood* 1996;88:645–656.
5. Rooney CM, Loftin SK, Holladay MS, Brenner MK, Krance RA, Heslop HE. Early identification of Epstein-Barr virus-associated post-transplantation lymphoproliferative disease. *Br J Haematol* 1995;89:98–103.
6. Hanto DW, Frizzera G, Purtilo DT, Sakamoto K, Sullivan JL, Saemundsen AK, et al. Clinical spectrum of lymphoproliferative disorders in renal transplant recipients and evidence for the role of Epstein-Barr virus. *Cancer Res* 1981;41:4253–4261.
7. SEER cancer statistics review, 1973-1997. Bethesda MD: National Cancer Institute, 2000.
8. Burkitt DP. A sarcoma involving the jaws in African children. *Br J Surg* 1958;46:218–223.
9. Knowles DM, Cesarman E, Chadburn A, Frizzera G, Chen J, Rose EA, et al. Correlative morphologic and molecular genetic analysis demonstrates three distinct categories of posttransplantation lymphoproliferative disorders. *Blood* 1995;85:552–565.
10. Ho M, Miller G, Atchison RW, Breinig MK, Dummer JS, Andiman W, et al. Epstein-Barr virus infections and DNA hybridization studies in posttransplantation lymphoma and lymphoproliferative lesions: the role of primary infection. *J Infect Dis* 1985; 152:876–886.
11. Chang Y, Cesarman E, Culpepper J, Knowles DM, Moore PS. Identification of Herpes-like DNA in AIDS-associated Kaposi's sarcoma. *Science* 1994;266:1865–1869.
12. Soulier J, Grollet L, Oksenhendler E, Cacoub P, Cazals-Hatem D, Babinet P, et al. Kaposi's sarcoma-associated Herpesvirus-like DNA sequences in multicentric Castleman's disease. *Blood* 1995;86:1276–1280.
13. Rappaport H, Winter WJ, Hicks EB. Tumors of the hematopoietic system. In: Washington DC US Armed Forces Institute of Pathology: 1966. Section 3, Fascicle 8.
14. Lukes R, Collins R. Immunologic characterization of human malignant lymphomas. *Cancer* 1974;34:1488–1503.
15. Non-Hodgkin's lymphoma pathologic classification project. National Cancer Institute sponsored study of classifications of non-Hodgkin's lymphomas: summary and description of a Working Formulation of clinical usage. *Cancer* 1982;49:2112–32135.
16. NCI non-Hodgkin's Classification Project Writing Committee. Classification of non-Hodgkin's lymphomas. Reproducibility of major classification systems. *Cancer* 1985; 55:91–95.
17. Harris NL, Jaffe ES, Diebold J, Flandrin G, Muller-Hermelink H-K, Vardiman J, et al. World Health Organization classification of neoplastic diseases of the hematopoietic and lymphoid tissues: report of the clinical advisory committee meeting-Arlie House, Virginia, November 1997. *J Clin Oncol* 1999;17:3835–3849.

18. Harris NL, Jaffe ES, Stein H, Banks PM, Chan JKC, Cleary ML, et al. A revised European-American classification of lymphoid neoplasms: a proposal from the international lymphoma study group. *Blood* 1994;84:1361–1392.
19. O'Hara C, Said JW, Pinkus GS. Non-Hodgkin's lymphoma, multilobated B cell type. *Hum Pathol* 1986;17:593–599.
20. Hill ME, MacLennan KA, Cunningham DC, Hudson BV, Burke M, Clarke P, et al. Prognostic significance of BCL-2 expression and bcl-2 major breakpoint region rearrangement in diffuse large cell non-Hodgkin's lymphoma: a British National Lymphoma Investigation Study. *Blood* 1996;88:1046–1051.
21. Akasaka T, Akasaka H, Ueda C, Yonetani N, Maesako Y, Shimizu A, et al. Molecular and clinical features of non-Burkitt's, diffuse large-cell lymphoma of B-cell type associated with the c-MYC/immunoglobulin heavy-chain fusion gene. *J Clin Oncol* 2000;18:510–518.
22. Flynn KJ, Dehner LP, Gajl-Peczalska KJ, Dahl MV, Ramsay N, Wang N. Regressing atypical histiocytosis: a cutaneous proliferation of atypical neoplastic histiocytes with unexpectedly indolent biologic behaviour. *Cancer* 1982; 49:959–970.
23. Benharroch D, Meguerian-Bedoyan Z, Lamant L, Amin C, Brugieres L, Terrier-Lacombe MJ, et al. ALK-positive lymphoma: a single disease with a broad spectrum of morphology. *Blood* 1998;91:2076–2084.
24. Piris M, Brown DC, Gatter KC, Mason DY. CD30 expression in non-Hodgkin's lymphoma. *Histopathology* 1990;17:211–218.
25. Mason DY, Bastard C, Rimokh R, Dastugue N, Huret JL, Kristoffersson U, et al. CD30-positive large cell lymphomas ('Ki-1 lymphoma') are associated with a chromosomal translocation involving 5q35. *Br J Haematol* 1990;74:161–168.
26. O'Connor NTJ, Stein H, Gatter KC, Wainscoat JS, Crick J, Al Saati T, et al. Genotypic analysis of large cell lymphomas which express the Ki-1 antigen. *Histopathology* 1987;11:733–740.
27. Herbst H, Tippelmann G, Anagnostopoulos I, Gerdes J, Schwarting R, Boehm T, et al. Immunoglobulin and T-cell receptor gene rearrangements in Hodgkin's disease and Ki-1-positive anaplastic large cell lymphoma: dissociation between phenotype and genotype. *Leuk Res* 1989;13:103–116.
28. Kuefer MU, Look AT, Tripp R, Behm FG, Pattengale PK, Morris SW. Retrovirus mediated gene transfer of NPM-ALK causes lymphoid malignancy in mice. *Blood* 1996;88:450 (abst. 1788).
29. Krenacs L, Wellman A, Sorbara L, Himmelmann AW, Bagdi E, Jaffe ES, et al. Cytotoxic cell antigen expression in anaplastic large cell lymphomas of T- and null-cell type and Hodgkin's disease: evidence for distinct cellular origin. *Blood* 1997;89:980–989.
30. Lepretre S, Buchonnet G, Stamatoullas A, Lenain P, Duval C, d'Anjou J, et al. Chromosome abnormalities in peripheral T-cell lymphoma. *Cancer Genet Cytogenet* 2000; 117:71–79.
31. Lazzarino M, Orlandi E, Paulli M, Strater J, Klersy C, Gianelli U, et al. Treatment outcome and prognostic factors for primary mediastinal (thymic) B-cell lymphoma: a multicenter study of 106 patients. *J Clin Oncol* 1997;15:1646–1653.
32. Fraternali-Orcioni G, Falini B, Quaini F, Campo E, Piccioli M, Gamberi B, et al. Beta-HCG aberrant expression in primary mediastinal large B-cell lymphoma. *Am J Surg Pathol* 1999;23:717–721.
33. Bishop PC, Wilson WH, Pearson D, Janik J, Jaffe ES, Elwood PC. CNS involvement in primary mediastinal large B-cell lymphoma. *J Clin Oncol* 1999;17:2479–2485.
34. The International Non-Hodgkin's Lymphoma Prognostic Factors Project. A predictive model for aggressive non-Hodgkin's lymphoma. *N Engl J Med* 1993;329:987–994.
35. Abou-Elella AA, Weisenburger DD, Vose JM, Kollath JP, Lynch JC, Bast MA, et al. Primary mediastinal large B-cell lymphoma: a clinicopathologic study of 43 patients from the Nebraska Lymphoma Study Group. *J Clin Oncol* 1999;17:784–790.

36. Cazals-Hatem D, Lepage E, Brice P, Ferrant A, d'Agay MF, Baumelou E, et al. Primary mediastinal large B-cell lymphoma. A clinicopathologic study of 141 cases compared with 916 nonmediastinal large B-cell lymphomas, a GELA ("Groupe d'Etude des Lymphomes de l'Adulte") study. *Am J Surg Pathol* 1996;20:877–888.

37. Chen HS, Shen MC, Tien HF, Su IJ, Wang CH. Leptomeningeal seeding with acute hydro-cephalus-unusual central nervous system presentation during chemotherapy in Ki-1-positive anaplastic large cell lymphoma. *Acta Haematol* 1996;95:135–139.

38. Tsukamoto N, Morita K, Maehara T, Mitsuhashi M, Karasawa M, Murakami H, et al. Ki-1-positive large cell anaplastic lymphoma with protean manifestations including central nervous system involvement. *Acta Haematol* 1992;88:147–150.

39. Abdulkader I, Cameselle-Teijeiro J, Fraga M, Rodriguez-Nunez A, Allut AG, Forteza J. Primary anaplastic large cell lymphoma of the central nervous system *Hum Pathol* 1999; 30:978–981.

40. Falini B, Pileri S, Zinzani PL, Carbone A, Zagonel V, Wolf-Peeters C, et al. ALK+ lymphoma: clinico-pathological findings and outcome. *Blood* 1999; 93:2697–2706.

41. Bostwick DG, Iczkowski KA, Amin MB, Discigil G, Osborne B. Malignant lymphoma involving the prostate: report of 62 cases. *Cancer* 1998;83:732–738.

42. Froberg MK, Hamati H, Kant JA, Addya K, Salhany KE. Primary low-grade T-helper cell testicular lymphoma. *Arch Pathol Lab Med* 1997;121:1096–1099.

43. Zaja F, Russo D, Silvestri F, Fanin R, Damiani D, Infanti L, et al. Retrospective analysis of 23 cases with peripheral T-cell lymphoma, unspecified: clinical characteristics and outcome. *Haematologica* 1997;82:171–177.

44. Ansell SM, Habermann TM, Kurtin PJ, Witzig TE, Chen MG, Li CY, et al. Predictive capacity of the International Prognostic Factor Index in patients with peripheral T-cell lymphoma. *J Clin Oncol* 1997;15:2296–2301.

45. Melnyk A, Rodriguez A, Pugh WC, Cabanillas F. Evaluation of the Revised European-American Lymphoma classification confirms the clinical relevance of immunophenotype in 560 cases of aggressive non-Hodgkin's lymphoma. *Blood* 1997;89:4514–4520.

46. Gisselbrecht C, Gaulard P, Lepage E, Coiffier B, Briere J, Haioun C, et al. Prognostic significance of T-cell phenotype in aggressive non-Hodgkin's lymphomas. Groupe d'Etudes des Lymphomes de l'Adulte (GELA). *Blood* 1998;92:76–82.

47. Liang R, Chiu E, Loke SL. Secondary central nervous system involvement by non-Hodgkin's lymphoma: the risk factors. *Hematol Oncol* 1990;8:141–145.

48. Bashir RM, Bierman PJ, Vose JM, Weisenburger DD, Armitage JO. Central nervous system involvement in patients with diffuse aggressive non-Hodgkin's lymphoma. *Am J Clin Oncol* 1991;14:478–482.

49. Cheson BD, Horning SJ, Coiffier B, Shipp M, Fisher RI, Conners JM, et al. Report of an International workshop to standardize response criteria for non-Hodgkin's lymphomas. *J Clin Oncol* 1999;17:1244–1253.

50. Kaminski MS, Coleman CN, Colby TV, Cox RS, Rosenberg SA. Factors predicting survival in adults with stage I and II large-cell lymphoma treated with primary radiation therapy. *Ann Intern Med* 1986;104:747–756.

51. Hallahann DE, Farah R, Vokes EE, Bitran JD, Ultman JE, Glolomb HM, et al. The patterns of failure in patients with pathological stage I and II diffuse histiocytic lymphoma treated with radiation therapy alone. *Int J Radiat Oncol Biol Phys* 1989;17:767–771.

52. Longo DL, Glatstein E, Duffey PL, Ihde DC, Hubbard SM, Fisher RI, et al. Treatment of localized aggressive lymphomas with combination chemotherapy followed by involved-field radiation therapy. *J Clin Oncol* 1989;7:1295–1302.

53. Fisher RI, DeVita-VT Jr, Hubbard SM, Longo DL, Wesley R, Chabner BA, et al. Diffuse aggressive lymphomas: increased survival after alternating flexible sequences of proMACE and MOPP chemotherapy. *Ann Intern Med* 1983;98:304–309.

54. Jones SE, Miller TP, Connors JM. Long-term follow-up and analysis for prognostic factors for patients with limited-stage diffuse large-cell lymphoma treated with initial chemotherapy with or without adjuvant radiotherapy. *J Clin Oncol* 1989;7:1186–1191.
55. DeVita VT Jr, Canellos GP, Chabner B, Schein P, Hubbard SP, Young RC. Advanced diffuse histiocytic lymphoma, a potentially curable disease. *Lancet* 1975;1:248–250.
56. Nissen NI, Ersboll J, Hansen HS, Walbom-Jorgensen S, Pedersen-Bjergaard J, Hansen MM, et al. A randomized study of radiotherapy versus radiotherapy plus chemotherapy in stage I-II non-Hodgkin's lymphoma. *Cancer* 1983;52:1–7.
57. Miller TP, Dahlberg S, Cassady JR, Adelstein DJ, Spier CM, Grogan TM, et al. Chemotherapy alone compared with chemotherapy plus radiotherapy for localized intermediate- and high-grade non-Hodgkin's lymphoma. *N Engl J Med* 1998;339:21–26.
58. Schein PS, DeVita-VT Jr, Hubbard S, Chabner BA, Canellos GP, Berard C, et al. Bleomycin, adriamycin, cyclophosphamide, vincristine, and prednisone (BACOP) combination chemotherapy in the treatment of advanced diffuse histiocytic lymphoma. *Ann Intern Med* 1976;85:417–422.
59. Vose JM, Armitage JO, Weisenburger DD, Bierman PJ, Sorensen S, Hutchins M, et al. The importance of age in survival of patients treated with chemotherapy for aggressive non-Hodgkin's lymphoma. *J Clin Oncol* 1988;6:1838–1844.
60. Skarin AT, Canellos GP, Rosenthal DS, Case DC Jr, MacIntyre JM, Pinkus GS, et al. Improved prognosis of diffuse histiocytic and undifferentiated lymphoma by use of high dose methotrexate alternating with standard agents (M-BACOD). *J Clin Oncol* 1983;1:91–98.
61. Klimo P, Connors JM. MACOP-B chemotherapy for the treatment of diffuse large-cell lymphoma. *Ann Intern Med* 1985;102:596–602.
62. Longo DL, DeVitaVT Jr, Duffey PL, Wesley MN, Ihde DC, Hubbard SM, et al. Superiority of ProMACE-CytaBOM over ProMACE-MOPP in the treatment of advanced diffuse aggressive lymphoma: results of a prospective randomized trial. *J Clin Oncol* 1991;9:25–38.
63. Fisher RI, Gaynor ER, Dahlberg S, Oken MM, Grogan TM, Mize EM, et al. Comparison of a standard regimen (CHOP) with three intensive chemotherapy regimens for advanced non-Hodgkin's lymphoma. *N Engl J Med* 1993;328:1002–1006.
64. Verdonck LF, van Putten WLJ, Hagenbeek A, Schouten HC, Sonneveld P, van Imhoff GW, et al. Comparison of CHOP chemotherapy with autologous bone marrow transplantation for slowly responding patients with aggressive non-Hodgkin's lymphoma. *N Engl J Med* 1995;332:1045–1051.
65. Gianni AM, Bregni M, Siena S, Brambilla C, Di Nicola M, Lombardi F, et al. High-dose chemotherapy and autologous bone marrow transplantation compared with MACOP-B in aggressive B-cell lymphoma. *N Engl J Med* 1997;336:1290–1297.
66. Haioun C, Lepage E, Gisselbrecht C, Bastion Y, Coiffier B, Brice P, et al. Benefit of autologous bone marrow transplantation over sequential chemotherapy in poor-risk aggressive non-Hodgkin's lymphoma: updated results of the prospective study LNH87-2. *J Clin Oncol* 1997;15:1131–1137.
67. Link BK, Grossbard ML, Fisher RI, Czuczman MS, Gilman P, Lowe AM, et al. Phase II pilot study of the safety and efficacy of rituximab in combination with CHOP chemotherapy in patients with previously untreated intermediate- or high-grade NHL. *Proc ASCO* 1998;17:3a.
68. Coiffier B, Lepage E, Briére J, Herbrecht R, Tilly H, Bouabdalah R, et al. CHOP chemotherapy plus rituximab compared with CHOP alone in elderly patients with diffuse large B-cell lymphoma. *N Engl J Med* 2002;346:235–242.
69. Armitage JO, Weisenburger DD, Hutchins M, Moravec DF, Dowling M, Sorensen S, et al. Chemotherapy for diffuse large-cell lymphoma-rapidly responding patients have more durable remissions. *J Clin Oncol* 1986;4:160–164.
70. Haioun C, Lepage E, Gisselbrecht C, Salles G, Coiffier B, Brice P, et al. Survival benefit of high-dose therapy in poor-risk aggressive non-Hodgkin's lymphoma: final analysis of the

prospective LNH87-2 protocol—a Groupe d'Etude des Lymphomes de l'Adulte study. *J Clin Oncol* 2000;18:3025–3030.

71. Santini G, Salvagno L, Leoni P, Chisesi T, De Souza C, Sertoli MR, et al. VACOP-B versus VACOP-B plus autologous bone marrow transplantation for advanced diffuse non-Hodgkin's lymphoma: results of a prospective randomized trial by the non-Hodgkin's lymphoma Cooperative Study Group. *J Clin Oncol* 1998;16:2796–2802.

72. Philip T, Armitage JO, Spitzer G, Chauvin F, Jagannath S, Cahn JY, et al. High-dose therapy and autologous bone marrow transplantation after failure of conventional chemotherapy in adults with intermediate-grade or high-grade non-Hodgkin's lymphoma. *N Engl J Med* 1987;316:1493–1498.

73. Bosly A, Coiffier B, Gisselbrecht C, Tilly H, Auzanneau G, Andrien F, et al. Bone marrow transplantation prolongs survival after relapse in aggressive lymphoma patients treated with the LNH-84 regimen. *J Clin Oncol* 1992;10:1615–1623.

74. Vose JM, Anderson JR, Kessinger A, Bierman PJ, Coccia P, Reed EC, et al. High-dose chemotherapy and autologous hematopoietic stem cell transplantation for aggressive non-Hodgkin's lymphoma. *J Clin Oncol* 1993;11:1846–1851.

75. Philip T, Guglielmi C, Hagenbeek A, Somers R, van der Lelie H, Bron D, et al. Autologous bone marrow transplantation as compared with salvage chemotherapy in relapses of chemotherapy-sensitive non-Hodgkin's lymphoma. *N Engl J Med* 1995;333:1540–1545.

76. Blay J-Y, Gomez F, Sebban C, Bachelot T, Biron P, Guglielmi C, et al. The international prognostic index correlates to survival in patients with aggressive lymphoma in relapse: analysis of the PARMA trial. *Blood* 1998;92:3562–3568.

77. Liu SY, Eary JF, Petersdorf SH, Martin PJ, Maloney DG, Appelbaum FR, et al. Follow-up of relapsed B-cell lymphoma patients treated with iodine-131-labeled anti-CD20 antibody and autologous stem-cell rescue. *J Clin Oncol* 1998;16:3270–3278.

78. Coiffier B, Haioun C, Ketterer N, Engert A, Tilly H, Ma D, et al. Rituximab (anti-CD20 monoclonal antibody) for the treatment of patients with relapsing or refractory aggressive lymphoma: a multicenter phase II study. *Blood* 1998;92:1927–1932.

79. Jones RJ, Ambinder RF, Piantadosi S, Santos G. Evidence of a graft-versus-lymphoma effect associated with allogeneic bone marrow transplantation. *Blood* 1991;77:649–653.

80. van Besien KW, de Lima M, Giralt SA, Moore DF, Khouri IF, Rondon G, et al. Management of lymphoma recurrence after allogeneic transplantation: the relevance of graft-versus-lymphoma effect. *Bone Marrow Transplant* 1997;19:977–982.

12 Hodgkin's Disease

Steven M. Horwitz, MD
and Sandra J. Horning, MD

CONTENTS

INTRODUCTION

Hodgkin's disease is a unique cancer of the lymphoid system, first described by Thomas Hodgkin in 1832 and later, independently by Samuel Wilks in 1856. Despite its relative rarity, Hodgkin's disease is one of the most intensively studied of all malignancies. These studies have led to a detailed understanding of the clinical and pathologic features of the disease and have rendered Hodgkin's disease one of the most curable cancers. It is now generally accepted that the characteristic malignant cell of Hodgkin's disease, the Reed-Sternberg cell, is of

From: *Current Clinical Oncology: Chronic Leukemias and Lymphomas:*
Biology, Pathophysiology, and Clinical Management
Edited by: G. J. Schiller © Humana Press Inc., Totowa, NJ

Table 1
Classification of Hodgkin's Disease

WHO Classification (Proposed)

Nodular lymphocyte predominance
Classical Hodgkin's disease
      Nodular sclerosis
      Mixed cellularity
      Lymphocyte depletion
      Lymphocyte-rich

B-lymphoid lineage. Continually improved and refined treatment regimens, often tested in randomized controlled trials, result in a cure for more than 80% of newly diagnosed patients. Moreover, these improvements in treatment have been accompanied by reductions in the late effects of the therapy.

CLASSIFICATION

The Rye classification, a modification of that proposed by Lukes, Butler, and Hicks, described four histopathologic subtypes of Hodgkin's disease: lymphocyte predominance, nodular sclerosis, mixed cellularity, and lymphocyte depletion. The recently proposed World Health Organization (WHO) Classification of Lymphoid Neoplasms includes Hodgkin's disease under the synonym Hodgkin's lymphoma. Nodular lymphocyte predominance subtype is delineated from classical Hodgkin's disease on the basis of its unique clinical and pathologic features. A newly described entity, lymphocyte-rich Hodgkin's disease, is included as a subtype of classical Hodgkin's lymphoma (Table 1).

PATHOLOGY

Identification of the characteristic multinucleated giant cells, Reed-Sternberg cells or their mononuclear variants (RS-H), with the appropriate cellular background is the hallmark of the histologic diagnosis of Hodgkin's disease. However, Reed-Sternberg cells may represent only 1–10% of the total cellularity and are not entirely specific to Hodgkin's disease. On immunophenotypic analysis, Reed-Sternberg cells show varied antigen expression and no single marker is specific for Hodgkin's disease. Typical patterns are observed, making immunophenotyping studies of paraffin-embedded tissues very useful in the diagnosis of Hodgkin's disease. Approximately 85% of cases of nodular sclerosis and mixed cellularity express the CD30 antigen (Ki-1), a marker of lymphocyte activation *(1,2)*. The majority of RS-H cells in classical Hodgkin's disease express the CD15 antigen as well *(3,4)*. The B-cell antigens CD 19 and CD20 are expressed by RS-H cells in only about 25% of classical Hodgkin's disease but are nearly uniformly expressed on the lymphocyte and histiocytic (L&H) variants of lymphocyte predominant Hodgkin's disease *(5–9)*. CD45 (LCA) is usually negative in Hodgkin's disease but positive in non-Hodgkin's lymphoma.

CLINICAL AND PATHOLOGIC CORRELATION

There is a strong correlation between age at onset, the anatomic extent of disease, and histologic subtype of Hodgkin's disease. About 10% of patients present with nodular lymphocyte predominance (NLPHD) which, as stated previously, is considered to be a unique subtype. Progressive transformation of germinal centers may precede or follow NLPHD in other sites *(10,11)*. The cellular composition is predominantly benign B-lymphocytes with or without histiocytes. The characteristic multilobated L&H cells are relatively abundant. Patients most commonly present with stage I disease (70%), particularly in peripheral lymph nodes, and there is a 4:1 male predominance *(12)*. This subtype has been associated with large cell non-Hodgkin's lymphoma as a composite tumor or the large-cell lymphoma may occur at a later date *(13,14)*.

Nodular sclerosis (NSHD) is noted for its distinctive histologic features and frequent involvement of the lower cervical, supraclavicular and mediastinal lymph nodes in adolescents and young adults, particularly females. Approximately 70% of patients present with limited-stage disease. Nodular sclerosis constitutes the majority of Hodgkin's disease cases, ranging from 40–70%. One of the distinguishing histologic features is the lacunar cell, an RS variant that results from retraction of the cytoplasm of RS-H cells during formalin fixation. Another is the thickened capsule and fibrous bands which divide the lymphoid tissue into nodules. NSHD can be subclassified as grade 1 or 2, based on the frequency of malignant cells and normal lymphocytes. The malignant cells are numerous in grade 2 subtype, also referred to as the syncytial variant. The clinical and prognostic significance of NSHD subtypes is controversial *(15,16)*.

Mixed-cellularity Hodgkin's disease involves both pediatric and older age groups and is more commonly associated with advanced-stage disease, constitutional symptoms and immunodeficiency. About 30% of patients in Western countries present with this histology. Classic RS-H cells are easily found amid a cellular background composed of lymphocytes, eosinophils, plasma cells, and histiocytes. A worse prognosis has been characteristic of this subtype in the historical literature, but these differences have been largely erased by modern therapy.

The incidence of lymphocyte-depletion Hodgkin's disease is much lower than originally reported, as many cases have been reclassified as non-Hodgkin's lymphoma *(17)*. Two subtypes have been described: reticular and diffuse fibrosis. The reticular variant contains abundant pleomorphic neoplastic cells. The more common diffuse fibrosis variant, as the name implies, has a prominent fibroblastic proliferation with few normal lymphocytes. RS-H cells are sparse. The disease presents in the older age group with symptomatic, extensive disease. Peripheral and mediastinal adenopathy is much less common than in other cases of Hodgkin's disease (18). Presentation with fever of unknown origin, jaundice, hepatosplenomegaly, or pancytopenia is not rare. This subtype is also associated with the acquired immunodeficiency syndrome.

The 1999 WHO classification of lymphoma introduces a new subtype for the first time in 25 yr. "Lymphocyte-rich" Hodgkin's disease was discovered during an expert pathology review of cases of lymphocyte predominance (19). The two subtypes differ subtly on morphologic grounds, but the major difference is that the RS-H cells in lymphocyte-rich Hodgkin's disease have a classic immunophenotype. The presenting features are very similar to cases of NLPHD, although patients with the lymphocyte-rich subtype tend to be older (19). A higher rate of multiple relapses and a more favorable prognosis upon relapse are characteristic of NLPHD.

EPIDEMIOLOGY

The incidence of Hodgkin's disease in the United States has been stable at a rate of approx 7500 new diagnoses/year (20). The incidence is higher in men than women, and higher in whites than blacks. Hodgkin's disease has a bimodal age-incidence curve: rates rise through early life, peaking in the third decade and declining until age 45, after which the incidence increases steadily (21–23). There appear to be three distinct forms of Hodgkin's disease: a childhood form (ages 0–14), a young adult form (15–34 yr) and an older adult form (55–74 yr). The nodular sclerosis subtype predominates in young adults, and the mixed cellularity subtype is more common in the pediatric population and at older ages. There is a male predominance at all ages, but this is most marked in childhood cases (85%).

An increased risk of Hodgkin's disease in the young adult population has been associated with high socioeconomic status (21,24,25). High intelligence, small family size, single family dwelling and high educational attainment of patients, and their immediate families have all been associated with increased risk.

Geographic patterns vary for the three major age groups. In less developed countries, the incidence of Hodgkin's disease is greater in childhood, and there is a predominance of mixed cellularity histology, whereas in developed nations, the incidence peaks in young adulthood and is associated with the more favorable histologic subtypes (26). Together, these data suggest an interesting association between socioeconomic and environmental factors in the incidence of Hodgkin's disease.

ETIOLOGY

The etiology of Hodgkin's disease is unknown, yet evidence points toward a viral causation and genetic susceptibility. The demographic features have long supported the concept that one or more subtypes of Hodgkin's disease have an infectious etiology. Several reports of clusters of Hodgkin's disease at the time of diagnosis suggested the possibility of infectious transmission (27,28). Some population-based studies have found significant case aggregation (shared exposure) in schools, but these results have been questioned on the basis of methodology (29–32).

Several large studies have demonstrated that a prior history of serologically confirmed infectious mononucleosis confers a threefold increased risk of young adult Hodgkin's disease (33–35). Elevated titers of Epstein-Barr virus (EBV), the etiologic agent of infectious mononucleosis, have been reported in people diagnosed with Hodgkin's disease. A large population study showed that people who developed Hodgkin's disease had abnormally high titers of anti-EBV antibodies in prediagnostic sera (36). The presence of EBV genomes, detectable in nearly half of classical Hodgkin's disease tissues, was confirmed in 1987 (37). However, the relationship remains perplexing as the young adult, nodular sclerosis type is associated with the EBV-related epidemiologic factors, and the proportion of EBV-positive cases are higher in the mixed-cellularity category (38,39). A higher incidence of EBV-positive cases is found in pediatric and HIV-infected individuals with Hodgkin's disease (40–44).

Evidence supporting a genetic basis for increased susceptibility to Hodgkin's disease includes the increased risk among siblings and close relatives and an association with other tumor types, particularly non-Hodgkin's lymphomas (45–48). Hodgkin's disease has been described in monozygous twins (49–51). However, in support of an environmental influence, the interval between diagnoses in affected siblings in Hodgkin's disease-prone families is shorter than their age differences (52). The increased incidence in same-sex siblings (nine-fold) vs opposite-sex siblings (fivefold) may also support an environmental influence (53).

CLINICAL FEATURES

History and Physical Examination

Constitutional symptoms, some of which confer a less favorable prognosis, may accompany the diagnosis of Hodgkin's disease. Patients with fever higher than 38°C, drenching night sweats, and weight loss exceeding 10% of baseline body wt during the 6 mo preceding diagnosis are designated as having "B" disease. Fevers, which are present in 27% of patients at diagnosis in the Stanford series, are usually low-grade and irregular (54). Rarely, a cyclic pattern of high fevers for 1–2 wk alternating with afebrile periods of similar duration, is present at diagnosis. This classic Pel-Ebstein fever is virtually diagnostic *(55,56)*. Generalized pruritus—often accompanied by marked excoriation—may be present at diagnosis, but it is not prognostically significant *(57)*. Pain in the affected lymph nodes immediately after the ingestion of alcohol is a peculiar complaint that is very specific to Hodgkin's disease. It occurs in less than 10% of patients, and has no prognostic significance *(58)*. The etiology of these symptoms has been the subject of speculation, but remains largely unexplained. Patients with extensive intrathoracic disease may present with cough, chest pain, dyspnea, and, rarely, hemoptysis. Rarely, patients present with bone pain, including the constellation of back pain accompanied by signs and symptoms of spinal-cord compression.

Detection of an unusual mass or swelling in the superficial lymph nodes is the most common presentation of Hodgkin's disease. Lymphadenopathy is usually nontender, and has a "rubbery" consistency. A diffuse swelling rather than a discrete mass may be apparent in the supraclavicular, infraclavicular, or anterior chest-wall regions. Rarely, compression of the superior vena cava will result in facial swelling and engorgement of the veins in the neck and upper chest. Auscultation of the chest may reveal a pleural effusion. Palpation is an insensitive method for the detection of intra-abdominal adenopathy or organ enlargement, but examination should be oriented toward the liver, spleen, and upper retroperitoneal area. Although parenchymal or meningeal involvement of the central nervous system (CNS) is rare, a variety of paraneoplastic syndromes have been described in Hodgkin's disease. Patients have presented with signs of progressive multifocal leukoencephalopathy *(59)*, subacute cerebellar degeneration *(60,61)*, necrotizing myelopathy *(62)*, subacute sensory or motor neuropathy *(63)*, episodic neurologic dysfunction *(64)*, memory loss *(65)*, the Guillain-Barré syndrome *(66)*, and granulomatous angiitis of the CNS *(67)*.

Radiographic Features

Intrathoracic disease is present at diagnosis in two-thirds of patients. Mediastinal adenopathy is common in Hodgkin's disease, particularly in young women with nodular sclerosis histology *(68)*. Hilar adenopathy, pulmonary parenchymal involvement, pleural effusions, pericardial effusions, and chest-wall masses may be appreciated by plain chest X-ray, although a more precise definition of the extent of disease can be made by computed tomography (CT) of the chest. CT scans of the chest, abdomen, and pelvis are routinely used in the diagnostic evaluation of Hodgkin's disease. CT is a valuable tool in detecting lymph nodes in the celiac, portal, splenic hilar, and mesenteric areas, although the correlation with histologic involvement of the spleen has been disappointing. Bipedal lymphoangiograms are more sensitive than CT in evaluating the para-aortic, para-caval, and pelvic lymph nodes, because they can detect filling defects in otherwise normal-sized nodes. Extensive experience with lymphography has demonstrated that as many as 30–60% of patients with clinical disease limited to the supradiaphragmatic regions had involvement of the abdominal or pelvic lymph nodes *(69)*. Another advantage of this technique is that contrast material may remain for months to years, and can be used to assess the response to treatment and in follow-up. Despite its utility, lymphography is becoming less available, with the exception of specialized treatment centers *(70–72)*. Gallium-67 scintigraphy is useful in evaluating the mediastinum or areas that appear abnormal on a bone scan, and in the evaluation of residual masses following treatment. Single photon-emitted computed tomography (SPECT) increases the accuracy of the gallium scan. Whole-body positron emission tomography (PET) correlates well with CT evaluation, and may demonstrate additional areas of disease. PET, like gallium, is proving to be very useful in the evaluation of residual masses, and has an emerging role as an initial staging procedure. However, despite this increased sensitivity in detecting occult disease, changes in stage or therapy are rare *(73,74)*. Magnetic resonance imaging (MRI) has been disappointing in the evaluation of abdominal disease or residual mediastinal masses in treated patients *(75,76)*.

Anatomic Distribution of Disease

About 60–80% of clinical presentations are in the cervical nodes, 6–20% are in the axillary nodes, and 6–12% are in the inguinal nodes *(54)*. A minority of patients present with exclusive subdiaphragmatic disease, The frequency of splenic involvement at laparotomy in untreated patients averages 37% in 17 published series *(54)*. Involvement is strongly dependent on histologic sub-type; it is present in 35–60% of mixed cellularity and lymphocyte depletion cases compared with 17–34% of lymphocyte predominance or nodular sclerosis. Hepatic and bone-marrow disease are invariably associated with splenic involvement.

Staging

Peters described a clinical staging system in 1950, emphasizing the diagnostic evaluation of the anatomic extent of disease *(77,78)*. Modern concepts of staging were codified at the Rye, New York conference in 1965 *(79)* and further refined at the Workshop on the Staging of Hodgkin's Disease in Ann Arbor, Michigan in 1971 *(80)* (Table 2). Clinical stage refers to the results of physical, radiographic, and laboratory examination, and pathologic stage refers to the use of additional biopsy procedures. The classification is further characterized by the presence or absence of constitutional symptoms. Extranodal disease, representing extracapsular extension of lymph-node disease that can be treated with a curative dose of radiotherapy, is distinguished from disseminated stage IV disease. The correlation of this staging classification system with prognosis has

Table 2
Ann Arbor Staging System

Staging

The staging system used for non-Hodgkin's lymphomas is the Ann Arbor
    classification developed for the staging and treatment (primarily with radiation)
    of Hodgkin's disease.

Stage I	Involvement of a single lymph-node region (I), or localized involvement of a single organ or site other than lymph nodes (I_E).
Stage II	Involvement of two or more lymph-node regions on the same side of the diaphragm (stage II) or localized involvement of a single associated organ or site other than lymph nodes (extranodal) and its regional lymph nodes, with or without other lymph node regions on the same side of the diaphragm (II_E).
Stage III	Involvement of lymph node regions on both sides of the diaphragm (stage III) that may also be accompanied by localized involvement of an extranodal organ or site (III_E), involvement of the spleen (III_S), or both (III_S + E).
Stage IV	Diffuse or disseminated involvement of one or more extranodal sites with or without associated lymph-node involvement, or isolated extranodal organ involvement with distant lymph-node involvement.

Each stage may be subdivided into A or B according to the presence or absence of general
symptoms. "A" means the absence of "B" symptoms, which include any of: fevers over 38°C
(100.4°F), drenching night sweats, or the unexplained loss of more than 10 percent of body wt.

been extensively verified. Prognostic information such as mediastinal bulk,
other bulky nodal masses, and the extent of subdiaphragmatic nodal disease is
included in a modification of the Ann Arbor system, known as the Cotswold
classification *(81)*.

Recommended staging procedures for untreated patients have evolved with
changes in therapy. The use of staging laparotomy, a surgical diagnostic procedure in which the intra-abdominal and pelvic lymph nodes are sampled, the
spleen is removed and examined pathologically, the liver is biopsied by needle
and wedge technique and the bone marrow is biopsied, has become very
restricted. This procedure is currently used in selected centers to identify a small
subset of patients who are candidates for management with limited radiotherapy
only. Historically, staging laparotomy advanced about one-third of clinical stage
I and II patients to pathologic stage III and IV and reduced less than one-fourth
of clinical stage III patients to pathologic stage I or II *(82–85)*. Prognostic indicators of laparotomy findings have been described *(86,87)*. For instance, all of
the following have only a 5–10% risk of subdiaphragmatic disease: CS I women,
CS I intrathoracic-only disease, CS I high-neck disease and favorable histology,
and CS I men with lymphocyte predominance histology.

Bone-marrow involvement occurs in 5–20% of new patients and is more common in patients of older age, advanced stage, and less favorable histology, or those with constitutional symptoms or immunodeficiency. Because the bone marrow is almost never involved in young, asymptomatic patients with favorable clinical stage I or II presentations, bone-marrow biopsy may at times be omitted in their routine staging. Bone scans are indicated in patients with bone pain; skeletal X-rays may demonstrate osteolytic, osteoblastic, or mixed lesions.

Laboratory Features

There are no diagnostic laboratory features of Hodgkin's disease. A routine complete blood count may reveal granulocytosis *(88)*, eosinophilia *(89)*, lymphocytopenia *(90)*, thrombocytosis *(91)*, anemia *(92)*, or thrombocytopenia *(93–95)*. Cytopenias are particularly common in advanced-stage disease, and lymphocyte depletion histology. Elevation of the erythrocyte sedimentation rate (ESR), has been correlated with prognosis in limited disease, and may herald recurrance *(96–98)*. Serum lactate dehydrogenase and alkaline phosphatase levels may be elevated in Hodgkin's disease *(99–101)*. As discussed here, anemia, granulocytosis, lymphopenia, and low-serum albumin constitute four of seven adverse prognostic factors identified in advanced Hodgkin's disease *(102)*. Rare laboratory abnormalities and clinical presentations include hypercalcemia *(103)*, hypoglycemia *(104,105)*, inappropriate secretion of antidiuretic hormone *(106)*, and the nephrotic syndrome *(107,108)*.

Examination of pleural fluid in Hodgkin's disease may reveal transudative, exudative, or chylous properties, but cytology rarely yields diagnostic RS-H cells. The etiology is most often considered to be one of central lymphatic obstruction.

THERAPY, COURSE, AND PROGNOSIS
Radiotherapy

Hodgkin's disease first became a curable neoplasm through the systematic study of the spread of the disease and the use of supervoltage radiotherapy techniques. Pusey (1902) *(109)* and Senn (1903) *(110)* were the first to report dramatic regressions of lymphadenopathy with X-rays. Motivated by the nearly inevitable recurrences in untreated areas, Gilbert proposed the systematic treatment of both involved and uninvolved areas in 1939 *(111)*. Peters (1950) is credited for the first demonstration of the curative potential of radiotherapy *(77)*. The development of megavoltage radiotherapy (doses >4000 cGy), as reported by Kaplan in 1962 *(112)*, permitted the delivery of tumoricidal doses to virtually all lymphoid regions in the body within acceptable limits of normal tissue tolerance.

The classic regions of radiotherapy employed in Hodgkin's disease include the mantle, para-aortic region, and pelvis (Fig. 1). The mantle region encom-

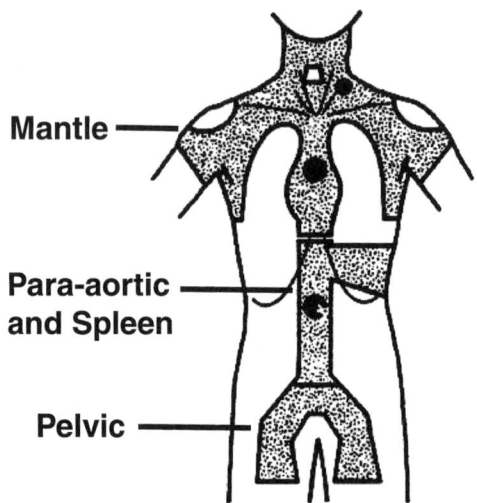

Fig. 1. Radiation fields.

passed the cervical, supraclavicular, infraclavicular, axillary, mediastinal, and hilar nodes. The para-aortic region included treatment to the pelvic brim and the splenic pedicle or the spleen, if still intact. Together, these regions were referred to as "subtotal lymphoid irradiation." The combination of the para-aortic region and the pelvic region was called an "inverted Y," and total lymphoid irradiation referred to the combined mantle and inverted Y regions. In the current management of Hodgkin's disease, wide-field irradiation is rarely used. In the setting of combined chemotherapy and radiotherapy treatment, modifications of the mantle field have been made to address adverse consequences of treatment. The axillae and the upper neck often are not included in the field. Lung blocks are shaped to ensure adequate irradiation of the tumor volume. The whole heart is not treated unless there is evidence of pericardial involvement. A pericardial block is placed at 1500 cGy, and a subcarinal block is placed at 3000 cGy. The technical aspects of radiotherapy—including fractionation, simulators, individually constructed blocks, detailed positioning, beam definition, and dosimetry—are extremely important.

Chemotherapy

From 1942 through 1963, a number of single chemotherapy drugs, including nitrogen mustard, vinca alkaloids, corticosteroids, and procarbazine became available for clinical use *(113,114)*. Although responses were observed, there was no evidence of cure. The first modern combination chemotherapy program was devised by DeVita and colleagues *(115)*. The MOPP (nitrogen mustard, vincristine, procarbazine, and prednisone) program differed from previous attempts in its curative intent, longer treatment program, and the introduction of a sliding scale for dose adjustment based upon hematologic toxicity. The national mortality figures for Hodgkin's disease decreased by more than 60% in the decade that followed the introduction of MOPP chemotherapy *(116)*.

Bonadonna and colleagues developed the next important alternative regimen. ABVD (adriamycin, bleomycin, vinblastine, and dacarbazine) was effective in the treatment of patients who had failed MOPP. ABVD was subsequently employed alone, in combination with radiotherapy, and used together with MOPP in alternating or "hybrid" programs *(117–123)* (Table 3).

Recently, two chemotherapy regimens have been introduced as part of combined modality approaches with radiotherapy for the treatment of Hodgkin's disease. The German Hodgkin Lymphoma Study Group (GHSG) developed the BEACOPP (bleomycin, etoposide, doxorubicin, cyclophosphamide, vincristine, prednisone, and procarbazine) combination, which has been tested in standard and escalated doses with radiotherapy to bulky and residual masses *(124,125)*. The Stanford group developed an abbreviated 12-wk combination, Stanford V (doxorubicin, vinblastine, vincristine, bleomycin, nitrogen mustard, etoposide, and prednisone) with radiation to bulky sites *(126,127)*. Table 3 describes the drugs, doses, and schedules of combination chemotherapy programs effective in the management of Hodgkin's disease.

FAVORABLE LIMITED-STAGE DISEASE

Favorable, limited-stage disease may be defined as asymptomatic stage I or II supradiaphragmatic disease with no bulky sites and ≤1 extranodal site. Extended-field (subtotal lymphoid) radiotherapy was the treatment of choice for these patients in the United States for many years. This treatment was based on the results of clinical trials, including one conducted at Stanford University in which stage I–IIA patients were randomized to involved-field or extended-field radiotherapy *(128)*. Extended-field radiotherapy yielded a highly significant advantage in freedom from relapse, 80%, compared with 32% for involved field. The overall survival rate was the same for the two groups because of effective treatment at relapse. Subsequent reports from multiple institutions have confirmed the high rate of cure in stage I and II with extended-field radiotherapy. A recent meta-analysis concluded that more extensive radiotherapy increased the chance of cure by more than 30%, although no survival benefit was seen at 10 yr *(129)*. An exception is for very favorable patients (≤40 yr with nodular sclerosis or lymphocyte predominance, laparotomy-stage (PS) I, and IIA with mediastinal disease and ESR less than 70), in which no difference was seen between mantle radiotherapy or subtotal lymphoid radiotherapy for treatment failure or overall survival *(130–132)*.

The treatment of early-stage disease is so successful that at 15–20 yr, the overall mortality rate from other causes exceeds deaths caused by Hodgkin's

Table 3
Common Combination Chemotherapy Regimens for Hodgkin's Disease

Drug	Dose mg/m^2	Route	Schedule	Cycle length
MOPP				**28 days**
Nitrogen mustard	6	IV	Days 1,8	
Vincristine	1.4*	IV	Days 1,8	
Procarbazine	100	PO	Days 1–14	
Prednisone	40	PO	Days 1–14	
ChlVPP				**28 days**
Chlorambucil	6**	PO	Days 1–14	
Vinblastine	6**	IV	Days 1,8	
Procarbazine	100	PO	Days 1–14	
Prednisone	40	PO	Days 1–14	
ABVD				**28 days**
Adriamycin	25	IV	Days 1,15	
Bleomycin	10 U/m^2	IV	Days 1,15	
Vinblastine	6	IV	Days 1,15	
Dacarbazine	375	IV	Days 1,15	
MOPP/ABV hybrid				**28 days**
Nitrogen mustard	6	IV	Day 1	
Vincristine	1.4*	IV	Day 1	
Procarbazine	100	PO	Days 1–7	
Prednisone	40	PO	Days 1–14	
Adriamycin	35	IV	Day 8	
Bleomycin	10 U/m^2	IV	Day 8	
Vinblastine	6	IV	Day 8	
MOPP/ABVD alternating				
Alternating months of MOPP and ABVD, as above				
STANFORD V				**8 wk (12 wk)**
Nitrogen mustard	6	IV	Wk. 1,5,(9)	
Doxorubicin	25	IV	Wk 1,3,5,7,(9,11)	
Vinblastine	6	IV	Wk 1,3,5,7,(9,11)	
Vincristine	1.4*	IV	Wk 2,4,6,8,(10,12)	
Bleomycin	5 U/m^2	IV	Wk 2,4,6,8,(10,12)	
Etoposide	60 × 2	IV	Wk 3,7,(11)	
Prednisone	40	PO	Q.O.D. Wk 1–6 (1–10), taper	
G-CSF	For dose reduction or delay			
BEACOPP (escalated)				**21 days**
Bleomycin	10 U/m^2	IV	Day 8	
Etoposide	100 (200)	IV	Days 1–3	
Doxorubicin	25 (35)	IV	Day 1	
Cyclophosphamide	650 (1250)	IV	Day 1	
Vincristine	1.4*	IV	Day 8	
Procarbazine	100	PO	Days 1–7	
Prednisone	40	PO	Days 1–14	
G-CSF	(+)	SC	Day 8—leukocyte recovery	

*Vincristine usually capped at a maximun of 2 mg per dose.
**Some stuides cap at 10 mg.

disease *(133)*. The largest cause of mortality is second cancers, which appears to be most closely linked to the extent of radiotherapy. Thus, there is considerable interest in reducing the volume and dose of radiotherapy. In sequential clinical trials, Stanford University investigators demonstrated that involved-field radiotherapy with adjuvant chemotherapy could substitute for extended-field radiotherapy in stage I and II patients *(128,134,135)*. Each of these trials demonstrated equivalent or superior results for combined modality therapy. The EORTC showed improved event-free survival (EFS) in a randomization of favorable CS I-IIA patients between six cycles of EBVP (epirubicin, bleomycin, vinblastine, and prednisone) plus involved-field radiotherapy vs subtotal radiotherapy *(136)*.

In recent years, clinical trials have sought to test the optimal number of cycles of chemotherapy and the volume and dose of radiotherapy. The Milan Tumor Institute described more than 95% disease control with four cycles of ABVD and either extended-field or involved-field radiotherapy *(137)*. Preliminary data from the GHSG trial in favorable I–II patients indicate that two cycles of ABVD followed by subtotal radiotherapy are superior to subtotal radiotherapy alone *(138)*. The Manchester group has shown a 91% progression-free survival with 4 wk of VAPEC-B (vinblastine, doxorubicin, prednisone, etoposide, cyclophosphamide, and bleomycin) and limited radiotherapy *(139)*. An 8-wk course of Stanford V and limited-field and dose radiotherapy yields a 95% EFS in favorable CS I-IIA *(140)*. These outstanding results with relatively modest therapy are encouraging, although longer follow-up is required before a true reduction in late effects can be assessed.

Several subsets of limited patients deserve further mention. Subdiaphragmatic presentations of Hodgkin's disease are best managed with combined modality therapy or chemotherapy alone. Stage IIB patients are generally managed with chemotherapy or combined modality. Early-stage NLPHD patients may be considered for treatment with involved-field radiotherapy alone.

LOCALLY EXTENSIVE LIMITED-STAGE HODGKIN'S DISEASE

Extensive mediastinal Hodgkin's disease is frequently accompanied by extranodal extension to the lungs, pericardium, and chest wall. Pleural effusions may also be seen. The used of combined chemotherapy and radiation (combined modality therapy) results in freedom from relapse in 80% or more of such patients compared with only 40–55% following radiation alone *(141)*, although effective salvage with chemotherapy after radiation failure resulted in similar overall survival. In question are the optimal chemotherapy regimen and its duration, the radiation dose, and the sequence of therapy for combined treatment. The Milan group randomized 232 patients with subtotal lymphoid irradiation sandwiched between six courses of MOPP or ABVD *(119,142)*. A portion of these patients had extensive mediastinal disease. The ABVD/RT combination was significantly superior to MOPP/RT, as measured by both freedom from progression and survival. The major concerns in the choice of chemotherapy relate to late effects, specifically the concern for sterility and acute leukemia ascribed to alkylating agents and the potential for enhanced cardiopulmonary toxicity with ABVD, especially when combined with radiotherapy. Subsequently, the Milan group has reported the efficacy of four cycles of ABVD and involved-field radiotherapy in stage I–II patients, many of whom had massive mediastinal disease *(138)*. The 12-wk Stanford V program, together with modified mantle radiotherapy, was also very effective in these patients *(124)*. There is relatively little experience with the use of chemotherapy alone for bulky mediastinal Hodgkin's disease. A retrospective report of the results with MOPP alone or MOPP with adjuvant radiotherapy in this subset described cure of less than one-half of these patients with MOPP alone *(143)*.

ADVANCED DISEASE

Chemotherapy forms the basis of current treatments for stage III–IV classical Hodgkin's disease. Twenty-year follow-up of the original NCI MOPP series demonstrated that the actuarial freedom from progression was 54%, and 48% had survived *(144)*. Constitutional symptoms, male sex, advanced-stage disease, and administration of vincristine lower than the projected rate were prognostic for complete response. Bonadonna and colleagues tested a program of MOPP alternating with ABVD vs MOPP for 12 mo in stage IV patients *(118)*. The 8-yr freedom from progression rates significantly favored MOPP/ABVD 65% vs 36%. Overall survival rates were superior, although not significant, for MOPP/ABVD (84%) compared with MOPP (64%). The Cancer and Acute Leukemia Group B (CALGB) compared MOPP for eight cycles, ABVD for eight cycles, and MOPP alternating with ABVD for 12 monthly cycles *(120)*. For patients with stages IIIA, IIIB, and IV disease, the ABVD and MOPP/ABVD results showed superior freedom from progression compared to MOPP (Table 4). An Intergroup study led by CALGB randomized patients to ABVD alone vs a MOPP/ABV hybrid regimen (Table 4). The study was stopped early because of excess deaths and second cancers in the hybrid arm. At the time the study was reported, there were no differences in efficacy with 65% of ABVD patients and 67% of hybrid patients failure-free *(145)*. In aggregate the multiple clinical trials indicate that 60–70% of patients with advanced Hodgkin's disease are cured with ABVD, hybrid, or alternating combinations. Of these, ABVD alone has emerged as the preferred treatment because it has a more favorable toxicity profile.

In an attempt to further improve outcomes in advanced Hodgkin's disease, the GHSG developed the BEACOPP regimen *(124,125)*. An escalated version incorporates higher doses of these drugs facilitated by a granulocyte colony-

Table 4
Selected Randomized Trials in Advanced Hodgkin's Disease

	F/U	FFP%	OS%	Comments
Milan *(118)*	8 yr			12 cycles of therapy. Due to small numbers (*n* = 88), significance for OS not met
MOPP		36	64	
MOPP/ABVD		65	84	
Milan *(119)*	7 yr			Difficulty in giving planned doses of MOPP after radiation
MOPP-RT-MOPP		63	68	
ABVD-RT-ABVD		91	77	
CALGB *(120)*	5 yr			Significant advantage of ABVD and ABVD/MOPP for FFP, trend for OS
	50	66		
ABVD		61	73	
MOPP/ABVD		65	75	
Intergroup *(145)*	3 yr			Greater toxicity with hybrid regimen
ABVD		65	87	
MOPP/ABV		67	84	
GHSG *(124)*	28 mo			
COPP/ABVD		69	86	BEACOPP regimens superior, longer follow-up needed to assess late effects
BEACOPP		79	90	
BEACOPP (escalated)		88	91	

stimulating factor (G-CSF). Patients with initial tumor bulk or residual radiographic disease received 36 gy radiation to these sites after chemotherapy. Interim analyses showed superior outcomes for BEACOPP compared with the standard alternating chemotherapy arm (Table 4). The results, with cure rates in greater than 80%, are the best recorded for a large phase III trial in advanced Hodgkin's disease. Secondary leukemias are reported in these early reports, and mature follow-up is required to determine the combined efficacy and toxicity of this approach. The Stanford V regimen shortens the duration of therapy, reducing the cumulative drug doses, and adding radiotherapy for patients with bulky (≥5 cm) nodal or macroscopic splenic disease. At the latest update, the 12 wk Stanford V regimen, rendered freedom from progression in excess of 85% and overall survival in excess of 95% *(146)*. The current Intergroup study in North America is testing ABVD vs Stanford V, including radiotherapy, in locally extensive and advanced Hodgkin's disease with 0–2 adverse international prognostic factors as defined here *(102)*.

Benefits of low-dose irradiation as a consolidation to combination chemotherapy were reported in single-arm experiences *(147,148)*. However, no sig-

Table 5
Prognostic Factors for Hodgkin's Disease

	Limited stage xs		Advanced stage
	GHSG	*EORTC*	*International collaborative study*
			Adverse prognostic factors
Very favorable (must meet all criteria)	CS-IA Female Age <40 yr LP/NS MMR< 0.35		Age ≥50 yr Stage IV
Favorable	All others	All others	Male sex White blood cell count $15,000 cells/μL
Unfavorable (If any criteria)	MMR ≥0.35 High ESR ≥4 sites Age ≥50 yr	MMR ≥0.35 High ESR ≥3 Sites Extranodal sites Massive Splenic Disease	Lymphocyte count <800 cells/μL or <6% Albumin <4 g/dL Hemoglobin <10.5 g/dL

LP=lymphocyte predominant; NS=nodular sclerosing; MMR=mediastinal mass ratio; ESR=erythrocyte sedimentation rate.

nificant advantage was seen when compared with chemotherapy alone in randomized trials, although these studies have been criticized because radiation was not delivered properly in a subset of patients *(149–152)* High-dose chemotherapy followed by autologous stem-cell transplant is currently being studied in poor-risk patients.

PROGNOSTIC FACTORS

A number of complex prognostic factor schemes have been developed for limited Hodgkin's disease treated with radiotherapy alone (Table 5). Massive mediastinal disease and constitutional symptoms were consistently identified as independent predictors of relapse, whereas only older age was predictive of inferior survival *(153,141,154,155)*. European and Canadian investigators incorporated gender, age, ESR, number of Ann Arbor disease sites, stage, and histology into stratifications for favorable, very favorable, and unfavorable disease categories *(131,156)*. When newer combined modality treatments are used for limited disease, the significance of these factors is unknown, but it is important to be aware of the variable eligibility criteria when interpreting the literature. Recently, an international consortium pooled patient data and identified a prognostic score for advanced Hodgkin's disease based on seven factors (Table 5) *(102)*. These include male sex, age ≥45 yr, stage IV, white blood count

≥15,000/μL, lymphocyte count <8% or <600/μL, hemoglobin <10. 5 g/dL, and albumin <4 g/dL. The presence of each factor reduced the freedom from progression by about 7%. Only 7% of patients were in the worst prognostic group (5–7 factors), and the freedom from progression in this subset was 42% at 5 yr. Consensus with regard to prognostic factors promotes uniformity in clinical trial design and provides a rationale for new approaches such as dose intensification and autologous bone-marrow transplantation in high-risk subsets *(157)*.

These clinical prognostic factors are surrogates for the underlying biology of Hodgkin's disease. Prognostic significance has been ascribed to a variety of biologic parameters including histopathologic grading of nodular sclerosis, immunophenotype, oncogene expression, and characteristics of the T-cell infiltrate *(7,15,158,159)*. In addition, serum levels of soluble CD30, Il-6, IL-10, and the IL-2 receptor have been reported to correlate with constitutional symptoms and advanced disease *(160–164)*.

TREATMENT OF RECURRENT DISEASE

Patients who relapse after radiotherapy alone have an excellent probability of cure with chemotherapy *(165,166)*. Patients with extensive disease at recurrence and those with constitutional symptoms have a less favorable prognosis *(167)*. The outlook is significantly less favorable for patients who relapse after chemotherapy alone or chemotherapy given in combination with radiotherapy. The length of prior remission—greater or less than 1 yr—has a significant effect on the ability of patients to respond to subsequent treatment and maintain their response *(168)*. The availability of autologous bone marrow or peripheral-blood stem cells has markedly increased the options for treatment of recurrent Hodgkin's disease. For patients in first relapse, disease-free survival rates of 50–60% are reported at 4–5 yr and, with early transplant-related mortality less than 5% *(169–172)*. Two randomized clinical trials provide compelling evidence for the superiority of transplantation in relapsed Hodgkin's disease. In the British National Lymphoma Investigation trial, patients were randomized to conventional or high-dose BEAM (carmustine, etoposide, cytosine arabinoside, melphalan), the latter with autologous stem-cell transplantation *(173)*. This study was stopped because the 3-yr EFS was markedly superior in the high-dose arm compared with standard BEAM, 53% vs 10%, respectively. The largest multicenter trial was conducted in Europe, where patients with relapsed Hodgkin's disease were randomly assigned to four cycles of Dexa-BEAM (dexamethasone and BEAM) or two cycles of Dexa-BEAM followed by autologous stem-cell transplantation *(174)*. Interim analysis of this trial demonstrated superior freedom from treatment failure in the transplant group (53%) vs 39% for patients receiving Dexa-BEAM alone ($p = 0.025$). No survival advantage was observed.

Primary treatment induction failures present a special challenge to clinicians. Single-institution and registry data indicate that a subset of refractory patients, as many as 38–49%, were alive and disease-free after high-dose therapy and transplantation with follow-up of 3–4yr *(175–177)*.

COMPLICATIONS OF TREATMENT

The treatment of Hodgkin's disease is associated with a wide array of acute and chronic side effects. Although the acute complications of chemotherapy and radiotherapy may be troublesome, they are relatively easily managed. Late treatment effects in the form of sterility, cardiopulmonary disease, and second malignancy are more serious.

Acute leukemia and myelodysplasia were the initial second malignancies to be observed after successful treatment for Hodgkin's disease with MOPP chemotherapy *(178–180)*. The risk is proportional to the cumulative dose of alkylating agents, which in some cases included maintenance therapy, prolonged treatment, or salvage therapy *(181,182)*. Actuarial risks of 1–10% with relative risks in excess of 100 have been reported over a 7–10-yr period *(183,184)*. In a multi-institutional, case-control study of 29,552 Hodgkin's disease patients, the relative risk of acute leukemia was increased in patients who received more than six cycles of MOPP chemotherapy, and no increased risk was found with combined radiation and chemotherapy *(181)*. The risk of acute leukemia is significantly less after ABVD chemotherapy.

There is an increased relative risk of non-Hodgkin's lymphomas after treatment for Hodgkin's disease *(184,185)*. These are diffuse, aggressive B-cell lymphomas that may occur early or late after treatment. There is no clear relationship to the type of primary treatment. Some have considered the non-Hodgkin's lymphomas to be a result of the ongoing immunodeficiency, and others have suggested a common cell of origin.

An increased risk of solid cancers after treatment for Hodgkin's disease has been identified *(184,186,187)*. The risk is related to radiotherapy exposure, with tumors occurring infield or at the edges of the radiotherapy field. In the Stanford series, the overall actuarial risk of second solid-cancer malignancy at 15 yr was about 18% *(184)*. Cancers of the lung, stomach, bone, and soft tissue were observed. An increased risk of breast cancer and thyroid cancer was only appreciated when mean follow-up was 10 or more years *(188–190)*. Breast cancer is increased in women treated before age 30, and is markedly increased in children and adolescents *(188,190,191)*.

Mediastinal radiotherapy is associated with an increased risk of cardiac disease. An increased risk of death from coronary artery disease and acute myocardial infarction has been identified in adults and children *(133,192,193)*. Other types of cardiac disease following chest radiotherapy include valvular disease, constrictive pericarditis, and cardiomyopathy. It is unclear whether the risks of radiation-related heart disease can be significantly influenced by the addition of chemotherapy. The onset of increased risk is within 5–10 yr.

About 90% of males are permanently sterilized by six cycles of MOPP chemotherapy *(194)*. Female fertility after MOPP is related to age at treatment as well as cumulative alkylating agent dose *(195,196)*. Women over age 25 at treatment have an 80% probability of sterility following six courses of MOPP. The ABVD combination is associated with temporary amenorrhea and azoospermia, with full recovery noted in 50–90% of patients *(197,198)*. No increase in birth defects has been seen in the offspring of patients previously treated for Hodgkin's disease *(196)*.

Lhermitte's sign, a transient complaint of an "electric shock" sensation produced by head flexion is a common sequela of mantle radiotherapy *(199)*. An elevated thyroid-stimulating hormone level, with or without a low T3 or T4, is seen in about 30% of patients following mantle radiotherapy *(189)*. Rarely, hyperthyroidism, Grave's ophthalmopathy, or thyroid neoplasms occur after neck radiotherapy *(189)*. The incidence of radiation pneumonitis depends on the volume of lung irradiated and the total dose. Symptoms include cough, dyspnea, and fever. Although the prospective assessment of pulmonary function demonstrates reduction of lung volumes following mantle radiotherapy, recovery is seen in 12–24 mo and symptomatic radiation pneumonitis is unusual *(200,201)*.

Full-dose radiation therapy interferes with normal growth and development in children. Current pediatric therapy programs use low dose or no radiotherapy for all stages of disease. Overwhelming sepsis is a rare event in patients who have been splenectomized and treated for Hodgkin's disease, particularly children *(202,203)*. Vaccination against encapsulated organisms 10–14 d prior to the onset of treatment is advised. However, it must be recognized that neither vaccines nor antibiotic prophylaxis may provide adequate protection, and patients must be educated about this risk. Psychosocial sequelae of treatment for Hodgkin's lymphoma deserve further study *(204)*. With the high rates of cure currently attained in the management of Hodgkin's disease, reduction in late effects and quality of life assume even greater importance.

REFERENCES

1. Miettinen M. CD30 distribution. Immunohistochemical study on formaldehyde-fixed, paraffin-embedded Hodgkin's and non-Hodgkin's lymphomas. *Arch Pathol Lab Med* 1992; 116:1197.
2. Penny RJ, Blaustein JC, Longtine JA, Pinkus GS. Ki-1-positive large cell lymphomas, a heterogenous group of neoplasms. Morphologic, immunophenotypic, genotypic, and clinical features of 24 cases. *Cancer* 1991; 68:362.
3. Schienle HW, Stein N, Muller RW. Neutrophil granulocytic cell antigen defined by a monoclonal antibody—its distribution within normal haemic and non-haemic tissue. *J Clin Pathol* 1982; 35:959.
4. Stein H, Uchánska-Ziegler B, Gerdes J, Ziegler A, Wernet P. Hodgkin and Sternberg-Reed cells contain antigens specific to late cells of granulopoiesis. *Int J Cancer* 1982; 29:283.

5. Schmid C, Pan L, Diss T, Isaacson PG. Expression of B-cell antigens by Hodgkin's and Reed-Sternberg cells. *Am J Pathol* 1991; 139:701.

6. Lauritzen AF, Moller PH, Nedergaard T, Guldberg P, Hou-Jensen K, Ralfkiaer E. Apoptosis-related genes and proteins in Hodgkin's disease. *APMIS* 1999; 107:636.

7. von Wasielewski R, Mengel M, Fischer R, et al. Classical Hodgkin's disease. Clinical impact of the immunophenotype. *Am J Pathol* 1997; 151:1123.

8. Papadimitriou CS, Bai MK, Kotsianti AJ, Costopoulos JS, Hytiroglou P. Phenotype of Hodgkin and Sternberg-Reed cells and expression of CD57 (LEU7) antigen. *Leuk Lymphoma* 1995; 20:125.

9. Pinkus GS, Said JW. Hodgkin's disease, lymphocyte predominance type, nodular—further evidence for a B cell derivation. L & H variants of Reed-Sternberg cells express L26, a pan B cell marker. *Am J Pathol* 1988; 133:211.

10. Poppema S, Kaiserling E, Lennert K. Nodular paragranuloma and progressively transformed germinal centers. Ultrastructural and immunohistologic findings. *Virchows Arch B Cell Pathol* 1979; 31:211.

11. Burns BF, Colby TV, Dorfman RF. Differential diagnostic features of nodular L & H Hodgkin's disease, including progressive transformation of germinal centers. *Am J Surg Pathol* 1984; 8:253.

12. Hansmann ML, Zwingers T, Boske A, Loffler H, Lennert K. Clinical features of nodular paragranuloma (Hodgkin's disease, lymphocyte predominance type, nodular). *J Cancer Res Clin Oncol* 1984; 108:321.

13. Miettinen M, Franssila KO, Saxen E. Hodgkin's disease, lymphocytic predominance nodular. Increased risk for subsequent non-Hodgkin's lymphomas. *Cancer* 1983; 51:2293.

14. Sundeen JT, Cossman J, Jaffe ES. Lymphocyte predominant Hodgkin's disease nodular subtype with coexistent "large cell lymphoma." Histological progression or composite malignancy? *Am J Surg Pathol* 1988; 12:599.

15. MacLennan KA, Bennett MH, Tu A, et al. Relationship of histopathologic features to survival and relapse in nodular sclerosing Hodgkin's disease. A study of 1659 patients. *Cancer* 1989; 64:1686.

16. Masih AS, Weisenburger DD, Vose JM, Bast MA, Armitage JO. Histologic grade does not predict prognosis in optimally treated, advanced-stage nodular sclerosing Hodgkin's disease. *Cancer* 1992; 69:228.

17. Kant JA, Hubbard SM, Longo DL, Simon RM, DeVita VJ, Jaffe ES. The pathologic and clinical heterogeneity of lymphocyte-depleted Hodgkin's disease. *J Clin Oncol* 4:284, 1986.

18. Neiman RS, Rosen PJ, Lukes RJ. Lymphocyte-depletion Hodgkin's disease. A clinicopathological entity. *N Engl J Med* 1973; 288:751.

19. Diehl V, Sextro M, Franklin J, et al. Clinical presentation, course, and prognostic factors in lymphocyte-predominant Hodgkin's disease and lymphocyte-rich classical Hodgkin's disease: report from the European Task Force on Lymphoma Project on Lymphocyte-Predominant Hodgkin's Disease. *J Clin Oncol* 1999; 17:776.

20. Landis SH, Murray T, Bolden S, Wingo PA. Cancer statistics, 1999. *CA Cancer J Clin* 1999; 49:8.

21. MacMahon B. Epidemiology of Hodgkin's disease. *Cancer Res* 1966; 26:1189.

22. Grufferman S, Duong T, Cole P. Occupation and Hodgkin's disease. *J Natl Cancer Inst* 1976; 57:1193.

23. Young JJ, Percy CL, Asire AJ, et al. Cancer incidence and mortality in the United States, 1973–77. *Natl Cancer Inst Monogr* 1981; 57:1.

24. Abramson JH, Pridan H, Sacks MI, Avitzour M, Peritz E. A case-control study of Hodgkin's disease in Israel. *J Natl Cancer Inst* 1978; 61:307.

25. Gutensohn N, Cole P. Childhood social environment and Hodgkin's disease. *N Engl J Med* 1981; 304:135.

26. Grufferman S, Delzell E. Epidemiology of Hodgkin's disease. *Epidemiol Rev* 1984; 6:76.

27. Vianna NJ, Greenwald P, Davies JN. Extended epidemic of Hodgkin's disease in high-school students. *Lancet* 1971; 1:1209.
28. Klinger RJ, Minton JP. Case clustering of Hodgkin's disease in a small rural community, with associations among cases. *Lancet* 1973; 1:168.
29. Vianna NJ, Greenwald P, Davies JNP. Epidemiologic evidence for transmission of Hodgkin's disease: the lymphoid tissue barrier. *N Engl J Med* 1974; 10:499.
30. Cuneo JM. Infectious aspects of Hodgkin's disease. *N Engl J Med* 1974; 290:345.
31. Pike MC, Henderson BE, Casagrande J. Infectious aspects of Hodgkin's disease. *N Engl J Med* 1974; 290:341.
32. Grufferman S, Cole P, Levitan TR. Evidence against transmission of Hodgkin's disease in high schools. *N Engl J Med* 1979; 300:1006.
33. Rosdahl N, Larsen SO, Clemmesen J. Hodgkin's disease in patients with previous infectious mononucleosis: 30 years' experience. *Br Med J* 1974; 2:253.
34. Munoz N, Davidson RLJ, Witthoff B. Infectious mononucleosis and Hodgkin's disease. *Int J Cancer* 1978; 22:10.
35. Kvale G, Hoiby EA, Pedersen E. Hodgkin's disease in patients with previous infectious mononucleosis. *Int J Cancer* 1979; 23:593.
36. Mueller N, Evans A, Harris N. Altered antibody titers to Epstein-Barr virus before the diagnosis of Hodgkin's disease. *N Engl J Med* 1989; 320:689.
37. Weiss LM, Strickler JG, Warnke RA, Purtilo DT, Sklar J. Epstein-Barr viral DNA in tissues of Hodgkin's disease. *Am J Pathol* 1987; 129:86.
38. Boiocchi M, De RV, Dolcetti R, Carbone A, Scarpa A, Menestrina F. Association of Epstein-Barr virus genome with mixed cellularity and cellular phase nodular sclerosis Hodgkin's disease subtypes. *Ann Oncol* 1992; 3:307.
39. Herbst H, Pallesen G, Weiss LM, et al. Hodgkin's disease and Epstein-Barr virus. *Ann Oncol* 1992; 4:27.
40. Armstrong AA, Alexander FE, Paes RP, et al. Association of Epstein-Barr virus with pediatric Hodgkin's disease. *Am J Pathol* 1993; 142:1683.
41. Ambinder RF, Browning PJ, Lorenzana I, et al. Epstein-Barr virus and childhood Hodgkin's disease in Honduras and the United States. *Blood* 1993; 81:462.
42. Chang KL, Albújar PF, Chen YY, Johnson RM, Weiss LM. High prevalence of Epstein-Barr virus in the Reed-Sternberg cells of Hodgkin's disease occurring in Peru. *Blood* 1993; 81:496.
43. Weinreb M, Day PJ, Murray PG, et al. Epstein-Barr virus (EBV) and Hodgkin's disease in children: incidence of EBV latent membrane protein in malignant cells. *J Pathol* 1992; 168:365.
44. Herndier BG, Sanchez HC, Chang KL, Chen YY, Weiss LM. High prevalence of Epstein-Barr virus in the Reed-Sternberg cells of HIV-associated Hodgkin's disease. *Am J Pathol* 1993; 142:1073.
45. Lynch HT, Saldivar VA, Guirgis HA, et al. Familial Hodgkin's disease and associated cancer. A clinical-pathologic study. *Cancer* 1976; 38:2033.
46. Creagan ET, Fraumeni JJ. Familial Hodgkin's disease. *Lancet* 1972; 2:547.
47. Buehler SK, Firme F, Fodor G, Fraser GR, Marshall WH, Vaze P. Common variable immunodeficiency, Hodgkin's disease, and other malignancies in a Newfoundland family. *Lancet* 1975; 1:195.
48. Manigand G, Macrez C, Chome J. Maladie de Hodgkin's familial. *Presse Med* 1964; 72:1871.
49. Bohunicky L, Poliakova L, Krizan Z, Cerny V, Hal'ko J. The incidence of lymphogranulo-matosis in single-ovum twins. *Neoplasma* 1971; 18:283.
50. Gracz K, Kofman S, Economou SG. Hodgkin disease in monozygotic twins: a case report. *J Surg Oncol* 1979; 12:221.
51. Razis DV, diamond HD, Craver LF. Familial Hodgkin's disease—Its signficance and implications. *Ann Intern Med* 1953; 51:933.

52. Vianna NJ, Davies JN, Polan AK, Wolfgang P. Familial Hodgkin's disease: an environmental and genetic disorder. *Lancet* 1974; 2:854.

53. Grufferman S, Cole P, Smith PG, Lukes RJ. Hodgkin's disease in siblings. *N Engl J Med* 1977; 296:248.

54. Kaplan HS. Hodgkin's Disease. Harvard University Press, Cambridge, MA, 1980.

55. Pel PK. Zur symptomatolgie der sogennanten pseudoleukamie. II. Pseudokeukamie oder chronisches Ruckfallsfieber? *Berlin Klin Wochenschr* 1887; 24:844.

56. Ebstein WV. Das chronische Ruckfallsfieber, eine neu infectionskrankheit. *Berlin Klin Wochenshr* 1887; 24:565.

57. Tubiana M, Attie E, Flamant R, Gerard MR, Hayat M. Prognostic factors in 454 cases of Hodgkin's disease. *Cancer Res* 1971; 31:1801.

58. Atkinson K, Austin DE, McElwain TJ, Peckham MJ. Alcohol pain in Hodgkin's disease. *Cancer* 1976; 37:895.

59. Bjerrum OW, Hansen OE. Progressive multifocal leucoencephalopathy in Hodgkin's disease. *Scand J Haematol* 1985; 34:442.

60. Trotter JL, Hendin BA, Osterland CK. Cerebellar degeneration with Hodgkin disease. An immunological study. *Arch Neurol* 1976; 33:660.

61. Greenberg HS. Paraneoplastic cerebellar degeneration. A clinical and CT study. *J Neurooncol* 1984; 2:377.

62. Dansey RD, Hammond TG, Lai K, Bezwoda WR. Subacute myelopathy: an unusual paraneoplastic complication of Hodgkin's disease. *Med Pediatr Oncol* 1988; 16:284.

63. Sagar HJ, Read DJ. Subacute sensory neuropathy with remission: an association with lymphoma. *J Neurol Neurosurg Psychiatry* 1982; 45:83.

64. Feldmann E, Posner JB. Episodic neurologic dysfunction in patients with Hodgkin's disease. *Arch Neurol* 1986; 43:1227.

65. Carr I. The Ophelia syndrome: memory loss in Hodgkin's disease. *Lancet* 1982; 1:844.

66. Julien J, Vital C, Aupy G, Lagueny A, Darriet D, Brechenmacher C. Guillain-Barré syndrome and Hodgkin's disease—ultrastructural study of a peripheral nerve. *J Neurol Sci* 1980; 45:23.

67. Rewcastle NB, Tom MI. Non-infectious granulomatis angiitis of the nervous system associated with Hodgkin's disease. *J Neurol Neurosurg Psychiatry* 1962; 25:51.

68. Filly R, Bland N, Castellino RA. Radiographic distribution of intrathoracic disease in previously untreated patients with Hodgkin's disease and non-Hodgkin's lymphoma. *Radiology* 1976; 120:277.

69. Kaplan HS. Survival and relapse rates in Hodgkin's disease: Stanford experience 1961–1971. *Natl Cancer Inst Monogr* 1973; 36:489.

70. Mansfield CM, Fabian C, Jones S, et al. Comparison of lymphangiography and computed tomography scanning in evaluating abdominal disease in stages III and IV Hodgkin's disease. A Southwest Oncology Group study. *Cancer* 1990; 66:2295.

71. Castellino RA, Hoppe RT, Blank N, et al. Computed tomography, lymphography, and staging laparotomy: correlations in initial staging of Hodgkin disease. *Ajr Am J Roentgenol* 1984; 143:37.

72. Castellino RA. Imaging techniques for staging abdominal Hodgkin's disease. *Cancer Treat Rep* 1982; 66:697.

73. Jerusalem G, Warland V, Najjar F, et al. Whole-body 18F-FDG PET for the evaluation of patients with Hodgkin's disease and non-Hodgkin's lymphoma. *Nucl Med Comm* 1999; 20:13.

74. Bangerter M, Moog F, Buchmann I, et al. Whole-body 2-[18F]-fluoro-2-deoxy-D-glucose positron emission tomography (FDG-PET) for accurate staging of Hodgkin's disease. *Ann Oncol* 1998; 9:1117.

75. Skillings JR, Bramwell V, Nicholson RL, Prato FS, Wells G. A prospective study of magnetic resonance imaging in lymphoma staging. *Cancer* 1991; 67:1838.

76. Gasparini MD, Balzarini L, Castellani MR, et al. Current role of gallium scan and magnetic resonance imaging in the management of mediastinal Hodgkin lymphoma. *Cancer* 1993; 72:577.

77. Peters M. A study of survivals in Hodgkin's disease treated radiologically. *Am J Roentgenol* 1950; 63:299.

78. Peters M. A study of Hodgkin's disease treated by irradiation. *Am J Roetgenol* 1958; 79:114.

79. Rosenberg S. Report of the committee on the staging of Hodgkin's disease. *Cancer Res* 1966; 26:1310.

80. Carbone P, Kaplan H, Musshoff K. Report of the committee on the Hodgkin's disease staging. *Cancer Res* 1971; 31:1860.

81. Lister TA, Crowther D, Sutcliffe SB, et al. Report of a committee convened to discuss the evaluation and staging of patients with Hodgkin's disease: Cotswolds meeting. *J Clin Oncol* 1989; 7:1630.

82. Piro AJ, Hellman S. Invited discussion: laparotomy alters treatment in Hodgkin's disease. *Natl Cancer Inst Monogr* 1973; 36:307.

83. Kaplan HS, Dorfman RF, Nelsen TS, Rosenberg SA. Staging laparotomy and splenectomy in Hodgkin's disease: analysis of indications and patterns of involvement in 285 consecutive, unselected patients. *Natl Cancer Inst Monogr* 1973; 36:291.

84. Desser RK, Golomb HM, Ultmann JE, et al. Prognostic classification of Hodgkin disease in pathologic stage III, based on anatomic considerations. *Blood* 1977; 49:883.

85. Stein RS, Golomb HM, Diggs CH, et al. Anatomic substages of stage III-A Hodgkin's disease. A collaborative study. *Ann Intern Med* 1980; xx:159.

86. Leibenhaut MH, Hoppe RT, Efron B, Halpern J, Nelsen T, Rosenberg SA. Prognostic indicators of laparotomy findings in clinical stage I-II supradiaphragmatic Hodgkin's disease. *J Clin Oncol* 1989; 7:81.

87. Mauch P, Larson D, Osteen R, et al. Prognostic factors for positive surgical staging in patients with Hodgkin's disease. *J Clin Oncol* 1990; 8:257.

88. Simmons AV, Spiers AS, Fayers PM. Haematological and clinical parameters in assessing activity in Hodgkin's disease and other malignant lymphomas. *Q J Med* 1973; 42:111.

89. Tauro GP. Hodgkin's disease associated with raised eosinophil counts. *Med J Aust* 1966; 2:604.

90. MacLennan KA, Hudson BV, Jelliffe AM, Haybittle JL, Hudson GV. The pretreatment peripheral blood lymphocyte count in 1100 patients with Hodgkin's disease: the prognostic significance and the relationship to the presence of systemic symptoms. *Clin Oncol* 1981; 7:333.

91. Ultmann JE, Cunningham JK, Gellhorn A. The clinical picture of Hodgkin's disease. *Cancer Res* 1966; 26:1047.

92. MacLennan KA, Vaughan HB, Easterling MJ, Jelliffe AM, Vaughan HG, Haybittle JL. The presentation haemoglobin level in 1103 patients with Hodgkin's disease (BNLI report no. 21). *Clin Radiol* 1983; 34:491.

93. Sonnenblick M, Kramer R, Hershko C. Corticosteroid responsive immune thrombocytopenia in Hodgkin's disease. *Oncology* 1986; 43:349.

94. Cohen JR. Idiopathic thrombocytopenic purpura in Hodgkin's disease: a rare occurrence of no prognostic significance. *Cancer* 1978; 41:743.

95. Kedar A, Khan AB, Mattern JQ, Fisher J, Thomas PR, Freeman AI. Autoimmune disorders complicating adolescent Hodgkin's disease. *Cancer* 1979; 44:112.

96. Le Bourgeois J, Tubiana M. The erythrocyte sedimentation rate as a monitor for relapse in patients with previously treated Hodgkin's disease. *Int J Radiat Oncol Biol Phys* 1977; 2:241.

97. Haybittle JL, Hayhoe FG, Easterling MJ, et al. Review of British National Lymphoma Investigation studies of Hodgkin's disease and development of prognostic index. *Lancet* 1985; 1:967.
98. Tubiana M, Henry AM, van dW, et al. A multivariate analysis of prognostic factors in early stage Hodgkin's disease. *Int J Radiat Oncol Biol Phys* 1985; 11:23.
99. Schilling RF, McKnight B, Crowley JJ. Prognostic value of serum lactic dehydrogenase level in Hodgkin's disease. *J Lab Clin Med* 1982; 99:382.
100. Friedenberg WR, Gatlin PF, Mazza JJ, et al. Prognostic value of serum lactic dehydrogenase level in Hodgkin's disease. *J Lab Clin Med* 1984; 103:489.
101. Aisenberg AC, Kaplan MM, Rieder SV. Serum alkaline phosphatase at the onset of Hodgkin's disease. *Cancer* 1970; 26:318.
102. Hasenclever D, Diehl V. A prognostic score for advanced Hodgkin's disease. International Prognostic Factors Project on Advanced Hodgkin's Disease. *N Engl J Med* 1998; 339:1506.
103. Mercier RJ, Thompson JM, Harman GS, Messerschmidt GL. Recurrent hypercalcemia and elevated 1,25-dihydroxyvitamin D levels in Hodgkin's disease. *Am J Med* 1988; 84:165.
104. Braund WJ, Naylor BA, Williamson DH, et al. Autoimmunity to insulin receptor and hypoglycaemia in patient with Hodgkin's disease. *Lancet* 1987; 1:237.
105. Walters EG, Tavare JM, Denton RM, Walters G. Hypoglycaemia due to an insulin-receptor antibody in Hodgkin's disease. *Lancet* 1987; 1:241.
106. Eliakim R, Vertman E, Shinhar E. Syndrome of inappropriate secretion of antidiuretic hormone in Hodgkin's disease. *Am J Med Sci* 1986; 291:126.
107. Moorthy AV, Zimmerman SW, Burkholder PM. Nephrotic syndrome in Hodgkin's disease. Evidence for pathogenesis alternative to immune complex deposition. *Am J Med* 1976; 61:471.
108. Routledge RC, Hann IM, Jones PH. Hodgkin's disease complicated by the nephrotic syndrome. *Cancer* 1976; 38:1735.
109. Pusey W. Cases of sarcoma and of Hodgkin's disease treated by exposures to x-rays: a preliminary report. *JAMA* 1902; 38:166.
110. Senn N. Therapeutical value of rontgen ray in treatment of pseudoleukemia. *NY Med J* 1903; 77:665.
111. Gilbert R. Radiotherapy in Hodgkin's disease (malignant granulomatosis): anatomic and clinical foundations, governing principles, results. *Am J Roentgenol* 1939; 41:198.
112. Kaplan H. The radical radiotherapy of regionally localized Hodgkin's disease. *Radiology* 1962; 78:553.
113. Goodman L, Wingtrobe M, Dameshek W. Nitrogen mustard therapy: use of methyl bis (β-chloroethyl)amine hydrochloride and tris-(β-chloroethyl)amine hydrochloride for Hodgkin's disease, lymphosarcoma, leukemia, and certain allied and miscellaneous disorders. *JAMA* 1946; 132:126.
114. Jacobson L, Spurr C, Baron EG. Nitrogen mustard therapy: use of methyl bis (β-chloroethyl)amine hydrochloride on neoplastic disorders of the hematopietic system. *JAMA* 1946; 132:263.
115. DeVita V, Serpick A, Carbone P. Combination chemotherapy in the treatment of advanced Hodgkin's disease. *Ann Intern Med* 1970; 73:881.
116. Feuer EJ, Kessler LG, Baker SG, Triolo HE, Green DT. The impact of breakthrough clinical trials on survival in population based tumor registries. *J Clin Epidemiol* 1991; 44:141.
117. Santoro A, Bonadonna G, Bonfante V, Valagussa P. Alternating drug combinations in the treatment of advanced Hodgkin's disease. *N Engl J Med* 1982; 306:770.
118. Bonadonna G, Valagussa P, Santoro A. Alternating non-cross-resistant combination chemotherapy or MOPP in stage IV Hodgkin's disease. A report of 8-year results. *Ann Intern Med* 1986; 104:739.

119. Santoro A, Bonadonna G, Valagussa P, et al. Long-term results of combined chemotherapy-radiotherapy approach in Hodgkin's disease: superiority of ABVD plus radiotherapy versus MOPP plus radiotherapy. *J Clin Oncol* 1987; 5:27.

120. Canellos GP, Anderson JR, Propert KJ, et al. Chemotherapy of advanced Hodgkin's disease with MOPP, ABVD, or MOPP alternating with ABVD. *N Engl J Med* 1992; 327:1478.

121. Klimo P, Connors JM. MOPP/ABV hybrid program: combination chemotherapy based on early introduction of seven effective drugs for advanced Hodgkin's disease. *J Clin Oncol* 1985; 3:1174.

122. Connors JM, Klimo P, Adams G, et al. Treatment of advanced Hodgkin's disease with chemotherapy—comparison of MOPP/ABV hybrid regimen with alternating courses of MOPP and ABVD: a report from the National Cancer Institute of Canada clinical trials group. *J Clin Oncol* 1997; 15:1638.

123. Viviani S, Bonadonna G, Santoro A, et al. Alternating versus hybrid MOPP and ABVD combinations in advanced Hodgkin's disease: ten-year results. *J Clin Oncol* 1996; 14:1421.

124. Diehl V, Franklin J, Hasenclever D, et al. BEACOPP, a new dose-escalated and accelerated regimen, is at least as effective as COPP/ABVD in patients with advanced-stage Hodgkin's lymphoma: interim report from a trial of the German Hodgkin's Lymphoma Study Group. *J Clin Oncol* 1998; 16:3810.

125. Diehl V, Sieber M, Rüffer U, et al. BEACOPP: an intensified chemotherapy regimen in advanced Hodgkin's disease. The German Hodgkin's Lymphoma Study Group. *Ann Oncol* 1997; 8:143.

126. Horning SJ, Rosenberg SA, Hoppe RT. Brief chemotherapy (Stanford V) and adjuvant radiotherapy for bulky or advanced Hodgkin's disease: an update. *Ann Oncol* 1996; 7(Suppl 4):105.

127. Bartlett NL, Rosenberg SA, Hoppe RT, Hancock SL, Horning SJ. Brief chemotherapy, Stanford V, and adjuvant radiotherapy for bulky or advanced-stage Hodgkin's disease: a preliminary report. *J Clin Oncol* 1995; 13:1080.

128. Rosenberg SA, Kaplan HS: The evolution and summary results of the Stanford randomized clinical trials of the management of Hodgkin's disease: 1962–1984. *Int J Radiat Oncol Biol Phys* 1985; 11:5.

129. Specht L, Gray RG, Clarke MJ, Peto R. Influence of more extensive radiotherapy and adjuvant chemotherapy on long-term outcome of early-stage Hodgkin's disease: a meta-analysis of 23 randomized trials involving 3,888 patients. International Hodgkin's Disease Collaborative Group. *J Clin Oncol* 1998; 16:830.

130. Carde P, Burgers JM, Henry AM, et al. Clinical stages I and II Hodgkin's disease: a specifically tailored therapy according to prognostic factors. *J Clin Oncol* 1988; 6:239.

131. Tubiana M, Henry AM, Carde P, et al. Toward comprehensive management tailored to prognostic factors of patients with clinical stages I and II in Hodgkin's disease. The EORTC Lymphoma Group controlled clinical trials: 1964–1987. *Blood* 1989; 73:47.

132. Wirth A, Byram D, Chao M, Corry J, Davis S. Long term results of mantle irradiation alone in 261 patients with clinical stage I-II supradiaphragmatic Hodgkin's disease. *Int J Radiat Oncol Biol Phys* 1997; (abst 78):174.

133. Hancock SL, Hoppe RT, Horning SJ, Rosenberg SA. Intercurrent death after Hodgkin disease therapy in radiotherapy and adjuvant MOPP trials. *Ann Intern Med* 1988; 109:183.

134. Horning SJ, Hoppe RT, Hancock SL, Rosenberg SA. Vinblastine, bleomycin, and methotrexate: an effective adjuvant in favorable Hodgkin's disease. *J Clin Oncol* 1988; 6:1822.

135. Horning SJ, Hoppe RT, Mason J, et al. Stanford-Kaiser Permanente G1 study for clinical stage I to IIA Hodgkin's disease: subtotal lymphoid irradiation versus vinblastine, methotrexate, and bleomycin chemotherapy and regional irradiation. *J Clin Oncol* 1997; 15:1736.

136. Noordijk EM, Carde P, Hagenbeek A, Mandard A-M, Kluin-Nelemans JC. Combination of radiotherapy and chemotherapy is advisable in all patients with clinical stage I-II Hodgkin's

disease. Six year results of the EORTC-GPMC controlled clinical trials 'H7-VF, 'H7-F', and 'H7-UF'. *Int J Radiat Oncol Biol Phys* 1997; 173(abst 77).

137. Bonfante V, Santoro A, Vivani S, Devizzi L. ABVD plus radiotherapy (subtotal nodal vs involved field) in early-stage Hodgkin's disease (HD). *Proc Am Soc Clin Oncol* 1994; 373(abst 1262).

138. Tesch H, Sieber M, Ruffer JU, Franklin J. 2 cycles ABVD plus radiotherapy is more effective than radiotherapy alone in early stage HD- Interim analysis of the HD7 trial of the GHSG. *Proc Am Soc Hematol* 1998; (abst 2001).

139. Radford JA, Cowan RA, Ryder WDJ, Deakin DP, James RD. Four weeks of neo-adjuvant chemotherapy significantly reduces the progression rate in patients treated with limited field radiotherapy for clinical stage IA/IIA Hodgkin's disease. Results of a randomized trial. *Ann Oncol* 1996; 21(abst 066).

140. Horning SJ, Hoppe RT, Breslin S, Baer DM, Mason J, Rosenberg SA. Very brief (8 week) chemotherapy and low dose (30 Gy) radiotherapy for limited stage Hodgkin's disease: preliminary results of the Stanford-Kaiser G4 study of Stanford V + RT. *Proc Am Soc Hematol* 1999.

141. Hoppe RT, Coleman CN, Cox RS, Rosenberg SA, Kaplan HS. The management of stage I-II Hodgkin's disease with irradiation alone or combined modality therapy: the Stanford experience. *Blood* 1982; 59:455.

142. Bonfante V, Santoro A, Viviani S, Valagussa P, Bonadonna G. ABVD in the treatment of Hodgkin's disease. *Semin Oncol* 1992; 19:38.

143. Longo DL, Russo A, Duffey PL, et al. Treatment of advanced-stage massive mediastinal Hodgkin's disease: the case for combined modality treatment. *J Clin Oncol* 1991; 9:227.

144. Longo DL, Young RC, Wesley M, et al. Twenty years of MOPP therapy for Hodgkin's disease. *J Clin Oncol* 1986; 4:1295.

145. Duggan D, Petroni G, Johnson J. MOPP/ABV vs ABVD for advanced Hodgkin's disease: a preliminary report of CALGB 8952. *Proc Am Soc Clin Oncol* 1997; (abst 12a):41.

146. Horning SJ, Williams J, Bartlett NL, et al. E1492: Assessment of the Stanford V regimen and consolidative radiotherapy for bulky and advanced Hodgkin's disease. *J Clin Oncol* 1999; (in press).

147. Prosnitz LR, Farber LR, Kapp DS, et al. Combined modality therapy for advanced Hodgkin's disease: 15-year follow-up data. *J Clin Oncol* 1988; 6:603.

148. Donaldson SS, Link MP. Combined modality treatment with low-dose radiation and MOPP chemotherapy for children with Hodgkin's disease. *J Clin Oncol* 1987; 5:742.

149. Meerwaldt JH, Coleman CN, Fischer RI, Lister TA, Diehl V. Role of additional radiotherapy in advanced stages of Hodgkin's disease. *Ann Oncol* 1992; 4:83.

150. Fabian CJ, Mansfield CM, Dahlberg S, et al. Low-dose involved field radiation after chemotherapy in advanced Hodgkin disease. A Southwest Oncology Group randomized study. *Ann Intern Med* 1994; 120:903.

151. Diehl V, Loeffler M, Pfreundschuh M, et al. Further chemotherapy versus low-dose involved-field radiotherapy as consolidation of complete remission after six cycles of alternating chemotherapy in patients with advance Hodgkin's disease. German Hodgkins' Study Group (GHSG). *Ann Oncol* 1995; 6:901.

152. Weiner MA, Leventhal B, Brecher ML, et al. Randomized study of intensive MOPP-ABVD with or without low-dose total-nodal radiation therapy in the treatment of stages IIB, IIIA2, IIIB, and IV Hodgkin's disease in pediatric patients: a Pediatric Oncology Group study. *J Clin Oncol* 1997; 15:2769.

153. Mauch P, Gorshein D, Cunningham J, Hellman S. Influence of mediastinal adenopathy on site and frequency of relapse in patients with Hodgkin's disease. *Cancer Treat Rep* 1982; 66:809.

154. Specht L, Nordentoft AM, Cold S, Clausen NT, Nissen NI. Tumor burden as the most important prognostic factor in early stage Hodgkin's disease. Relations to other prognostic factors and implications for choice of treatment. *Cancer* 1988; 61:1719.

155. Mauch PM. Controversies in the management of early stage Hodgkin's disease. *Blood* 1994; 83:318.

156. Gospodarowicz MK, Sutcliffe SB, Clark RM, et al. Analysis of supradiaphragmatic clinical stage I and II Hodgkin's disease treated with radiation alone. *Int J Radiat Oncol Biol Phys* 1992; 22:859.

157. Carella AM, Carlier P, Congiu A, et al. Autologous bone marrow transplantation as adjuvant treatment for high-risk Hodgkin's disease in first complete remission after MOPP/ABVD protocol. *Bone Marrow Transplant* 1991; 8:99.

158. Brink AA, Oudejans JJ, van den Brule AJ, et al. Low p53 and high bcl-2 expression in Reed-Sternberg cells predicts poor clinical outcome for Hodgkin's disease: involvement of apoptosis resistance? *Mod Pathol* 1998; 11:376.

159. Oudejans JJ, Jiwa NM, Kummer JA, et al. Activated cytotoxic T cells as prognostic marker in Hodgkin's disease. *Blood* 1997; 89:1376.

160. Pizzolo G, Vinante F, Chilosi M, et al. Serum levels of soluble CD30 molecule (Ki-1 antigen) in Hodgkin's disease: relationship with disease activity and clinical stage. *Br J Haematol* 1990; 75:282.

161. Nadali G, Vinante F, Ambrosetti A, et al. Serum levels of soluble CD30 are elevated in the majority of untreated patients with Hodgkin's disease and correlate with clinical features and prognosis. *J Clin Oncol* 1994; 12:793.

162. Kurzrock R, Redman J, Cabanillas F, Jones D, Rothberg J, Talpaz M. Serum interleukin 6 levels are elevated in lymphoma patients and correlate with survival in advanced Hodgkin's disease and with B symptoms. *Cancer Res* 1993; 53:2118.

163. Pizzolo G, Chilosi M, Vinante F, et al. Soluble interleukin-2 receptors in the serum of patients with Hodgkin's disease. *Br J Cancer* 1987; 55:427.

164. Sarris AH, Kliche KO, Pethambaram P, et al. Interleukin-10 levels are often elevated in serum of adults with Hodgkin's disease and are associated with inferior failure-free survival. *Ann Oncol* 1999; 10:433.

165. Portlock CS, Rosenberg SA, Glatstein E, Kaplan HS. Impact of salvage treatment on initial relapses in patients with Hodgkin disease, stages I-III. *Blood* 1978; 51:825

166. Timothy AR, Sutcliffe SB, Wrigley PF, Jones AE. Hodgkin's disease: combination chemotherapy for relapse following radical radiotherapy. *Int J Radiat Oncol Biol Phys* 1979; 5:165.

167. Roach MD, Brophy N, Cox R, Varghese A, Hoppe RT. Prognostic factors for patients relapsing after radiotherapy for early-stage Hodgkin's disease. *J Clin Oncol* 1990; 8:623.

168. Fisher RI, DeVita VT, Hubbard SP, Simon R, Young RC. Prolonged disease-free survival in Hodgkin's disease with MOPP reinduction after first relapse. *Ann Intern Med* 1979; 90:761.

169. Chopra R, McMIllan AK, Linch DC, et al. The place of high-dose BEAM therapy and autologous bone marrow transplantation in poor-risk Hodgkin's disease. A single-center eight-year study of 155 patients. *Blood* 1993; 81:1137.

170. Bierman PJ, Anderson JR, Freeman MB, et al. High-dose chemotherapy followed by autologous hematopoietic rescue for Hodgkin's disease patients following first relapse after chemotherapy. *Ann Oncol* 1996; 7:151.

171. Horning SJ, Chao NJ, Negrin S, et al. High-dose therapy and autologous hematopoietic progenitor cell transplantation for recurrent of refractory Hodgkin's disease: analysis of the Stanford University results and prognostic indices. *Blood* 1997; 89:801.

172. Reece DE, Connors JM, Spinelli JJ, et al. Intensive therapy with cyclophosphamide, carmustine, etoposide +/− cisplatin, and autologous bone marrow transplantation for Hodgkin's disease in first relapse after combination chemotherapy. *Blood* 1994; 83:1193.

173. Linch DC, Winfield D, Goldstone AH, et al. Dose intensification with autologous bone-marrow transplantation in relapsed and resistant Hodgkin's disease; results of a BNLI randomized trial. *Lancet* 1993; 341:1051.

174. Schmitz N, Sextro M, Pfistner B, Hasenclever D, Tesch H. High dose therapy followed by hematopoietic stem cell Transplantation for relapsed chemosensitive Hodgkin's disease: final results of a randomized GHSC and EBMT atrial (HDR-1) *Proc Am Soc Clin Oncol* 1999; 2a (abst 5).

175. Lazarus HM, Rowlings PA, Zhang MJ, et al. Autotransplants for Hodgkin's disease in patients never achieving remission: a report from the Autologous Blood and Marrow Transplant Registry. *J Clin Oncol* 1999; 17:534.

176. Horning SJ. Primary refractory Hodgkin's disease. *Ann Oncol* 1998; (9 Suppl 5): S97.

177. Reece DE, Barnett MJ, Shepherd JD, et al. High-dose cyclophosphamide, carmustine (BCNU), and etoposide (VP16-213) with or without cisplatin (CBV +/−P) and autologous transplantation for patients with Hodgkin's disease who fail to enter a complete remission after combination chemotherapy. *Blood* 1995; 86:451.

178. Arseneau JC, Sponzo RW, Levin DL, et al. Nonlymphomatous malignant tumors complication Hodgkin's disease. Possible association with intensive therapy. *N Engl J Med* 1972; 287:1119.

179. Canellos GP, Arseneau JC, De Vita VT, Whang PF, Johnson RE. Second malignancies complicating Hodgkin's disease in remission. *Lancet* 1975; 1:947.

180. Coleman CN, Williams CJ, Flint A, Glatstein EJ, Rosenberg SA, Kaplan HS. Hematologic neoplasia in patients treated for Hodgkin's disease. *N Engl J Med* 1977; 297:1249.

181. Kaldor JM, Day NE, Clarke EA, et al. Leukemia following Hodgkin's disease. *N Engl J Med* 1990; 322:7.

182. Levine EG, Bloomfield CD. Leukemias and myelodysplastic syndromes secondary to drug, radiation, and environmental exposure. *Semin Oncol* 1992: 19:47.

183. Blayney DW, Longo DL, Young RC, et al. Decreasing risk of leukemia with prolonged follow-up after chemotherapy and radiotherapy for Hodgkin's disease. *N Engl J Med* 1987; 316:710.

184. Tucker, MA, Coleman CN, Cox RS, Varghese A, Rosenberg SA. Risk of second cancers after treatment for Hodgkin's disease. *N Engl J Med* 1988; 318:76.

185. Van LF, Somers R, Taal BG, et al. Increased risk of lung cancer, non-Hodgkin's lymphoma, and leukemia following Hodgkin's disease. *J Clin Oncol* 1989; 7:1046.

186. Boivin JF, Hutchison GB, Lyden M, Godbold J, Chorosh J, Schottenfeld D. Second primary cancers following treatment of Hodgkin's disease. *J Natl Cancer Inst* 1984; 72:233.

187. Henry AM. Second cancers after radiotherapy and chemotherapy for early stages of Hodgkin's disease. *J Natl Cancer Inst* 1983; 71:911.

188. Hancock SL, Tucker MA, Hoppe RT. Breast Cancer after treatment of Hodgkin's disease. *J Natl Cancer Inst* 1993: 85:25.

189. Hancock SL, Cox RS, McDougall IR. Thyroid diseases after treatment of Hodgkin's disease. *N Engl J Med* 1991; 325:599.

190. Shapiro CL, Mauch PM. Radiation-associated breast cancer after Hodgkin's disease: risks and screening in perspective. *J Clin Oncol* 1992; 10:1662.

191. Bhatia S, Robison LL, Oberlin O, et al. Breast cancer and other second neoplasms after childhood Hodgkin's disease. *N Engl J Med* 1996; 334:745.

192. Hancock SL, Donaldson SS, Hoppe RT. Cardiac disease following treatment of Hodgkin's disease in children and adolescent. *J Clin Oncol* 1993; 11:1208.

193. Boivin JF, Hutchison DB, Lubin JH, Mauch P. Coronary artery disease mortality in patients treated for Hodgkin's disease. *Cancer* 1992; 69:1241.

194. Chapman RM, Sutcliffe SB, Rees LH, Edwards CR, Malpas JS. Cyclical combination chemotherapy and gonadal function. Etrospective study in males. *Lancet* 1979; 1:285.

195. Chapman RM, Sutcliffe SB, Malpas JS. Cytotoxic-induced ovarian failure in women with Hodgkin's disease. I. Hormone function. *JAMA* 1979; 242:1877.
196. Horning SJ, Hoppe RT, Kaplan HS, Rosenberg SA. Female reproductive potential after treatment for Hodgkin's disease. *N Engl J Med* 1981; 304:1377.
197. Anselmo AP, Cartoni C, Bellantuono P, Maurizi ER, Aboulkair N, Ermini M. Risk of infertility in patients with Hodgkin's disease treated with ABVD vs MOPP vs ABVD/MOPP. *Haematologica* 1990; 75:155.
198. Viviani S, Santoro A, Ragni G, Bonfante V, Bestetti O, Bonadonna G. Gonadal toxicity after combination chemotherapy for Hodgkin's disease. Comparative results of MOPP vs ABVD. *Eur J Cancer Oncol* 1985; 21:601.
199. Carmel RJ, Kaplan HS. Mantel irradiation in Hodgkin's disease. An analysis of technique, tumor eradication, and complications. *Cancer* 1976; 37:2813.
200. Smith LM, Mendenhall NP, Cicale MJ, Block ER, Carter RL, Million R. Results of a prospective study evaluation the effects of mantle irradiation on pulmonary function. *Int J Radiat Oncol iol Phys* 1989; 16:79.
201. Horning SJ, Adhikari A, Rizk N, Hoppe RT, Olshem RA. Effect of treatment for Hodgkin's disease on pulmonary function: results of a prospective study. *J Clin Oncol* 1994: 12;297.
202. Donaldson SS, Kaplan HS. Complications of treatment of Hodgkin's disease in children. *Cancer Treat Rep* 1982; 66:977.
203. Rosner F, Zarrabi MH. Late infections following splenectomy in Hodgkin's disease. *Cancer Invest* 1983; 1:57.
204. Bloom JR, Fobair P, Gritz E, et al. Psychosocial outcomes of cancer: a comparative analysis of Hodgkin's disease and testicular cancer. *J Clin Oncol* 1993; 11:979.

Index

A

ABVD (adriamycin, bleomycin, vinblastine, dacarbazine)
adverse effects, 317
Hodgkin's disease, 309, 310, 311–312
Acetone, 12
Acute lymphoblastic leukemias (ALL)
differential diagnosis, 32
Acute monoblastic leukemia
differential diagnosis, 83
Acute myelogenous leukemia (AML)
cause, 38
occupational risk factors, 12
Adriamycin. *See also* ABVD
Sezary syndrome, 140
Adult T-cell leukemia-lymphoma
differential diagnosis, 32
Age
CLL, 35
essential thrombocythemia, 194
Aggressive large-cell lymphomas, 277–293
clinical features, 282–283
prognostic factors, 285–286
staging, 285–286
treatment, 287–293
Agnogenic myeloid metaplasia with myelofibrosis (AMMM), 197–203
clinical features, 199–200
diagnosis, 198–199
natural course, 200–201
pathogenesis, 197

therapy, 201–202
Agricultural workers, 12
AIHA, 24
CLL, 47
Alemtuzumab
CLL, 4
Alkylator-based multi-agent therapy
CLL, 39–40
ALL
differential diagnosis, 32
Allogeneic bone-marrow transplantation (Allo-BMT)
CMML, 99–100
low-grade lymphoma, 256–257, 261–262
Allogeneic stem-cell transplantation (Allo-SCT)
CLL, 45–46
low-grade lymphoma, 261–262
All trans retinoic acid (ATRA), 134
AML
cause, 38
occupational risk factors, 12
AMMM. *See* Agnogenic myeloid metaplasia with myelofibrosis
Anagrelide
essential thrombocythemia, 196
PCV, 192
Anaplastic large-cell lymphoma, 280–282
clinical features, 283–284
Ann Arbor staging system, 306
Anthracycline
CLL, 40
Anti-CD20. *See* Rituxan